GERIATRIC
NURSING CARE PLANS

GERIATRIC NURSING CARE PLANS

WITHDRAWN

Edited by

FRANCES F. ROGERS-SEIDL, R.N., M.N.

Nurse Consultant,
Gerontology Department,
HCA/Wesley Medical Center,
Wichita, Kansas

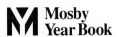
Mosby
Year Book

St. Louis Baltimore Boston Chicago London Philadelphia Sydney Toronto

26.95

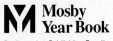
Mosby
Year Book
Dedicated to Publishing Excellence

Editor: Linda Duncan
Developmental editor: Linda Stagg
Assistant editor: Rebecca Sweeney
Project manager: Mark Spann
Production editor: Stephen C. Hetager
Design: Laura Steube

Printed in the United States of America

Mosby–Year Book, Inc.
11830 Westline Industrial Drive, St. Louis, Mo 63146

Library of Congress Cataloging in Publication Data
Geriatric nursing care plans / edited by Frances F. Rogers-Seidl.
     p.   cm.
    Includes bibliographical references and index.
    ISBN 0-8016-5210-3
    1. Geriatric nursing. 2. Nursing care plans. I. Rogers-Seidl.
Frances F.
    [DNLM: 1. Geriatric Nursing. 2. Nursing Assessment. 3. Patient
Care Planning.   WY 152 G3697]
RC954.G46   1991
610.73′65—dc20
DNLM/DLC
for Library of Congress   91-6365
                                                                            CIP

GW/VH 9 8 7 6 5 4 3 2 1

Contributors

MARY E. ALLEN, R.N., C.S., Ph.D.

Associate Professor, College of Nursing,
University of Oklahoma,
Oklahoma City, Oklahoma

JANET T. BARRETT, R.N., B.S.N., M.S.N., Ph.D.

Administration, Barnes College,
St. Louis, Missouri

ROBERTA PURVIS BARTEE, R.N., M.S.

Formerly Assistant Professor, Louisiana State
University Medical Center School of Nursing,
New Orleans, Louisiana

TALLY N. BELL, R.N., M.N., C.C.R.N.

Manager, Clinical Education,
HCA/Wesley Medical Center,
Wichita, Kansas

JO EVA ZIEGLER BLAIR, R.N., M.N.

Director of Allied Health and Continuing Education,
Butler County Community College,
El Dorado, Kansas

DOROTHY E. BOOTH, R.N., Ph.D.

Assistant Professor of Gerontological Nursing,
University of Michigan School of Nursing,
Ann Arbor, Michigan

SHARON BOWLES, R.N., M.N.

Manager, Clinical Education,
HCA/Wesley Medical Center,
Wichita, Kansas

CHRISTINE CLARKIN, R.N.C., C.D.E.

Program Coordinator, Diabetes Learning Center,
Stormont Vail Regional Medical Center,
Topeka, Kansas

RHONDA W. COMRIE, R.N., M.S.N.

Instructor, Barnes College,
St. Louis, Missouri

THE REVEREND KAREN OSTERMAN FIESER,
R.N., B.S.N., M.Div.

Chaplain, HCA/Wesley Medical Center,
Wichita, Kansas

DIXIE M. FLYNN, R.N., B.S.N., M.A.

Nursing Administrator,
John Knox Village Care Center,
Lee's Summit, Missouri

ANN PENDLEBURY HUNTER, A.B.D., R.D., C.D.E.

Assistant Professor,
The Wichita State University,
Wichita, Kansas

NANCY KAUFMANN, R.N., M.S.Ed., M.S.N.

Special Care Unit Coordinator,
Clayton House Healthcare,
Ballwin, Missouri

MARILEE KUHRIK, R.N., M.S.N.

Nurse Educator, Barnes Hospital School of Nursing,
St. Louis, Missouri

NANCY KUHRIK, R.N., M.S.N.

Nurse Educator, Jewish Hospital School of Nursing,
St. Louis, Missouri

VIRGINIA G. LEVIN, R.N., B.S.

Assistant Director of Nursing I,
Kaiser Permanente,
Panorama City, California

LISA LOGAN, R.D., C.N., S.D.

Nutritional Support Dietitian Consultant
Presbyterian Denver Hospital,
Denver, Colorado

SUE E. MEINER, R.N., M.S.N.

Doctoral Candidate, Southern Illinois University,
Edwardsville, Illinois

SHARYN L. MILLS, M.S., C.C.C.

Director of Speech Pathology-Audiology,
Baptist Medical Center,
Kansas City, Missouri

SHIRLEY MOORE, R.N., B.S.N., M.S.N., M.S.

Instructor, Barnes College,
St. Louis, Missouri

CAROLYN L. MORRIS, R.N.C., M.S.N.

Lecturer, Clinical Nurse Specialist,
University of Michigan School of Nursing,
Ann Arbor, Michigan

MARGHERITA P. NAHRUP, R.N., M.S.H.S.A.

Faculty, Barnes College,
St. Louis, Missouri

JEAN NELSON, R.N., M.Ed.

Instructor, Barnes Hospital School of Nursing,
St. Louis, Missouri

JOAN D. NELSON, R.N., M.S.N.

Geriatric Nurse Educator and Consultant,
Hockessin, Delaware

LOIS ROBINSON, R.N., M.Ed., M.N.

Assistant Professor, Kansas Newman College,
Wichita, Kansas

SUSAN A. RUZICKA, R.N., M.S.N.

In-Service Coordinator, Barnes Long-Term Care,
St. Louis, Missouri

SHIRLEY A. SAUNDERS, R.N., M.S.N.

Nursing Instructor, Barnes Hospital School of
Nursing,
St. Louis, Missouri

ELAINE E. STEINKE, R.N., Ph.D.

Associate Professor of Nursing,
Kansas Newman College,
Wichita, Kansas

To my Parents
who are my role models for aging

To all the Elders
who have been my teachers

To my Husband
Floyd Seidl
our children
and their children
who give light to my days

To all my Friends
who provided the encouragement to continue

Preface

Nurses have always cared for elders, but often in the same way that they have cared for younger clients. Research has generated a body of knowledge about age-related changes and the unique response elders have to health problems. Conventional wisdom dictates that those caring for elders need specialized knowledge and skills to give the most effective care. *Geriatric Nursing Care Plans* is designed to meet that need by combining a geriatrics-focused knowledge base and assessment guide with "real world" application through the nursing process. The overall purpose of the book is that elders receive the help to maintain or regain their optimal levels of mental and physical health, function, and autonomy—the best life possible. A second purpose is to provide a resource for nurses to develop a "need model" for care delivery, as contrasted with the "routine service" one that has been seen in the past. Care plans that address the specific needs of the elder with interventions designed in light of current knowledge will certainly produce a specialty practice.

The term "client" was chosen as a label for the person receiving care; it is seen as a more neutral title than "patient" or "resident." It is hoped that semantics do not become a block to health care professionals in the hospital, physician's office, or nursing facility setting, since the care plans are translatable to any setting.

Part I consists of care plans based on individual nursing diagnoses. The diagnoses used are the ones established by the North American Nursing Diagnosis Association (NANDA). Each care plan includes the following components:

Knowledge base: This section is intended to give the reader the knowledge background to adequately intervene in the client's problem. This section should help the nurse to understand the reasons for performing the nursing actions.

Assessment criteria: Physical, psychosocial, and spiritual realms of a person's being are considered, both in an objective way and in a subjective way. Signs and symptoms related to the particular diagnosis are included. To acknowledge that the care of elders clearly demonstrates the integral nature of body, mind, and spirit, the assessment criteria are categorized in this way.

Common contributing factors or etiologies, expected client outcomes, and suggested strategies for care: A nursing care plan table demonstrates the use of the nursing process in planning care. Client-centered outcomes are cited for each contributing factor. The expected outcomes can be used as quality improvement and dismissal planning criteria. The

nursing strategies contain the priority assessments that should be made throughout the care. They also indicate when referrals to other disciplines are indicated. Education and dismissal planning strategies are also included.

Evaluation: Summary statements reflect attainment of the expected outcomes and are indicators of the quality and appropriateness of care and whether care has resulted in positive client outcomes. Physical, psychosocial, and spiritual criteria indicate the commitment to care for the total person. Since the client is the customer, these statements become performance standards for the nurse.

Nursing alerts: These are "red flag" situations of which the nurse practitioner and other staff members should be aware. Some alerts are the result of age-related changes; others result from the interactive nature of the client's disease with other conditions, treatments, or medications.

Bibliography: Selected readings related to the nursing diagnosis are provided.

Part II consists of care plans that focus on diseases or traumatic conditions frequently seen in older adults. Each care plan contains a case study, which is necessarily brief but which illustrates how to identify a group of nursing diagnoses that lead to appropriate care. The other components of each care plan are similar to those of the care plans in Part I:

Knowledge base: In addition to the type of information found in this section in each care plan in Part I, pathophysiology, pertinent laboratory and diagnostic tests, and medical treatment regimens are discussed.

Assessment criteria: The criteria focus on the specific medical or surgical problem presented in the case study. Since the elder may have more than one medical or surgical problem, the assessments would necessarily need to be broadened to monitor for those conditions or other complications or to identify the collaborative problems.

Nursing diagnoses, expected client outcomes, and nursing strategies: A nursing care plan table illustrates the use of the nursing process based on the assessment data and the case study.

Evaluation: As in the care plans in Part I, this section consists of a list of statements that reflect the attainment of expected outcomes.

Nursing alerts: As in Part I, these are potentially dangerous situations of which the nurse should be aware.

Bibliography: Selected readings related to the disease or traumatic condition are provided.

The target population for this book includes nursing students, nurses who work with the aged, and other health professionals in any health care setting who are involved in the care of elders.

There are many who have contributed to this book. The contributors named on the preceding pages have shared their knowledge and expertise so well. I also wish to thank Linda Duncan and Linda Stagg for their knowledge, skill, judgment, and patience throughout the development of the book. My special thanks to Annette Lueckenotte and Jan Burggrabe for their editorial help. All have contributed to this book becoming a reality.

Frances F. Rogers-Seidl

Contents

Standard Nursing Care Plans

Activity Intolerance

Sharon Bowles

KNOWLEDGE BASE

1. Activity intolerance is a state in which an individual has insufficient physiological or psychological energy to endure or complete required or desired daily activities. Degenerative changes affect the elderly's mobility and activity tolerance. In the absence of disease, mobility and activity remain unimpaired. Activity can be compromised by disorders of the central nervous system, skeleton, muscles, cardiovascular system, or lungs, or by drug therapy, or environment.
2. Ingestion of a large meal is to be avoided before exercise. The personality type of the older adult may affect his or her reaction to activity intolerance and ultimate activity progression. One elderly client may, for instance, be open to new stimuli, whereas another will have strong dependency needs and seek help and support from others.
3. Undesirable consequences can result from unrecognized and untreated causes of activity intolerance, such as disuse atrophy, impaired physical mobility, poor nutrition, altered self-esteem, role change, and perceived powerlessness.
4. Progression of activities in a slow, methodical manner promotes a return to normal activity level without undue fatigue and/or complications.
5. Overexertion can lead to complications such as cardiac or respiratory compromise. The daily schedule must be adjusted to balance activity with rest.
6. Encouragement and emotional support with each progressive stage of activity help the client recognize his or her achievements.
7. Mobility and/or ambulation aids such as cane, walker, or wheelchair allow greater ease of mobility, conserve energy, and may be indicated for client safety.
8. Lean muscle mass is lost and muscle cells atrophy when there is decreased use of muscles.
9. Collagen and connective tissues have decreased elasticity, resulting in less flexibility and increased stiffness.
10. Limitation in joint activity and range of motion can occur because of deterioration of the cartilage surfaces of joints and because of a decrease in collagen and connective tissue elasticity.
11. The lungs lose elasticity and there are fewer alveoli, along with thickening of the aveolar membranes.
12. A 10% to 15% decrease in arterial blood oxygen level occurs as the maximum breathing capacity decreases.
13. With progression of the atherosclerotic process, effects on the aorta, coronary arteries, and carotid arteries are especially apparent.
14. Cardiac output per minute for elders is lower; this value is affected by the heart rate and the amount of ventricular filling during diastole, the contractility of the myocardium, and the degree of peripheral resistance.
15. An elderly person requires a longer time for pulse rate, respiratory rate, and blood pressure to return to baseline after an activity.
16. Cardiac output is increased by exercise and physical activity, making the heart more efficient. Elderly people respond to regular exercise up to their toleration levels.
17. Fatigue is a common complaint of aging clients and indicates activity intolerance.
18. Thermoregulatory mechanisms involving perspiration and vasodilatation are diminished.
19. The energy needed to perform basic activities of daily living (ADLs) increases when there is any impairment to movement.

ASSESSMENT CRITERIA
Physical

History of contributing factors
History of ADLs/activity intolerance
    Type/amount of exercise per day/week
    Coordination
    Changes in stamina
    Use of leisure time
    Socialization/lack of socialization
Musculoskeletal
    Muscle strength/size
    Endurance
    Range of motion
    Muscle tone
    Skeletal abnormalities
Cardiovascular
    Heart rate and rhythm
    Blood pressure

Skin color
Time required to return to baseline
Respiratory
   Rate
   Depth
   Lung sounds
Neurological
   Level of consciousness
   Orientation
   Mentation
   Motor status
   Sensory status
Hepatorenal
   Fluid retention

Subjective data
   Report of pain with activity
   Dyspnea with activity
   Fatigue with activity
   Weakness with activity
Physical/psychological findings before, during, and
   after activity

Psychosocial

Knowledge of the following:
   Contributing factors
   Activity limitations
   Activity progression
Desire to increase level of activity
Support from family or significant others

 NURSING CARE PLAN: ACTIVITY INTOLERANCE

Common contributing factors	Expected patient outcomes	Nursing strategies
Disorders of central nervous, skeletal, muscular, pulmonary, cardiorespiratory, hepatorenal systems	Client will discuss any known contributing factors that may influence and potentiate activity intolerance	Correlate the contributing factors with activity intolerance and activity limitations in order to plan nursing strategies accordingly.
Decreased level of activity	Client will discuss present status of mobility	Discuss with client his or her present mobility status and related factors: Activity/need for activity Mobility range Stress Physical impairments Obesity Smoking Edema
	Client will report any symptoms of activity intolerance; client will demonstrate an increase in activity tolerance.	Observe and document before, during, and after response to activity, and instruct client to report symptoms of activity intolerance. *Physiological:* Blood pressure Heart rate Heart rhythm Respiration Symptoms of activity intolerance—chest pain, shortness of breath, dizziness, excessive fatigue *Psychological:* Satisfaction/dissatisfaction Willingness to participate Desire for increased level of activity
Compromised oxygenation/ neuromuscular limitations	Client will stop activity if indicated	Assess respiratory status, color; instruct client to stop the activity and rest if intolerance is noted, such as dyspnea, pain, fatigue
	Client will enhance pulmonary competence.	Encourage client to use adaptive breathing techniques
	Client will perform self-care activities to level of tolerance	Encourage client to participate in and complete all self-care activities as tolerated; assist with ADLs as necessary; establish gradual progression of activities.
Bed rest/immobility	Client will tolerate range of motion (ROM) and bed exercises	Assist with active or passive range-of-motion exercises and bed exercises as tolerated if on bed rest or immobile

NURSING CARE PLAN: ACTIVITY INTOLERANCE—cont'd

Common contributing factors	Expected patient outcomes	Nursing strategies

Fatigue/generalized weakness	Client will have adequate rest periods
	Client will tolerate a progression of activities and will understand the need for gradual increases
		Organize nursing care to allow adequate periods of rest
		Request consultation with physical therapist; assist with progression of activity and document responses; explain the progression; progression example:
		  Active range of motion
		  Assist with self-care activities
		  Dangling
		  Dangling for meals
		  Bedside commode
		  Chair
		  Ambulation for short distances
		  Shower/bath
		  Up and around ad lib

Psychological impediments to activity progression	Client will verbalize a sense of accomplishment with each step in progression of activity	Provide encouragement and emotional support with each step in progression of activity; assist with goal setting.
Lack of knowledge	Client will discuss any activity limitations Client will identify necessary aids to increase/assist in level of activity Client will comprehend health status and accept referrals, if indicated Family and/or significant other will gain knowledge of client's level of activity	Teach the rationale for any activity limitations; teach energy conservation methods Assess the need for mobility or ambulation aids such as cane, walker, wheelchair Initiate health teaching and/or referrals, if indicated Provide the family members an opportunity to share their concerns and comprehend indicated activity limitations

EVALUATION

1. The client demonstrates diminishment in or management of contributing factors.
2. The client discusses his or her present mobility status and related factors that may limit or hinder a progression of activity levels.
3. The client reports and demonstrates toleration of increased activity, as evidenced by blood pressure within 20 mm Hg of baseline, heart rate within 20 beats/min of resting rate, respiratory rate less than 24 breaths/min, heart rhythm regular and in normal sinus rhythm, and no complaints of chest pain, shortness of breath, dizziness, or excessive fatigue.
4. The client expresses a desire to increase his or her level of activity and displays satisfaction when this goal is accomplished.
5. The client participates in and demonstrates an ability to perform desired self-care activities.
6. The client reports no complaints of fatigue and demonstrates no physiological signs of intolerance to increased levels of activity.
7. The client expresses a sense of accomplishment as activity progresses.
8. The client comprehends activity limitations.
9. The client utilizes mobility or ambulation aids as necessary.
10. The client comprehends health status and uses referrals as appropriate.
11. The family and/or significant others recognize and support the client's level of activity.

NURSING ALERTS

1. Clients taking vasodilators, diuretics, or beta blockers can exhibit orthostatic hypotension from vasodilation, fluid shifts from diuresis, and compromised cardiac function from lowered heart rate and blood pressure as activity levels are increased.
2. The older adult should not start an exercise program without consulting his or her physician. The physician can determine what, if any, limitations are needed in an exercise program.
3. Caution should be taken with large meals and exercise, especially if there are cardiac or pulmonary problems.

Bibliography

Eliopoulos C: A guide to the nursing of the aging, Baltimore, 1987, The Williams & Wilkins Co.

Esberger KK and Hughes ST Jr: Nursing care of the aged, Norwalk, Conn, 1989, Appleton & Lange.

Gulanick M, Klopp A, and Galanes S: Nursing care plans: nursing diagnosis and intervention, St Louis, 1986, The CV Mosby Co.

Kim MJ, McFarland GK, and McLane AM: Pocket guide to nursing diagnoses, ed 3, St Louis, 1989, The CV Mosby Co.

Long BC and Phipps WJ: Medical-surgical nursing: a nursing process approach, St Louis, 1989, The CV Mosby Co.

Matteson MA and McConnell ES: Gerontological nursing: concepts and practice, Philadelphia, 1988, WB Saunders Co.

McLane AM: Classification of nursing diagnosis: proceedings of the Seventh Conference, St Louis, 1987, The CV Mosby Co.

Murray RB and Zentner JP: Nursing assessment and health promotion strategies through the life span, ed 4, Norwalk, Conn, 1989, Appleton & Lange.

Swearingen PL, Somers S, and Miller K: Manual of critical care: applying nursing diagnosis to adult critical illness, St Louis, 1988, The CV Mosby Co.

Adjustment, Impaired (Depressed Mood)

Nancy Kaufmann

KNOWLEDGE BASE

1. Depression has been referred to as the "common cold" of the elderly but is the least treated, since it is frequently misdiagnosed as dementia or hypochrondriasis. Alcoholism may contribute to a chronic depressed mood.
2. Impaired adjustment refers to the state in which an individual is unable to modify his or her lifestyle or behavior in a manner consistent with a change in health status.
3. Impaired adjustment is most likely to occur when multiple stressors occur within a short period of time.
4. An older person may have a chronic depressed mood because losses are never fully resolved before another loss occurs.
5. A depressed mood can be either a reaction to stress or an indicator of inability to adapt to stressors.
6. Symptoms of depression in elders include the following:
   a. Dysphoric mood, including crying, looking sad, reporting being blue, and sounding sad
   b. Suicidal behavior and ideas
   c. Pessimism and feelings of inadequacy, hopelessness, dependent behavior, indecisiveness, worry
   d. Guilt, shame, or feelings of worthlessness
   e. Fatigue and lack of energy
   f. Apathy and social withdrawal
   g. Poor memory, bewildered

   h. Poor attention span
   i. Sleep disturbances
   j. Anorexia
   k. Decrease in sexual interest or sexual pleasure
   l. Somatic complaints such as headaches, constipation, dry mouth, stomach pains, nausea, or dyspepsia
7. Early awakening in the morning is a normal physiological change of aging as well as a symptom of depression.
8. One must be careful to assess for suicide risk, since suicide rates increase with age, especially among the ill and older, single, white men.
9. One needs to recognize the subtle suicide attempts of the elderly client: starvation, accidental overdose, and noncompliance with the treatment regime.
10. It is important to obtain a careful drug history, since many drugs produce depressed mood (e.g., hypotensives, psychotropics, cardiotonics, analgesics, antianxiety agents, cancer chemotherapeutic agents, steroids, cimetidince [Tagamet]). Decreased kidney and liver function causes early medication toxicity.
11. A complete physical assessment must be performed to rule out a physiological cause for a depressed state. The symptoms of hypothyroidism mimic depression. Depression is one of the first symptoms of Parkinson's disease, multiinfarct dementia, and cancer of the pancreas, or it may be a response to chronic pain.

12. Common psychosocial causes of depression are anticipated or actual loss of health, loss of autonomy, loss of significant others, loss of roles, and decreased self-concept, with resultant social isolation.
13. Symptoms of depression in later life are different from those of younger clients:

Younger clients	Elderly clients
Have more psychological complaints	Have more somatic than psychological complaints
Experience more feelings of guilt, anger, self-dislike	Experience less guilt
	Are more apathetic and withdrawn
	Deny feeling depressed

14. Environmental factors that lead to isolation of the elderly, with resulting depression, are decreased mobility, lack of transportation, and decreased financial security.
15. Some research has shown that the elderly may experience depressive moods related to a decrease in catecholamine neurotransmission caused by an increase in monoamine oxidase (MAO) production.

ASSESSMENT CRITERIA
Physical

Vital signs
Nutritional status
Sleep pattern disturbances (insomnia or early morning awakening)
Change in activity patterns
Fatigue/weakness
Slowed speech and movements
Slumped posture

Laboratory results: thyroid-stimulating hormone (TSH), triiodothyronine (T_3), thyroxine (T_4), hemoglobin, hematocrit, creatinine, total protein
Current medications

Psychosocial

Loss of interest in hobbies/activities
Decreased libido
Confusion
Inability to concentrate
Inability to make decisions
Withdrawn
Apathetic
Helplessness
Hopelessness
Despair
Sad affect/tearfulness
Guilt
Lack of affect
Feelings of emptiness
Negativism regarding self and future
Somatic preoccupation
Suicidal ideation
Covert anger or irritability
Inattention to activities of daily living (ADLs)
Past/present illnesses
Coping patterns
Environmental or life-style changes
Stressors
Losses, current and past

Spiritual

Sense of trust in self, God, and others
Misdirected anger toward God
Sense of worthlessness

Assessment Tools

Zung Self-Rating Depression Scale
Beck Depression Scale
Geriatric Depression Scale (Brink)

 ## NURSING CARE PLAN: IMPAIRED ADJUSTMENT (DEPRESSED MOOD)

Common contributing factors	Expected client outcomes	Nursing strategies
Suicidal thoughts	Client will not attempt suicide	Assess for suicidal risk (suicidal feelings or ideas)
	Client will seek out staff if begins to have suicidal ideas	Ask how the client feels about the future; ask if he or she has ever felt life was not worth living
		Determine if there is a definite suicide plan (the more detailed the plan, the higher the risk)
		Assess for subtle suicide attempts, such as anorexia, overdose, noncompliance
		Implement suicide precautions if necessary; this may mean hospitalization

Continued.

NURSING CARE PLAN: IMPAIRED ADJUSTMENT (DEPRESSED MOOD)—cont'd

Common contributing factors	Expected client outcomes	Nursing strategies
Actual or perceived losses	Client will verbalize feelings about normal changes of aging Client will discuss feelings regarding loss of health Client will discuss feelings regarding losses Client will state that his self-awareness has increased Client will discuss and identify coping styles that have worked in the past Client will actively participate in the planning and completing of ADL's Client will interact with others on the unit or in the community Client will demonstrate problem-solving and decision-making abilities Client will make positive statements about himself or herself Client will make plans for the future Client will substitute new roles for lost ones	Assess for suicide risk If client is in severe depression, sit quietly with him or her for short periods of time throughout the day; do not expect conversation, since the client has no energy to talk or feels unworthy of conversation During severe depression ensure all physical needs are met, since the depressed client has no energy to eat, dress, or groom himself or herself. The nurse may have to perform total client care in the beginning Assess premorbid abilities and life-style. As depression lifts, encourage the client to resume as many ADLs as tolerated As the mood improves, allow the client a more active role in the decision-making process As the depressed mood lifts, encourage the client to ventilate feelings Explore the client's feelings about a loss Discuss with the client the process of normal aging; allow the client to verbalize feelings regarding growing old and to discuss losses experienced and anticipated (declining health, the death of more of their family members or friends, increased dependence on others) Acknowledge the losses and changes that have occurred Assist the client in increasing his or her level of self-awareness by exploring how he or she has successfully coped with losses in the past Offer opportunities to be successful (i.e., activity therapy) Discuss with the client activities and hobbies enjoyed in the past, and rekindle an interest if appropriate Encourage interactions with others to decrease the client's withdrawal from others Encourage the client to make positive statements about himself or herself Encourage the client to participate in the decision-making process; begin with small decisions (e.g., which blouse of two to wear today) and progress to more involved ones; this gives back to the client a measure of control Allow every opportunity for autonomy Encourage activity and exercise, which will increase the levels of serotonin, a catecholamine responsible for allowing one to experience pleasure
Hypothryoidism	Client will follow the recommended treatment regimen Client will report understanding of the relationship of thyroid levels to depression	Encourage a medical and psychological workup to accurately diagnose the client's condition Request a physician's order for blood work regarding thyroid function Arrange for medication and follow-up tests for thyroid levels according to physician order

NURSING CARE PLAN: IMPAIRED ADJUSTMENT (DEPRESSED MOOD)—cont'd

Common contributing factors	Expected client outcomes	Nursing strategies
Medications	Client will identify problems or behaviors that would indicate a drug-related cause Client will notify physician of these problems and obtain a change in medication	Review medications being taken by the client (both prescription and over-the-counter) Encourage consultations from physician to determine if symptoms are drug related Discuss with the client the side effects he or she needs to be aware of Consider divided-dose regimens
Poor nutritional status	Client will discuss the relationship of nutrituion to depressed mood Client will participate in planning for adequate nutrient intake Client will increase nutrient intake to premorbid levels	Assess the history and onset of the problem Assess likes and dislikes and offer preferred food Request consultation with dietician Assess nutrient intake and evaluate for adequacy Discuss importance of consuming adequate amounts of nutrients Encourage client to eat with others as tolerated Promote foods that are nutrient dense

EVALUATION

1. The client does not attempt suicide.
2. The client views himself or herself in an improved light.
3. The client verbalizes acceptance of losses.
4. The client engages in making plans for the future.
5. The client demonstrates a renewed interest in hobbies and activities previously enjoyed.
6. The client willingly interacts with others.
7. The client's problem-solving and decision-making abilities increase.
8. The client views the world and the future more optimistically.
9. The client is not experiencing a depressed mood from the medication.

NURSING ALERTS

1. Since many elderly people have decreased function of the liver and kidneys, elimination of drugs is prolonged, causing drug toxity or paradoxical effects.
2. Side effects of tricyclic antidepressants:
   a. Increased sedation
   b. Urinary retention
   c. Diaphoresis
3. There are many contraindications to the use of antidepressants:
   a. Cardiac dysfunction
   b. Narrow-angle glaucoma
   c. Urinary obstruction
4. Electroconvulsive therapy (ECT) is commonly used in elderly clients. Obtain a baseline to determine post ECT confusion.

Bibliography

Burnside I: Nursing and the aged, ed 3, New York, 1988, McGraw-Hill Book Co.

Cape R, Coe R, and Rossman I: Fundamentals of geriatric medicine, New York, 1983, Raven Press.

Ebersole P and Hess P: Toward healthy aging, ed 2, St Louis, 1985, The CV Mosby Co.

Kim MJ, McFarland GK, and McLane AM: Pocket guide to nursing diagnoses, ed 3, St Louis, 1989, The CV Mosby Co.

Stuart G and Sundeen S: Pocket guide to psychiatric nursing, St Louis, 1988, The CV Mosby Co.

Stuart G and Sundeen S: Principles and practices of psychiatric nursing, ed 3, St Louis, 1989, The CV Mosby Co.

Anxiety

Nancy Kaufmann

KNOWLEDGE BASE

1. Anxiety is defined as a subjective feeling of apprehension, dread, or foreboding in response to an unknown source.
2. Anxiety varies in intensity according to the severity of the threat perceived by the individual.
3. There are four levels of anxiety:
   a. Mild—one's perceptual field is increased; the senses sharpen; heart rate, respiratory rate, muscle tone increase; memory and motivation to problem solve are increased.
   b. Moderate—one's perceptual field narrows. The individual focuses on immediate concerns but can be redirected to attend to other areas.
   c. Severe—an individual is completely focused on a specific detail and is unable to take in messages from the periphery.
   d. Panic—the individual is no longer able to relate to the surrounding world. Behaviors are disorganized, and the person is disoriented. This last stage is incompatible with life and cannot be sustained over a great length of time.
4. Anxiety is a valuable warning system necessary for survival. High levels become life-threatening.
5. Coping mechanisms are developed to neutralize, deny, or counteract anxiety. When used to an extreme degree, they distort reality, interfere with relationships, limit one's productivity, and threaten ego integrity.
6. Utilization of coping mechanisms with past experiences may influence present behavior.
7. Situational crises that may place an elderly client at risk include medical illness, relocation, financial problems, and losses (through death or separation).
8. Maturational crises that may place an elderly client at risk include retirement; sensory deficits, which may affect one's perception of reality; and physiological changes, which may decrease one's independence.
9. Although an older person commonly will seek help for somatic complaints, he or she may be unwilling to share feelings of anxiety with caregivers, causing further isolation.
10. Fear of being abandoned or feeling unable to support and care for oneself and loved ones may increase the client's anxiety and uncover unresolved conflicts.
11. Society's negative perception of the elderly may threaten an elderly client's self-concept.
12. A decrease in sensory acuity and mobility can cause a loss of autonomy, which may increase feelings of powerlessness.
13. Symptoms such as forgetfulness, decreased concentration, or thought blocks frequently go untreated.

ASSESSMENT CRITERIA
Physical

Vital signs
Skin color, warmth, dryness or diaphoresis
Physiological response resulting from parasympathetic reaction:
    Increased urinary frequency
    Headache
    Nausea
    Diarrhea
    Shortness of breath
    Hives
Restlessness
Musculoskeletal discomfort and angina
Neurological assessment, especially eyes
Nutritional status
Sleep patterns
Muscle strength and endurance
Medications
Laboratory findings: white blood cell count and blood glucose level

Psychosocial

Verbal and nonverbal behaviors
Attention span/ability to concentrate
Ability to retain/understand information
Ability to follow commands
Constant need for reassurance
Feeling of apprehension/dread
Sense of control
Interaction skills
Orientation
Rumination
Egocentricity
Past coping mechanisms
Support systems

Ability to communicate
Rate of speech

Spiritual

Concerns about spirituality and religious activity
Verbalizations about the connection between stressors and God's will

Use of coping mechanisms of sublimation, including prayer

Assessment Tools

Zung's Self-Rating Anxiety Scale (SAS)
Anxiety Status Inventory

 NURSING CARE PLAN: ANXIETY

Common contributing factors	Expected client outcomes	Nursing strategies
Feelings of helplessness when faced with crises	Client will be able to discuss the crisis being experienced Client will discuss positive coping strategies utilized in the past Client will discuss new coping mechanisms he or she could use and list possible situations when their use would be appropriate	Assess level of anxiety Determine if the client is at risk for suicide Assist the client in intellectualizing the crisis (e.g., what brought him or her into counseling, events that led up to this point) Discuss with the client past coping mechanisms and why they are not helping now Explore with the client new coping mechanisms and times when they need to be implemented Refer the client to a therapist if the crisis does not resolve itself in 4-6 weeks (crises are usually time limited); the client may need long-term therapy and prescribed antianxiety drugs
Failure to diagnose anxiety	Client will verbalize feelings of anxiety rather than somatic complaints Client will be able to identify behaviors that indicate he or she is becoming anxious Client will be able to identify contributing factors that lead to these behaviors (before anxiety reaches a severe or panic stage) Client will be able to demonstrate effective coping mechanisms to reduce anxiety levels	Provide reassurance Assess client's level of anxiety Stay calm, since the client will be able to sense if you are also becoming anxious If the client is in the severe or panic level, decrease stimuli and provide for a safe environment Communicate with short, simple sentences Once anxiety is decreased, assist client in developing self-awareness of behaviors Encourage recognition of behaviors that indicate one is becoming anxious Explore with the client factors that increase his or her anxiety Assist in developing coping mechanisms the client can use to decrease anxiety levels (e.g., relaxation techniques, problem solving)
Threat to self-concept related to society's perception of the elderly and change in role function Unresolved conflicts when unmet goals and feelings of failure arise	Client will make statements indicative of a positive self-concept Client will list some substitute or new roles he or she can engage in Client will identify and work through these unresolved conflicts	Assist the client in recognizing positive elderly role models in society Discuss ways in which substitute or new roles may be available (e.g., retired business owners assisting new small businesses, volunteer work, a possible part-time job) Explore with the client those areas of conflict, using the techniques of reminiscence or life review therapy
Fears of abandonment or inability to support and care for self and loved ones	Client will verbalize frustration over inability to completely care for self and loved ones independently Client will identify areas where autonomy still is possible Client will list resources that can help maintain autonomy	Assist the client with the recognition and acceptance of his or her limitations Maintain familiar routines Assist in identifying resources and support services available to the client

EVALUATION

1. The client's vital signs return to baseline.
2. The client verbalizes decreased anxiety and apprehension.
3. The client has increased ability to concentrate, follow directions, and problem solve.
4. The client's irritability and restlessness decrease.
5. The client displays knowledge of behaviors that indicate an increase in anxiety.
6. The client utilizes appropriate coping mechanisms to decrease anxiety.

NURSING ALERTS

1. Many of the commonly prescribed medications for anxiety-related disorders—barbituates and benzodiazepines—are contraindicated or must be used cautiously with the elderly.
2. Barbituates:
   a. Increase in nocturnal restlessness
   b. Hangover effect in morning, resulting in decreased cognition, and balance problems
   c. Since excreted through the kidneys, need to be used cautiously with clients with decreased renal function
   d. May decrease respiration; need to observe those clients on bed rest and experiencing respiratory difficulties
3. Benzodiazepines:
   a. Are often misused and can be addictive
   b. If discontinued abruptly, complications can occur: seizures, increase in blood pressure, pulse rate, and repiratory rate

Bibliography

Beck C, Rawlins R, and Williams S: Mental health–Psychiatric nursing: a holistic life-cycle approach, ed 2, St Louis, 1988, The CV Mosby Co.
Cape R, Coe R, and Rossman I: Fundamentals of geriatric medicine, New York, 1983, Raven Press.
Ebersole P and Hess P: Toward healthy aging, ed 3, St Louis, 1990, The CV Mosby Co.
Stuart G and Sundeen S: Pocket guide to psychiatric nursing, ed 2, St Louis, 1991, The CV Mosby Co.
Stuart G and Sundeen S: Principles and practices of psychiatric nursing, ed 4, St Louis, 1991, The CV Mosby Co.

Body Image Disturbance

Lois Robinson

KNOWLEDGE BASE

1. Body image disturbance is a disruption in the way one perceives one's body.
2. Body image is one factor in a cluster of characteristics defining one's sense of self and is influenced by feelings, attitudes, and values.
3. One's body image is influenced by the family in early childhood and evolves throughout life.
4. Factors influencing body image include developmental changes, aging, environment, fads, culture, and appraisal by self and others.
5. An older person may view his or her body in a negative way because age-related changes have altered the body's structure, function, or appearance.
6. Paralysis, amputation, colostomy, trauma, or any body change may cause a sense of loss resulting in grief, denial, anger, and shame.
7. An elderly person's physical appearance is often used as an indicator of intelligence or competence. A negative appraisal jeopardizes the person's sense of self.
8. Body image will influence an elder's self-care routines, life-style, relationships, social interactions, and health practices.
9. Increased attention to health practices may be necessary to maintain the older body.
10. Altered mobility, elimination, and sleep patterns may intrude on valued activities, altering the perception of body competence and body image.
11. Gradual changes may be nontraumatic until a limitation occurs, but sudden alterations are always traumatic and produce a greater crisis in body image and identity.

12. Body image can be greatly affected by retirement if a fixed income does not allow money for attractive clothing, hair care, dental care, or suitable housing.
13. Interactions with others are affected by the older person's sense of body.
14. Behaviors indicating body image disturbance include:
    a. Negative evaluation of self as compared with peers
    b. Verbalization of anger, shame, and loss of self-trust regarding structure, function, or appearance of the body
    c. Denial of alteration in functioning or non-compliance with limitations
    d. Obsession with body functioning or hypochondriasis
    e. Excessive use of youth-oriented make-up, clothing styles, and fads
    f. Refusal to view self in mirror or look at body part
    g. Refusal to participate in rehabilitation
    h. Refusal to talk about a body change
    i. Avoidance of social contacts

ASSESSMENT CRITERIA
Physical

Mobility level and degree of change
Activity and functional status
Nutritional status
Sleep patterns
Elimination patterns
General physical appearance
Hearing and vision
Chronic and acute diseases or trauma (present and past)
Loss or deformity of body parts
Posture

Psychosocial

History of personal investment in and feelings about body image
Client's appraisal of his or her most significant indices of body acceptance
Body language
Eye contact
Adjustment to change in life-style necessitated by physical condition
Importance of and feelings about appraisal of others
Losses related to significant others, physical appearance, function, roles
Behaviors and emotions in response to change
Timing of the change (gradual or sudden, traumatic or anticipated)
Duration of change (temporary or permanent)
Locus of control
Past and present coping skills
Relationships and roles
Current level of self-esteem
Significance of affected body part
Sense of purpose and productivity
Available support
Availability and use of a confidant
Financial resources
Social interactions/isolation
Degree of social "fit" for age group and culture

Spiritual

Concerns about meaning of life and death
Values and beliefs about the body purpose and function, beauty, independence
Responsibility for situation; perception of the disorder as punishment
Spiritual comfort

NURSING CARE PLAN: ACTIVITY INTOLERANCE

Common contributing factors	Expected client outcomes	Nursing strategies
Change in physical appearance or function	Client will identify the meaning of body change	Assess the client's perception of the change and of self
	Client will report his concerns, feelings, and perceptions	Assess specific elements of the change that have significant meaning for the client
	Client will demonstrate adaptation in daily activities	Demonstrate unconditional acceptance of the client's appearance, function, and behavior
	Client will have increased knowledge of the condition	Validate the normalcy of the client's response to the change
	Client will be able to recognize his strengths	Help the client to acknowledge the change and identify his or her concerns
	Client will use strengths to compensate for changes	Assess the knowledge level of client and family
		Establish a trusting relationship
		Encourage questions; provide information to toleration level
		Encourage the client to discuss his or her feelings
		Use active listening

Continued.

NURSING CARE PLAN: BODY IMAGE DISTURBANCE—cont'd

Common contributing factors	Expected client outcomes	Nursing strategies
	Client will participate in planning care Client will increase autonomous behavior Client will discover a valuable self Client and family will know of available support groups	Accept coping behaviors Help the client identify remaining physical, social, emotional and spiritual strengths Assist in identifying ways to maximize strengths and remaining abilities Allow and encourage decision making Assist in setting realistic goals Help the client develop strategies to compensate for the change Encourage self-care and independence Maximize hygiene, grooming, use of prostheses such as dentures, wigs Encourage the client to dress in appropriate, comfortable, attractive clothing Help the client to view the body change when able, and provide support through the process Develop a teaching plan based on the client's grief response and readiness to learn Offer emotional support to client and family and establish consistent communication Help the family to focus on the client rather than the problem Encourage the client to seek opportunities for social interaction and new relationships Refer the client to support groups
Loss of body part	Client will be able to identify meaning and feelings related to the loss Client will maintain mild to moderate levels of anxiety Client will consciously select positive coping mechanisms Client will talk positively about his or her body and abilities Client will report increased comfort Client will have a reality-based body image Client will maintain maximum autonomy over care and treatment	Assess the meaning of the loss for client and family Assess coping mechanisms being used by both client and significant others Accept the client's behavior Encourage expression of feelings and sharing of feelings between client and others Promote an appropriate dependence-independence pattern of care Involve family if appropriate Promote positive self-talk; explore feelings underlying negative statements Assist patient in identifying unique qualities and abilities of self Expect phantom pain, especially when there was chronic pain in the body part before surgery Assess and care for phantom pain as for all other pain Explore how past experiences can be used as a current resource Assess readiness to view and touch site Provide privacy and support for exploring the surgical site Assist in developing self-care skills and mastery of dressings, pouches, or care regimens Involve significant other/family in care if permitted by client Develop an exercise program within the prescribed limits Refer to a support group See also care plan for spiritual distress, p. 83

EVALUATION

1. The client openly discusses his or her feelings about the change or loss.
2. The client identifies his or her strenghts and abilities and uses them to compensate for changes.
3. The client participates in planning care.
4. The client shows desire to increase autonomy.
5. The client is aware of available support groups.
6. The client talks more positively about his or her body and abilities.

NURSING ALERTS

1. Depersonalization of the body part or the loss may result in noncompliance with the treatment regimen.
2. Anger as a grief behavior may be directed at self, significant others, or staff, causing disruption in supportive relationships.

3. Helplessness, hopelessness, and powerlessness may predispose the older person to depression. Depression in the elderly may not be as recognizable as in others, and is less likely to be treated.
4. Memory may be altered by stress and anxiety, which poses problems for reality teaching and resolution of the loss.

Bibliography

Carpenito LJ: Nursing diagnosis: application to clinical practice, ed 2, Philadelphia, 1987, JB Lippincott Co.

Kim MJ, McFarland GK, and McLane AM: Pocket guide to nursing diagnoses, ed 3, St Louis, 1989, The CV Mosby Co.

Phipps WJ, Long BC, and Woods NF: Medical-surgical nursing: concepts and clinical practice, ed 3, St Louis, 1987, The CV Mosby Co.

Taylor CM, and Cress SS: Nursing diagnosis cards, Springhouse, 1987, Springhouse Corp.

Yurick AG et al: The aged person and the nursing process, Norwalk, Conn, 1989, Appleton & Lange.

Cardiac Output, Decreased

Sharon Bowles

KNOWLEDGE BASE

1. Decreased cardiac output is defined as the state in which the amount of blood pumped by the heart is inadequate to meet the needs of the body's tissues.
2. It is sometimes difficult to determine whether decreased cardiac function is due to the aging process or disease or both. Generally, the aging process produces a slow and insidious decrease in cardiac function, whereas disease produces a more acute decrease.
3. Normal cardiac output is 4 to 8 liters/min. Because cardiac output is decreased in the elderly, the lower limits of normal or a different range may need to be established.
4. Inadequate cerebral perfusion secondary to decreased cardiac output may occur. Sensorium changes may be the first indication of decreased perfusion.

5. Auscultation of lung sounds and observation for jugular vein distention are important in order to detect the presence of pulmonary congestion, which may result from decreased cardiac output.
6. Dyspnea is a cardinal manifestation of left-ventricular failure.
7. Invasive hemodynamic monitoring permits close examination of cardiovascular function, the heart's ability to pump blood, and the integrity of the vascular system while cardiac responses to therapeutic interventions are being assessed.
8. Not all researchers agree about the specific effects of aging on the heart.
9. Resting heart rate is unchanged with age. Maximal heart rate and stroke volume decrease with age, at an estimated rate of 1% per year.
10. Cardiac output decreases up to 40% between ages 25 and 45.

11. The heart works less in the aged because of decreased lean body mass. Overall, the elderly require less oxygen both at rest and during exercise.
12. As aging occurs, the heart muscle becomes less elastic and loses its efficiency and contractile strength. This results in decreased stroke volume.
13. Lessened elasticity of all vessels, including the aorta, and the presence of atrial atrophy produce problems in filling and emptying the heart.
14. Resolution or management of an acute disease process may not totally reestablish previous cardiac output, since residual age-related cardiovascular changes are irreversible. The nurse's goal is to maximize functional abilities.
15. Rest periods are necessary to minimize exhaustion and promote a balance between oxygen demand and supply.
16. Beside commode or bathroom privileges for elimination are preferable to bedpan use. Using the bedpan can be exhausting and stressful and may increase oxygen demand and cardiac workload unnecessarily.

ASSESSMENT CRITERIA
General

See Table 1 for common etiologies of decreased cardiac output.

Physical

Detailed history
  Symptoms
    Precipitating factors
    Typical daily activities
Fatigue
Comparison of activities in last 5 to 10 years
Nutrition (especially sodium intake)
Smoking history
Family history for cardiovascular disease
History of dyspnea, dizzy spells, chest pain, heart irregularities and/or palpitations, coughing or wheezing
Medications
Other health problems
Life stressors
Physical findings
  Pulse: rate, regularity, pulse amplitude, pulse deficit; apical pulse should be taken for 1 minute with stethoscope; peripheral pulses
  Blood pressure: both arms, lying, sitting, standing
  Respiration: rate, dyspnea (exertional, orthopnea, paroxysmal nocturnal dyspnea at rest)
  Jugular vein distention and/or edema (pedal and sacral)
  Skin temperature, color, condition
  Heart sounds: auscultation with stethoscope for extra heart sounds and murmurs
  Heart rhythm: by electrocardiographic monitoring or telemetry
Signs and symptoms of decreasing cardiac function
  Abnormal data from invasive monitoring
  Blood oxygenation: by bedside pulse oximetry
Significant findings
  Abnormal physical findings
  Increased dyspnea, dizziness
  Onset of chest discomfort/pain
  Increased intolerance to activity
Signs and symptoms of complications
Level of activity intolerance; response to activity

Table 1 **Common etiologies for decreased cardiac output—partial listing**

Mechanical (alterations in preload, afterload, inotropic changes)	Electrical (alterations in rate, rhythm, and/or conduction)	Structural (age-related changes)
Myocardial disease/damage	Conduction defects	Decreased myocardial efficiency
Myocardial infarction	Heart block	Reduced elasticity of vessels
Ischemia	Bundle-branch block	Poor tolerance of tachycardia
Cardiomyopathy	Bradycardia	Increased thickness and rigidity of valves
Pericarditis	Tachycardia	Weaker contractile force
Bacterial endocarditis	Digitalis toxicity	
Valvular disease/damage		
Stenosis		
Insufficiency		
Rupture		
Severe hypertension		
Congestive heart failure/pulmonary edema		
Fluid and electrolyte imbalance		
Shock, sepsis, allergic response		
Chronic obstructive pulmonary disease		

Psychosocial

Client's perception of and reaction to heart condition, assessment and treatment modalities

Client's knowledge related to heart condition, diet, medications, and activity in preparation for discharge

Clients health beliefs and practices

Spouse/signficant other socialization patterns and support systems

Spiritual

Client's need for spriritual care

Source of comfort and hope

 ## NURSING CARE PLAN: DECREASED CARDIAC OUTPUT

Common contributing factors	Expected client outcomes	Nursing strategies
Mechanical, electrical, structural disorders (see Table 1)	Client will maintain hemodynamic stability Regular pulse and in normal range Blood pressure normal for client Respiratory rate in normal range	Monitor apical and radial pulse, blood pressure, respiration as indicated and report abnormal findings Assess for signs and symptoms of cardiogenic shock and report significant changes immediately: Mental confusion Systolic blood pressure less than 90 mm Hg Tachycardia Urine output less than 20 ml per hour Ensure that emergency equipment is available and functioning
	Client will display usual mental status Client's skin will be warm and dry; color will be pink Client's pulses will be present and full Client will maintain regular heart rate	Assess changes in sensorium such as confusion, disorientation, lethargy, restlessness Assess skin for warmness and dryness; observe color Note presence and quality of pulses Monitor heart rate and rhythm with cardiac monitor or telemetry, if indicated Document and report rate or rhythm disturbances, ectopy, or change in PR interval Observe for skin irritation from electrode placement; change electrodes often
	Client's lung sounds will be clear and respiration will be unlabored Client will have no abnormal heart sounds Client will demonstrate no edema or jugular vein distention Client will maintain normal invasive hemodynamic parameters	Auscultate breath sounds and assess patient for signs of dyspnea Auscultate heart sounds or review chart for presence of S_3 and/or S_4 gallop and murmurs Inspect for signs of peripheral or dependent edema and jugular vein distention Assess invasive hemodynamic parameters, if monitoring is indicated and available (e.g., central venous pressure, pulmonary arterial pressure, pulmonary capillary wedge pressure, cardiac output)
	Client will maintain optimal fluid balance Client will maintain initial bed rest and progress activity as tolerated	Weigh daily, before breakfast Monitor intake and output as indicated Administer intravenous fluids with caution; use microdrip or infusion pump; avoid saline solutions Provide a quiet, relaxed atmosphere and restriction of activity; assist with self-care activities Organize nursing care and treatments to allow adequate rest periods Assist in use of bedside commode or bathroom for elimination Encourage increased activity as tolerated

Continued.

NURSING CARE PLAN: DECREASED CARDIAC OUTPUT—cont'd

Common contributing factors	Expected client outcomes	Nursing strategies
	Client will immediately report any chest pain or discomfort	Instruct the client to report the development of chest pain immediately
	Client will communicate knowledge and understanding of signs and symptoms of decreased cardiac output, prescribed medications, and activity level	Educate the client and family regarding: Signs and symptoms to report, such as shortness of breath, chest pain, weakness, dizziness, syncope, palpitations Prescribed medications: name, dosage, frequency, therapeutic effects, side effects Prescribed diet Activity level Reinforce education through verbal repetition and written instructions for the client to take home
	Client will understand self-care adjustments to decreased cardiac output	Suggest ways to adjust to decreased cardiac output during activities of daily living; e.g., pace activities, drive instead of walking long distances, use elevator or escalator rather than walking stairs, rest between activities

EVALUATION

1. The client demonstrates vital signs within acceptable limits.
2. The client maintains optimal mentation.
3. The client's skin is warm and dry; the color is pink.
4. The client's pulse is regular; peripheral pulses are present and full; there is no pulse deficit.
5. The client's heart rate and rhythm are within the expected range.
6. The client's lung sounds are clear, with unlabored respiration.
7. The client's heart sounds are within an established range.
8. The client has a decrease in edema or jugular vein distention.
9. The client understands invasive monitoring.
10. The client reports no weight gain resulting from fluid volume overload.
11. The client reports fewer episodes of dyspnea and a decrease in or absence of chest pain.
12. The client demonstrates an increase in activity tolerance.
13. The client utilizes strategies to participate in activities that reduce cardiac workload.
14. The client verbalizes knowledge and understanding of his or her own heart condition, signs and symptoms to report, medication, dietary considerations, and activity level.
15. The client recognizes self-care adjustments related to decreased cardiac output.

NURSING ALERTS

1. The older person's cardiovascular system cannot compensate for excess fluid. Intravenous fluid administration must be used with extreme caution to prevent circulatory overload and ultimate cardiac compromise. Saline solutions promote water retention and should therefore be avoided or used cautiously. Daily weights are very important, to assess sudden changes in weight resulting from fluid loss or retention. Intake and output are also monitored to assess retention of water.
2. The elderly have an increase in adipose tissue as compared with their total body mass. Drugs that are stored in the adipose tissue may therefore accumulate and remain in the body for a longer time. Prescribed dosages should be adjusted accordingly, and signs of drug toxicity should be assessed.
3. In the elderly the number of functioning nephrons is reduced, the glomerular filtration rate is decreased, and blood flow to the kidneys is reduced. Therefore, the biologic half-lives of drugs are extended, increasing the time required for drugs to be filtered from the body. Age-adjusted dosages should be prescribed, and signs of drug toxicity should be assessed.
4. During assessment of heart sounds, abnormal heart sounds of S_3 and S_4 and murmurs are important to note. An S_4 is commonly seen in the elderly as a result of an age-related decrease in the compliance of the heart muscle. The onset of a new S_3 suggests increased heart failure. Systolic murmurs are often present in the elderly. A diastolic murmur is always abnormal.

Bibliography

Burnside I: Nursing and the Aged: a self-care approach, ed 3, New York, 1988, McGraw-Hill Book Co.

Carpenito LJ: Nursing diagnosis: application to clinical practice, ed 2, Philadelphia, 1987, J B Lippincott Co.

Doenges ME, Moorhouse MF, and Geissler AC: Nusing care plans: guidelines for planning patient care, ed 2, Philadelphia, 1989, FA Davis Co.

Eliopoulos C: Gerontological nursing, ed 2, Philadelphia, 1987, JB Lippincott Co.

Eliopoulos C: A guide to the nursing of the aging, Baltimore, 1987, The Williams & Wilkins Co.

Guzzetta CE and Dossey BM: Cardiovascular nursing: bodymind tapestry, St Louis, 1984, The CV Mosby Co.

Johanson BC and others: Standards for critical care, ed 3, St Louis, 1988, The CV Mosby Co.

Kim MJ, McFarland GK, and McLane AM: Pocket guide to nursing diagnoses, ed 3, St Louis, 1989, The CV Mosby Co.

Matteson MA and McConnell ES: Gerontological nursing: concepts and practice, Philadelphia, 1988, WB Saunders Co.

Murray RB and Zentner JP: Nursing assessment and health promotion strategies through the life span, ed 4, Norwalk, Conn, 1989, Appleton & Lange.

Schroeder CH: Pulse oximetry: a nursing care plan, Critical Care Nurse 8(8):50, 1989.

Taylor C and Cress S: Nusing '87 nursing diagnosis cards, Springhouse, Pa, 1987 Springhouse Corp.

Communication, Impaired Verbal

Dixie M. Flynn
Sharyn L. Mills

KNOWLEDGE BASE

1. Impaired verbal communication is the state in which an individual experiences a decreased or absent ability to use or understand language in human interaction.
2. Communication involves the sender of a message, the message itself, the receiver, and the environment in which the interaction occurs. When any one of the elements is disturbed, communication is impaired.
3. Communication occurs in numerous ways. In addition to spoken or written ideas, body language, voice tone, and other nonverbal communication are used. Communication can be intentional or unconscious. Understanding and using all communication forms greatly enhance the older person's life and the quality of care.
4. Verbal communication is a major means of interaction with one's environment.
5. Verbal communication is dependent on a person's ability to cognitively function, hear, read, recognize numerical relationships, and nonverbally communicate.
6. Speech/perception centers of the brain can be injured through disease processes (multiple sclerosis), through injury to the brain cells (cerebro-

vascular accident or blunt trauma), or through pressure (tumors, hydrocephalus).
7. Injury to the brain cells can result in the following speech abnormalities:
   a. Aphasia—partial or complete loss of the ability to speak or to comprehend the spoken word, because of injury, disease, or maldevelopment of the brain
   b. Expressive aphasia—the client can understand verbal and written communication but cannot organize ideas into words or phrases
   c. Receptive aphasia—the client cannot understand what is being said; it is as if he or she were hearing a foreign language; the client also has difficulty understanding written information and may or may not recognize objects
   d. Oral apraxia—loss of the ability to execute simple voluntary acts of the oral mechanism
   e. Verbal apraxia—loss of the ability to perform elementary units of action in the expression of language
   f. Dysarthria—a disorder of articulation caused by impairment of the part of the central nervous system that directly controls the muscles of the tongue and mouth

g. Verbal disorganization and nonexpansion—difficulty in sequencing verbal units and deleting detail

h. Lack of word fluency—loss of the power to name objects or to recall and recognize names

8. The neuromotor disturbances that cause impaired communication may be transient or long term, reversible or irreversible.

9. Diseases, tumors, or trauma may produce serious deficits in communication ability when superimposed upon age-related changes in the respiratory system, fibrotic changes in the larynx, and decreased neuromuscular effectiveness.

10. Aphasia is associated with brain damage involving the left hemisphere (posterior aspect of the inferior frontal gyrus). It has been held that a left-brain stroke will not result in aphasia in a left-handed person. Now it is known that between 33% and 50% of all left-brain strokes will produce some degree of aphasia, regardless of right- or left-sided dominance.

11. Fatigue, anxiety, and frustration reduce a client's ability to comprehend a message.

12. Clients with aphasia may have behavioral changes. The most common ones are mood swings, labile affect, and catastrophic reactions. Once the emotion is experienced, the neurological damage to the brain cortex results in an inability to inhibit or modify the behavior.

13. Impaired communication threatens a client's self-esteem and creates situations that produce feelings of anger, frustration, and powerlessness.

14. Depression is likely when a client has impaired communication.

15. Social isolation and alienation frequently are outcomes when an elder has difficulty communicating.

16. Staff education on techniques and care issues is critical. Aphasic clients may be mistakenly treated as hearing impaired, retarded, or demented.

ASSESSMENT CRITERIA
Physical

Verbal—client's ability to:
 Make utterances and produce oral movements volitionally
 Produce automatic series
  Words via sentence completion
  Initiate single words
 Spontaneously name objects
 Connect two or three words to express needs/thoughts
 Produce phrases without errors (with or without the use of gestures)
 Express needs in short sentences with high degree of accuracy

Auditory—client's ability to:
 Demonstrate a consistent yes/no system with 90% accuracy
 Comprehend single spoken words
 Comprehend one-step and multi-step commands
 Comprehend sentence-length material
 Comprehend phone conversations
 Understand conversational speech with one person
Reading—client's ability to:
 Recognize own name in print
 Match single written word to picture
 Recognize short one-step phrases, such as "make a fist"
 Locate emergency numbers in phone book (or use cue cards)
 Recognize settings on home appliances
 Recognize familiar signs
 Follow printed recipes on packaged foods
 Follow simple, multi-step recipes in cookbooks
 Understand directions on medicine lables
 Read/understand paragraph-length material
Cognition—client's ability to:
 Demonstrate awareness and responsiveness to environment
 Demonstrate orientation to environment and familiar people
 Sequence basic events of the day
 Adequately problem solve, especially cause-effect relationships
 Devise solutions and alternatives
 Integrate information and use effectively for logical reasoning and abstract verbal skills

Psychosocial

Client's ability to demonstrate:
 Situational coping skills
 Adjustment to disability
 Motivation
Other pertinent information:
 Prior verbal communication capability
 Cognitive status
 Anxiety level
 Presence of:
  Anger/agitation
  Depression
  Emotional lability
  Powerlessness
 Dependence/independence
 Educational level
 Social isolation
 Role relationships
 Coping ability of family
 Social/emotional support systems

Spiritual

Client's need to participate in a faith community
Patterns of practice related to religious rituals

NURSING CARE PLAN: IMPAIRED VERBAL COMMUNICATION

Common contributing factors	Expected client outcomes	Nursing strategies
Inability to form/ speak words	Client will be able to communicate needs Client will use alternative methods of communication Client will maximize communication ability Client will maximize ability to understand messages Client will be able to make needs known	Assess ability to understand by asking yes/no questions whose answers can be verified Obtain order for speech pathologist evaluation to determine severity of deficits contributing to client's inability to speak Establish alternative mechanism for communicating (e.g., picture board, spelling board, writing tablet, gesturing) Establish a positive, calm, permissive atmosphere; provide consistent approach Provide opportunity to hear speech between others and from radio or TV; encourage socialization Encourage any attempt at speech or communication by nodding and providing appropriate feedback Keep questions and instructions simple on an adult level (one idea or command at a time); give adequate time for response; do not rush the client or show impatience Teach staff/family to slow their rates of speech and use appropriate nonverbal communication Treat and speak to the client as a mature adult; avoid loud and/or childish language Avoid interruption of the client's attempts at speech; do not supply words Include family in education and therapy

Limited cognitive ability	Client will show his or her optimal level in:
	    Orientation
	    Attention span
	    Concentration
	    Memory
	    Organization
	    Internal control
	    Problem solving
	    Judgment
	    Visual perception
	Client will be able to make needs known
		Assess ability to make basic needs known
		Introduce self and function each time client's room is entered
		Present information in short units
		Eliminate distractions while communicating and turn off TV
		Restate information presented to client and, if appropriate, have patient repeat it
		For garbled language, listen to the context of the message (both verbal and nonverbal) rather than individual words
		Respond to the feeling expressed if the message is disoriented or not understandable
		Help with solutions and alternatives to problems
		Ask family to bring in a clock and a calendar if not provided by hospital
		Provide a schedule that is as routine as possible
		Avoid "overload" (too much stimulation at one time)
		Have client visually focus on side on which neglect exists; administer medications from side of neglect
		Place water glass and other frequently used items within sight and reach
		Be honest with client within reason
		Encourage group activities

Limited auditory capability	Client will demonstrate:
	    Increased auditory capability
	    Ability to lip read
	    Ability to understand gestures
	    Ability to use the telephone
		Turn TV/radio off when speaking to client
		Have client's attention before attempting to communicate; touch on shoulder to get attention
		Look directly at client while talking and speak at distance of approximately 3 feet
		Speak slowly and distinctly but without unneeded loudness
		Pair gestures with speech and other visual cues
		If client does not hear you first time, repeat/rephrase what you have said
		Request telephone amplification
		Assist in use of assistive listening device

Continued.

NURSING CARE PLAN: IMPAIRED VERBAL COMMUNICATION—cont'd

Common contributing factors	Expected client outcomes	Nursing strategies
Frustration, lack of motivation because of inability to talk or be understood	Client will have decreased level of frustration with inability to verbalize Client will have fewer and shorter episodes of frustration Client will demonstrate willingness to attempt speech and communication	Provide a quiet, relaxed environment, avoid noise and interruptions Determine strategies that decrease frustration Provide client with compensatory strategies; ask yes/no questions, use picture boards, writing tablets, etc. Give client time to respond in his or her most effective manner; if you do not have time to figure out what client is saying, tell him or her that you will return, and give a specific time; keep your promise Be honest with client if his or her message cannot be understood Use "I" messages: "I'm not understanding you today." Tolerate mistakes; do not correct; expect varying levels of performance from day to day and during a day Establish a predictable schedule of activities Avoid requiring speech/communication when client is tired, anxious, or frustrated

Family's lack of knowledge of communication plan of care	Family/significant other will:
	  Verbalize understanding of plan of care
	  Demonstrate knowledge of their role in the plan
	  Use compensatory communication mechanisms with client
	  Allow client to speak for self
		Daily log book of client's activities can be used
		Encourage family/significant other to attend treatment sessions with therapist's permission
		Provide handouts to family/significant other
		Reinforce support from family/significant other

EVALUATION

1. The client is able to communicate needs.
2. The client demonstrates use of alternate mechanisms to communicate needs.
3. The client demonstrates motivation to attempt to communicate and to participate in speech therapy.
4. With reversible cognitive impairment, the client demonstrates an increase in cognitive ability as demonstrated by improved orientation to time and place, attention span, concentration, memory, organization, internal control, problem solving, judgment, and perceptual skills (visual and auditory).
5. The client achieves improved auditory reception by demonstrating compensatory mechanisms (e.g., ability to read lips, understand gestures, or use phone).
6. The client demonstrates fewer and shorter episodes of frustration, allowing for improved compliance with plan of care.
7. The client's family/significant other demonstrates understanding of the plan of care and their role in implementing the plan.

NURSING ALERTS

1. A thorough assessment of a client's communication abilities must be completed to accurately diagnose to what degree the communications deficits exist.
2. Do not assume that in the presence of disease or injury to the brain, there are no communication deficits just because a client can communicate verbally.
3. All clients who have disease or injury to the brain should have a thorough speech and language evaluation by a speech pathologist and a hearing evaluation by an audiologist.
4. Responses to stimuli are slower with the older adult. Allow adequate time for the older adult to respond to questions and assessment mechanisms.
5. Deterioration of intellectual function should not be found unless the client has a disease of the central nervous system.
6. The plan of care must be developed through a multidisciplinary approach, including a qualified speech pathologist. All members of the health care team must be involved in assessment, planning, and implementation.

Bibliography

Bollinger RL, Waugh PF, and Zatz AF: Communication management of the geriatric patient, Danville, Ill, 1977, Interstate Printers & Publishers, Inc.

Glickstein: Aphasia: a pragmatic approach to management, Focus on Geriatric Care and Rehabilitation, 1(9):1, 1988.

Kim MJ, McFarland GK, and McLane AM: Pocket guide to nursing diagnoses, ed 3, St Louis, 1989, The CV Mosby Co.

Seidel H, Ball J, Dains J, and Benedict W: Mosby's guide to physical examination, St. Louis, 1987, The CV Mosby Co.

Travis LE, editor: Handbook of speech pathology and audiology, New York, 1971, Appleton-Century-Crofts.

Constipation

Margherita P. Nahrup

KNOWLEDGE BASE

1. Constipation is the state in which an individual experiences a change in normal bowel function characterized by a decrease in frequency and/or passage of hard, dry stools.
2. Clients' perceptions of what is normal bowel function may vary. Some elderly people believe that if they do not have a bowel movement daily, they are constipated. Normal bowel function may vary from three movements per day to only three per week. Some elders treat themselves unnecessarily.
3. The body's evacuation of feces depends upon an intact central nervous system and intact neural centers in the lower intestinal wall. The urge to defecate is caused by stimulation of nerves by the fecal mass.
4. Body time influences peristalsis, providing predictability to elimination schedules.
5. Adequate hydration allows the body to leave fluid within the feces.
6. Many older people have reduced smooth muscle tone of the intestines, resulting in slower peristalsis, and drier feces, which when combined with decreased strength of abdominal muscles, reduces the pressure that can be exerted during bowel evacuation.
7. Elderly people may use laxatives and enemas on a regular basis, resulting in habituation.
8. Chronic use of prescription medications can decrease bowel motility.
9. Prolonged inactivity or immobility resulting from a chronic illness may increase the risk of constipation.
10. Communication abilities may influence whether a person can report physical needs to caregivers.
11. Mental status changes resulting from the aging process may impair the client's ability to attend to or even recognize the need to defecate.
12. Anxiety inhibits peristalsis through the action of epinephrine and the sympathetic nervous system.
13. The presence of dementia or schizophrenia may be a factor.
14. Immobility can result in a loss of privacy during toileting.
15. Environmental factors that effect a change in normal daily routines (e.g., travel, use of a bedpan) may potentiate constipation.
16. Elderly people often live alone and do not have the energy or desire to eat a balanced diet. Or they eat highly refined and easily prepared foods that are low in fiber. Some older people do not eat regularly because of diminished appetite, poor dentition, financial problems, inability to prepare their own meals, changes in abilities to smell and taste, or anorexia.

ASSESSMENT CRITERIA
Physical

Use of routine medications such as:
  Antacids
  Laxatives
  Diuretics
  Anticholinergics
  Sedatives
  Tranquilizers
Comfort or pain with defecation
Usual defecation schedule
Description of feces
Specific bowel sounds
Distention/flatulence
Abdominal pain

Perianal problems, such as hemorrhoids
Nutritional status
Daily dietary habits, including fluid/fiber intake
Neurological deficits
Sensory/motor disorders
Past/present illnesses and treatments
Ability to assume optimal position for defecation
Relevant family history such as:
    Colorectal problems
    Ulcers
    Gastrointestinal malignancies
    Pernicious anemia

Psychosocial

Description of chief complaint
Mental status
Verbal/auditory skills
Activity level
Depression or stressors
Changes in environmental factors
Usual life-style and recent changes

Spiritual

Religious beliefs or practices

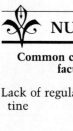

NURSING CARE PLAN: CONSTIPATION

Common contributing factors	Expected client outcomes	Nursing strategies
Lack of regular bowel routine	Client will establish routine bowel habit	Assess usual elimination patterns and surrounding events (e.g., hot coffee) Instruct client on the need for a daily routine for bowel elimination Assist client in establishing a toileting schedule (e.g., take 5-15 minutes every morning after breakfast and a hot drink to attempt to move bowels) Instruct client not to avoid the urge to defecate Instruct client on the hazards of prolonged use of irritant, stimulant type of laxatives
Excessive use of inappropriate laxatives or enemas	Client will defecate without routine use of laxatives or enemas	Assess for systemic allergic reactions to the laxative Insert glycerin suppository with concomitant anal stimulation Upright positioning for defecation is important; both feet should be flat on floor or supported on a footrest; knees and hips flexed to a semi-squatting position as possible; rocking motion of upper body will complete defecation if abdominal pressure cannot be forceful If glycerin suppository is not effective, repeat the routine on second day By third day, request order for bisacodyl suppository; if not effective, follow with a saline enema Request order for stool softener
Lack of dietary fluids and fiber	Client will alter dietary habits to include high-fiber foods and adequate fluids	Assess stool frequency and character, laxative use, diet, fluid, and activity Instruct client to eat foods high in fiber, such as bran, fruits, nuts, legumes, and root vegetables (fruit balls may be offered) Instruct client to drink at least six 6-ounce glasses of fluid per day, not including coffee, tea, or alcohol (unless contraindicated) Monitor output and edema Establish schedule and method for fluid intake; offer a glass of hot lemonade (an ounce of lemon juice, sweetened, in 6 ounces of water) 30 minutes before breakfast; three ounces of hot prune juice (nutmeg or cinnamon can be added) can also be suggested

NURSING CARE PLAN: CONSTIPATION—cont'd

Common contributing factors	Expected client outcomes	Nursing strategies
Environmental impediments to normal bowel function	Client will adapt his or her environment to make it more conducive to normal bowel function	Instruct client to locate public toilet facilities so they can be used readily when necessary Use of nightlights at home can be helpful; handrails by toilets can be installed to assist clients Instruct client to wear easily removable clothing Provide for privacy and comfort Instruct in relaxation exercises for anxious clients
Use of prescribed medications that cause constipation	Client will maintain a normal bowel routine when taking potentially constipating medications	Assess bowel sounds on regular basis; assess types of prescribed medications, especially analgesics, muscle relaxants, calcium and iron supplements Encourage client to talk with physician regarding prescribed medications when they are causing constipation; alternative drugs, doses, or dosage schedules can be utilized to avoid or relieve constipation Initiate preventive measures as soon as possible after medication is started
Inadequate activity or exercise	Client will increase activity within specified limits	Assess current level of activities and limitations Explain rationale for exercise or activity program If not contraindicated, establish walking program Teach bed or chair exercises to tolerance Teach abdominal and gluteal strengthening exercises Progress activity within restrictions and physician's medical plan Seek order for physical therapy consultation

EVALUATION

1. The client has achieved routine bowel function without excessive use of laxatives, straining, or pain.
2. The client's diet includes daily intake of high-fiber foods and adequate fluids.
3. The client has made adaptations to his or her environment to ensure maintenance of normal bowel function.
4. The client is able to avoid episodes of constipation even though he or she is still taking potentially constipating prescription medications.
5. The client has increased his or her activity level.

NURSING ALERTS

1. Chronic use of any laxative agent can cause dependence and ultimately impair the normal reflex to defecate.
2. Changes in a client's mental status can occur as a result of electrolyte imbalances, dehydration, or fecal impaction.
3. Older persons are at risk for paralytic ileus. Preventive measures should be initiated when analgesics or muscle relaxants are given.
4. Decreased activity or bed rest will cause a client to be at risk for constipation.

Bibliography

Eliopoulos C: Gerontological nursing, ed 2, Philadelphia, 1987, JB Lippincott Co.

Gioiella EC and Bevil CW: Nursing care of the aging client, Norwalk, Conn, 1985, Appleton-Century-Crofts.

Kasanof DM: Constipation: is it functional, or . . .? Patient Care 18(4):128, 1984.

Kim MJ, McFarland GK, and McLane AM: Pocket guide to nursing diagnoses, ed 3, St Louis, 1989, The CV Mosby Co.

Mager-O'Connor E: How to identify and remove fecal impactions, Geriatric Nursing, 5(3):158, 1984.

McShane RE et al: Constipation: consensual and empirical validation . . . nursing diagnoses, Nursing Clinics of North America, 20(4):801, 1985.

Meeroff JC: Approach to the patient with constipation, Hospital Practice, 20(1):148, 1985.

Resnick B: Constipation: common but not preventable, Geriatric Nursing 6(4):213, 1985.

Smith LE: Trouble in the anorectal: incontinence and constipation, part 5, Emergency Medicine Clinics of North America 18(6):132, 1986.

Wichita C: Treating and preventing constipation in nursing home residents, Journal of Gerontological Nursing 3(6):35, 1978.

Yurick AJ et al: The aged person and the nursing process, ed 3, Norwalk, Conn, 1989, Appleton & Lange.

Disuse Syndrome, Potential For

Frances F. Rogers-Seidl

KNOWLEDGE BASE

1. Disuse syndrome is defined as the state in which a person is at risk for deterioration of body systems as a result of inactivity.
2. Older people are at risk for complications of immobility because of age-related changes affecting all organs and tissues, which decrease efficiency and reserve.
3. There are predictable outcomes when an older person's movement is limited. The changes are a result of deconditioning caused by lack of use of body tissues and organs.
4. Disuse syndrome begins within the first day of inactivity. Disuse causes discomfort, since every system of the body is ultimately affected.
5. Cardiovascular function is decreased with disuse.
   a. The heart adapts to lessened demands, resulting in a less efficient pump. The recumbent position increases workload 30%.
   b. The autonomic nervous system is unable to equalize blood supply from the recumbent to the upright position.
   c. Vascular muscle tone decreases 10% to 15% per week, resulting in blood pooling in dependent vessels, predisposing the client to thrombus formation.
   d. Body position may put pressure on vessels; flexion may obstruct venous return
   e. Increased serum calcium from bone resorption increases the coagulability of the blood and thus increases risk of thrombus formation.
6. Respiratory function is decreased as a result of immobility.
   a. Chest expansion is limited by:
      (1) Resistance of the bed or chair
      (2) Sitting or lying posture
      (3) Abdominal distention
      (4) Decreased muscle power and coordination
      (5) Central nervous system depressing respiratory centers in medulla (tumor, medications, anesthesia)
      (6) Decreased elasticity of the chest muscles
   b. Depth of respiration is reduced because a decreased basal metabolism produces less carbon dioxide and decreases the need for oxygen.
   c. Stasis of secretions occurs with decreased physical movement. Tenacious secretions result from dehydration or anticholinergic drugs. Either situation causes the elder to be at risk for pneumonia.
7. Musculoskeletal integrity requires innervation and intermittent workloads on the skeletal muscles. Adequate exercise produces strength, endurance, and coordination. Disuse results in:
   a. Decrease in muscle strength and mass
   b. Decrease in endurance
   c. Loss of joint mobility/contractures
   d. Osteoporosis
8. Skin integrity requires an adequate supply of nutrients to skin cells and removal of waste materials. Continued pressure on the skin tissue results in tissue necrosis and pressure ulcers. Tissue made ischemic by one condition has less tolerance for other ischemia-inducing conditions.
9. The urinary tract is jeopardized by disuse.
   a. Altered gravity inhibits complete emptying of the kidney calyx and urinary bladder, predisposing the client to stone formation and infection.
   b. Increased excretion of calcium from the bone, combined with decreased fluid intake, increases the risk of stone formation.
10. The alimentary tract is altered by disuse.
    a. Catabolic activity increases during immobility, producing a rapid breakdown of cellular material, resulting in protein deficiency and anorexia.
    b. Peristalsis is slowed with disuse, accentuating an already existing problem of elderly people. Slower stomach emptying may cause distention or gastric reflux.
    c. Peristalsis of the small and large bowel is slowed during bed rest, thus compounding

age-related changes. Diminished expulsive power, loss of the defecation reflex, and decreased food and fluid intake cause constipation.

11. Psychosocial equilibrium is altered by disuse.
    a. Motivation, learning, retention, and transfer of learning are decreased.
    b. The motivation for problem solving is decreased.
    c. Drives and expectancies are greatly diminished.
    d. Apathy, withdrawal, frustration, aggression, and regression are common emotional behaviors.
    e. The quantity and quality of sensory information are reduced, which causes inaccurate interpretation of the environment. Time distortion, delusions, hallucinations, and disorientation are common experiences.

ASSESSMENT CRITERIA
Physical

Diseases, conditions, or treatment resulting in immobility:
  Neurological: cerebrovascular accident, amyotrophic lateral sclerosis, Parkinson's disease, brain tumor, Alzheimer's disease
  Cardiovascular: congestive heart failure, myocardial infarction, vascular disease
  Musculoskeletal: fractures, arthritis, osteoporosis
  Respiratory: chronic obstructive pulmonary disease, asthma, pneumonia
  Terminal disease: renal disease, cancer
Time frame: acute and traumatic or slowly progressive
Age at onset
System/part with limitations or imposed restriction in movement
Degree of physical mobility
  Self-care abilities; degree of dependence
  Realistic potentials
  Activity patterns, past and present

Activity limitation of part or system
Joint mobility
Assistive devices needed
Endurance
Weight bearing
Skin integrity
Respiratory function and secretions
Cardiovascular response and activity
  Orthostatic hypotension
  Signs and symptoms of thrombophlebitis
Urinary tract function
  Infection
  Pain
Nutrition and hydration status
Elimination
Health practices

Psychosocial

Response to condition causing immobility
Sensory stimulation or deprivation from the environment
Client's perception of prognosis
Motivation
Dependence/independence characteristics
Ability to learn
Hopefulness
Creativeness in acquiring new interests
Locus of control
Support systems, community resources available
Relationships; degree of participation by client and significant others
Life-style
Use of "sick role"
Self-concept
Value orientation
Mental status; orientation to time, place, person
Living environment
Economic conditions

Spiritual

Source of strength, hope, love
Meaning of illness or condition in relation to belief

 ## NURSING CARE PLAN: POTENTIAL FOR DISUSE SYNDROME

Common contributing factors	Expected client outcomes	Nursing strategies
Decreased physical activity related to chronic disease	Client will be active to the maximum level possible Client will participate in realistic goal setting in light of the prognosis Client and/or family will be able to explain rationale for activity Client will be able to demonstrate measures to maintain respiratory health	Assess usual activity level Assess degree of mobility possible and exercise restrictions Assess willingness to increase activity Provide comfort measures if pain limits activities Request consultation with physical therapist Develop activity and exercise plan congruent with limitations imposed by condition Educate client and family about effects of prolonged periods of joint flexion, lying supine, sitting, and lack of weight bearing

Continued.

NURSING CARE PLAN: POTENTIAL FOR DISUSE SYNDROME—cont'd

Common contributing factors	Expected client outcomes	Nursing strategies
	Client will have adequate bowel and bladder function Client will be able to explain the role that adequate nutrition plays in his well-being Client will demonstrate measures to enhance circulation	Teach client how to carry out respiratory toileting through use of position change, deep breathing, incentive spirometer, and adequate fluid intake Assess nutritional status If nutrition deficit is identified, consult with dietition to develop adequate nutrient intake plan Assess status of bowel and bladder elimination and develop plan for management (see care plans for constipation and incontinence, pp. 23 and 274) Help client to maintain circulation through frequent position changes, exercises, and avoidance of tight clothing, leg crossing, and dependent leg position
Limited movement related to casts or traction	Client will make decisions related to care Client will achieve maximum level of independence Client will change position, move, and exercise within limitations established by the physician Client will maintain or increase strength and endurance in muscle groups not limited by treatment orders Client will be willing to engage in movement within established limits	Assess and clarify with the physician movement restrictions in regard to body part, position, and joints Develop teaching plan about allowed activity, exercise, and necessary restrictions in movement Involve client in planning care Assist with care only to the degree needed Request consultation with physical therapist to establish a program of bed exercises congruent with physician orders Provide overhead trapeze to assist in position change Keep side rails up as safety and assistive device in changing position Maintain comfort by positioning, back rubs, correct alignment of the body, and use of proper traction Provide analgesics as necessary to achieve comfort Provide variety and stimulation in the environment to prevent sensory deprivation (see care plan for sensory-perceptual alterations, p. 67) For a client in traction, vary the environment by transporting him or her by bed outside the room
Total immobilization/total bed rest	Client will receive prompt treatment for complications of bed rest Muscle atrophy and joint contractures will be minimized Client will experience fewer episodes of hypostatic pneumonia and atelectasis Client will have maximum nutrient intake Client and family will participate in planning care to the extent possible	Establish regular schedule for assessment of skin, joint flexibility, muscle strength, lung sounds, circulation, thrombus formation, nutrition, bowel and bladder eliminations, and psychological status Establish a program of motion and exercise for all joints and muscles, from passive to active and within limits of the medical plan Position body in alignment; change position from side to side and supine to sitting on regular schedule, at least every 2 hours Establish schedule for respiratory excursion; if client cannot cooperate, use positioning and postural therapy when indicated Monitor intake and output; offer preferred fluids on a frequent schedule Monitor nutrient intake; offer variety of preferred foods in small, frequent feedings; provide pleasant social environment

NURSING CARE PLAN: POTENTIAL FOR DISUSE SYNDROME—cont'd

Common contributing factors	Expected client outcomes	Nursing strategies
		Request involvement of dietitian and family in client's nutrition
		Provide privacy and schedule for urinary and bowel elimination (see care plans for altered urinary elimination [p. 94] and constipation [p. 23])
		Position as upright as possible for urinary and bowel elimination
		Provide pressure-relief mattress and pads
		Keep skin clean and dry
		Encourage and allow self-care

EVALUATION

1. The client and/or family participates in planning preventive measures.
2. The client directs the preventive measures.
3. The client demonstrates a minimum of complications associated with immobility.
4. The client receives prompt treatment for any complication resulting from immobility.
5. The client verbalizes feelings about immobility.

NURSING ALERTS

1. To prevent disabilities, nursing measures must be initiated at the onset of immobilization. Physiological and psychological alterations can be observed within the first week.
2. Be aware that mobilizing any part of the body can provide benefits for all body systems.
3. Particular caution must be taken if a client who is at risk for thrombosis is immobilized. Increased coagulability resulting from increased serum calcium and circulatory stasis resulting from immobility would create a high-risk situation.
4. Nursing measures for hydration are especially important for the immobilized client because dehydration greatly increases the risk of renal stones, thrombosis, pressure ulcers, and constipation.

Bibliography

Burnside I: Nursing and the aged, ed 3, New York, 1988, McGraw-Hill Book Co.

Kim MJ, McFarland GK, and McLane AM: Pocket guide to nursing diagnoses, ed 3, St. Louis, 1989, The CV Mosby Co.

Long B and Phipps W: Medical-surgical nursing, ed 2, St Louis, 1989, The CV Mosby Co.

Olson E: The hazards of immobility, American Journal of Nursing 90(3):43, 1990.

Family Processes, Altered

Mary E. Allen

KNOWLEDGE BASE

1. Altered family processes is the state in which a family that normally functions effectively experiences a dysfunction.
2. The presence of physical problems could influence the severity, duration, or resolution of altered family processes.
3. Maturational and situational crises may precipitate or exacerbate altered family processes. An example of a maturational crisis is the unanticipated death of a spouse. An example of a situational crisis is the diagnosis of terminal cancer for a family member.
4. Economic hardship can precipitate a situational crisis that can impair family functioning.
5. Functional disability of an older person causes him or her to relinquish certain roles within the family. The family must form a new relationship with the person, preserving his or her optimal role function and autonomy.
6. Adult children may feel obliged to "take over" when parents have functional disabilities, and feel guilty if they fail to do so; the parents' autonomy becomes at risk.
7. Bereavement overload, or the experience of multiple losses over a relatively short period of time, will impair family members' ability to engage in grief work. The result is prolonged unresolved grieving that will lead to altered family processes.
8. Emotional reactions common to the elderly are loneliness, depression, anxiety, hopelessness, helplessness, and anger.
9. A common problem reported by families is difficulty of adult children to accept an elderly member's need for companionship, need for sexual activity, or plans to remarry.
10. Alcohol and prescribed drugs may be used excessively as a way to cope with depression, anxiety, or anger. The excessive use of chemicals as a coping mechanism can be an issue for both the family caregiver and the elderly member being cared for.
11. Long-established communication patterns within a family may cause difficulty in decision making and conflict resolution.
12. Values and beliefs held by a family are reflected in all behaviors and responses of the family.
13. If a family has never been close and supportive, parents' aging will not suddenly bring this situation about.
14. Family history, including sibling positions and relationships, is an important factor in understanding present relationships.
15. A long-term goal will be the establishment and maintenance of normal family processes. When developing nursing strategies, the nurse must consider age-related factors such as the presence of chronic, irreversible physical and mental changes and the developmental task stage of the family system before disequilibrium. This information will increase the probability that mutually agreed upon expected outcomes will be formulated realistically.

ASSESSMENT CRITERIA
Physical

Ability of the family system to meet the basic security needs of its members (e.g., food, clothing, shelter)

Psychosocial

Ability of the family system to:
  Meet the psychosocial needs of its members
  Communicate and accept thoughts/feelings among its members
  Examine family rules, rituals, and myths
  Sustain level-appropriate developmental tasks
  Negotiate family role function
  Function as an open system of the larger community, rather than as a closed system
  Manage family boundaries
  Engage in problem-solving techniques
  Use a logical decision-making process
  Adapt to change or cope with a crisis

Spiritual

Ability of the family system to:
  Meet the spiritual needs of its members
  Treat members with dignity and respect
  Promote the maximum potential of its members

NURSING CARE PLAN: ALTERED FAMILY PROCESSES

Common contributing factors	Expected client outcomes	Nursing strategies
Situational/maturational crises.	The family will return to a precrisis level of functioning within a certain length of time (specify) The family will verbalize an understanding of the maturational/developmental issues that contribute to the crisis state The family will formulate a plan for handling activities of daily living before a state of crisis is reached	Identify the family's decision-making style and who the decision makers are Approach the family in a calm and reassuring manner Assess the family rules and values Assess the degree to which the family is an open system rather than a closed system Assess family communication styles Encourage the expression of members' feelings Ask the family to identify the predisposing factors and precipitating event, if possible Ask the family members if they have experienced a similar crisis before and how they handled it Focus on a specific problem and assist the family in problem solving Ask the family members to explain how they normally handle stress List the family's approaches to handling crises that have worked in the past, and help apply them to the present situation Encourage the younger family members to maintain an adult-to-adult relationship with each other and the elderly member Help the client to regain or maintain the ability to perform activities of daily living; teach the family ways to assist in the process Help the family to recognize the elderly person's need for independence, and that care should be given only when the person cannot do something alone Identify with the family new approaches for managing crises, if necessary Teach assertive communication skills to family members, including the elderly person Support family members' expressions of increased ability to cope with the crisis situation Involve the elderly person in all decisions that affect him or her Identify with family members the need for referral to an ongoing family support group or service
Memory loss	The family members will be able to discuss the relationship between memory loss on the part of an elderly family member and their feelings of frustration and helplessness The family members will express an ability to cope with their feelings of frustration and helplessness by means of an identified action plan	Assess the family's knowledge about memory loss Identify problems as perceived by the family (e.g., asking repetitive questions, lowered inhibitions, accusations of stealing) Explore common erroneous interpretations of these problems (e.g., client could control this if he wanted to, client is doing this to annoy us) Ask the family members to explain how they usually handle these problems Encourage the family to verbalize feelings about the memory loss of the elder List problem-solving approaches that work and those that do not Engage in behavioral rehearsal of problem-solving approaches that work Teach alternative problem-solving approaches if necessary

EVALUATION

1. The family is able to return to the precrisis level of functioning within the specified time.
2. All family members can verbalize their ability to cope with the crisis situation.
3. The family members are able to express an understanding of maturational/developmental issues that contributed to the crisis state.
4. The family is able to formulate a plan for handling future activities of daily living before a state of crisis is reached.
5. The family members are able to understand the relationship between the elderly person's memory loss and their feelings of frustration and helplessness.
6. The family members can verbalize an ability to cope with their feelings of frustration and helplessness and can articulate an action plan.

NURSING ALERTS

1. Be aware that the elderly person may use manipulation as a coping mechanism. Avoid being part of his or her ploy to wield power within the family.
2. Avoid giving advice or being judgmental of the family dynamics. Rather, encourage conflict resolution and accept each family member as significant to the family system.

Bibliography

Butler RN and Lewis MI: Aging and mental health, St Louis, 1982, The CV Mosby Co.
Cenoweth B and Spencer B: Dementia: the experience of family caregivers, The Gerontologist 26(3):267, 1986.
de la Cruz L: On loneliness and the elderly, Journal of Gerontological Nursing 12(11):22, 1986.
Gearing B, Johnson M, and Heller T: Mental health problems in old age: a reader, New York, 1988, John Wiley & Sons, Inc.
Gilhooly, MLM: The impact of care-giving on caregivers: factors associated with the psychological well-being of people supporting a dementing relative in the community, British Journal of Medical Psychology 57:35, 1984.
Gulino D and Kadin M: Aging and reactive alcoholism, Geriatric Nursing 7(3):148, 1986.
Hurley ME, editor: Classification of nursing diagnoses: proceedings of the Sixth Conference, North American Nursing Diagnosis Association, St Louis, 1986, The CV Mosby Co, pp 521-522.
Kim MJ, McFarland GK, and McLane AM: Pocket guide to nursing diagnoses, ed 3, St Louis, 1989, The CV Mosby Co.
McCracken A: Emotional impact of possession loss, Journal of Gerontological Nursing 13(2):14, 1987.
Miller A: Nurse/patient dependency: a review of different approaches with particular reference to studies of the dependency of elderly patients, Journal of Advanced Nursing 9:479, 1984.
Reifler BV and Wu S: Managing families of the demented elderly, The Journal of Family Practice 14(6):1051, 1982.
Rigdon IS, Clayton DC and Dimond M: Toward a theory of helpfulness for the elderly bereaved: an invitation to a new life, Advanced Nursing Science 9(2):32, 1987.
Ruffing-Rahal MA: The spiritual dimension of well-being: implications for the elderly, Home Healthcare Nurse 2(2):12, 1984.
Slimmer L, Lopez M, LeSage J, and Elior J: Perceptions of learned helplessness, Journal of Gerontological Nursing 13(5):33, 1987.
Truglio-Londrigan M and Hayes P: Caregivers learn to cope, Geriatric Nursing 7(6):310, 1986.

Fear

Nancy Kaufmann

KNOWLEDGE BASE

1. Fear is defined as a reaction to an identifiable threat or danger, which evokes both a physiological reaction and a psychological response.
2. Fear is distinguished from anxiety in that fear has a definable source, anxiety an indefinable source.
3. Anxiety often is present when fear is experienced over a period of time.
4. Fear may be realistic or result from inadequate knowledge, altered perceptions, or mental incompetence.
5. When a fear is identified and results in problem solving, it is adaptive and enhances survival.
6. Past coping patterns will affect how an elderly client responds to a present situation.
7. Fears arise out of personal threat. Sources of fear for elderly people include threats to well-being, independence, life-style, comfort, and life.
8. Crime, falling, dependence, poverty, illness, loneliness, and death are frequent fears expressed by elders.

9. While some elderly persons openly voice their fears, others may be reluctant to talk about their fears because of pride.
10. Assessment skills are needed in order to recognize subtle clues that fear is the primary problem. Establishing a trusting relationship and an accepting attitude creates a supportive environment for identifying and resolving fears.
11. Resolution of a fear may involve one or more people, agencies, communities, or services.
12. The major focus in fear reduction is increasing the client's power or control, increasing his or her knowledge of the fear situation, and increasing his or her competence or necessary skills.

ASSESSMENT CRITERIA
Physical

Sympathetic response
    Vital signs
    Skin, color, warmth, moisture
    Pupils
    Nutritional intake
    Elimination; urine and feces
Ability for self-care
Potential for falls
Pain/comfort
Activity tolerance
Mobility
Medical, surgical, trauma history
Evidence of abuse
    Cuts, wounds, bruising
    Dehydration, malnourishment
    Poor hygiene
    Frequent emergency room visits

Psychosocial

Behaviors denoting fear
    Anxiety level
    Fright
    Apprehension
    Hypervigilance
    Suspiciousness
    Avoidance
    Attention deficit
    Aggressiveness/withdrawal
    Obsessive-compulsive rituals
    Distrust; questioning of caregivers
    Inflexibility
Coping patterns
Phobic reactions
    Refusal to leave home
    Refusal to see a physician
    Refusal to take medications
Past traumatic experiences (e.g., being mugged or robbed, falling in home)
Dependence/independence characteristics
Decision-making ability
Memory
Perception of aging
Personal meaning of death
Safety of home environment
Support systems
Potential for relocation of living site
Potential for or history of abuse

 NURSING CARE PLAN: FEAR

Common contributing factors	Expected client outcomes	Nursing strategies
Reluctance to leave home for fear of crime or possible injury	Client will identify the situations that make him or her fearful Client will discuss fears that are irrational or unfounded Client will discuss fears that have a base in reality Client will list the steps to take to provide for his or her safety Client will arrange to have a neighbor watch the house while he or she is gone Client will list the modes of transportation available to him or her within the community	Evaluate client's level of anxiety Explore client's perception of the fear, which may differ greatly from that of the caregiver Discuss the reality of the fear Discuss factors that can be controlled by the client and those that are out of his or her control (e.g., grocery shopping in the day versus at night; having Social Security check deposited directly into the bank; going out with others, not alone) Discuss ways to adapt life-style to regain control over fear (e.g., moving to a safer neighborhood, moving into a senior citizen center, living with another person, joining support group) Explain methods of crime prevention to protect oneself and one's home (joining a neighborhood watch program, having someone call and check on you daily)

Continued.

NURSING CARE PLAN: FEAR—cont'd

Common contributing factors	Expected client outcomes	Nursing strategies
Fear of rejection by others or society	Client will verbalize fears about being rejected Client will discuss behaviors of others Client will identify methods to maintain family and social contacts Client will list senior citizen centers near his or her home Client will become involved (if appropriate) in a foster grandparent program	Assess those who give the client acceptance Identify with client ways to maintain ties with family, friends, and community Assist client in developing a plan for continued involvement Discuss with client the various reactions one may encounter when dealing with the public Teach assertive communication skills Investigate with client those community resources he or she could utilize (senior centers, neighborhood groups, church groups, etc.)
Postponement of seeking health care for fear of diagnosis	Client will discuss reasons for not seeking medical care Client will list services available Client will seek medical consultation when experiencing problems Client will verbalize satisfaction with the care provided	Encourage client to discuss fears Discuss how important it is to diagnose problems early Encourage client to seek medical care when experiencing symptoms Explore alternative resources available to the client (e.g., if finances are a problem, is there a city or university-run clinic?) Suggest guided imagery through the process of diagnosis and learning of the outcome When providing care for client, always explain the purpose and describe the procedures before doing them Allow time for questions regarding illness or procedures Ask client about satisfaction or displeasure with care provided
Threats to well-being (i.e., pain)	Client will identify specific fears Client will demonstrate methods of pain control	Identify meaning of pain to client Identify pain characteristics and location Request prompt attention to source of pain for treatment purposes Teach client methods to control pain such as relaxation, massage; if client is mentally clear, support self-medication after education Develop program for pain management involving the client
Fear of falls	Client will have an increased sense of control and safety Client will participate in planning actions to alleviate fear	Assess previous fall patterns and influencing factors Discuss and identify specific fears related to falling Develop with client safety practices and assist in practice Identify threat to independence with client to establish realistic ideas Consider alert system for summoning help for client living in an independent setting Help client to obtain and use assistive aids such as grab bars and walkers or canes
Threats to life-style, independence, and personal space	Client will be able to identify the fear Client will demonstrate knowledge of the problem-solving process Client will identify expectations about the situation Client will be able to predict daily events Client will be able to express feelings to others	Identify with client the fear and the reality of the situation Identify specific options and possible solutions with client Allow client to make decisions to the extent of capabilities Be honest and supply needed information on rules, routines, and staff Orient client to new environment; help client to establish personal space and control over environment Assist in establishing a mutually satisfactory schedule for activities; staff to use a consistent approach and reassuring manner Assist in problem solving Teach assertive communication; assist in practice Provide emotional support and physical presence

EVALUATION

1. The client becomes more active in community activities.
2. The client states that feelings of fear have decreased.
3. The client can identify sources of fear.
4. The client demonstrates or describes the use of crime prevention methods.
5. The client utilizes available community resources.
6. The physiological symptoms of "fight or flight" response are absent.
7. The client seeks medical care when experiencing symptoms.
8. The client demonstrates problem solving when dealing with the fear source.

NURSING ALERTS

1. Identify client's perception of what is feared since the elderly persons views can be quite different from those of the caregiver.
2. It is important to take into account the elderly client's cultural, ethnic, and socioeconomic background.
3. As one ages, one goes back to a familiar way of responding (e.g., a person who had been a World War II refugee may not view an authority figure as a source of help).
4. Resolution of fears in elderly people may take a long time.
5. Some clients will reveal fears only after a trusting relationship has been established.

Bibliography

Cape R, Coe R, and Rossman I: Fundamentals of geriatric medicine, New York, 1983, Raven Press.

Ebersole P and Hess P: Toward healthy aging, ed 3, St Louis, 1990, The CV Mosby Co.

McLane A, editor: Classification of nursing diagnoses: proceedings of the Seventh Conference, North American Nursing Diagnosis Association, St Louis, 1987, The CV Mosby Co.

Townsend MC: Nursing diagnosis in psychiatric nursing, Philadelphia, 1988, FA Davis Co.

Fluid Volume Deficit

Christine Clarkin

KNOWLEDGE BASE

1. Fluid volume deficit is the state in which an individual experiences vascular, cellular, or intracellular dehydration related to active loss or failure of regulatory mechanisms.
2. Fluid volume deficit, or dehydration, is a problem often seen in the elderly.
3. Symptoms of fluid volume deficit commonly seen in older people include altered thought processes, weight loss, increased pulse and respiratory rates, decreased blood pressure, cool skin, delayed vein filling, shock, and decreased urinary output.
4. Laboratory findings associated with fluid deficit include increased red blood cell count, hematocrit, and hemoglobin, and urine specific gravity greater than 1.030.
5. Both renal mass and renal function decrease with aging. It is estimated that there is a 40% reduction in glomerular filtration rate between the ages of 20 and 70.
6. Although normal volume and composition of body fluids are usually maintained during aging, adaptation to demands placed on the body by illness or environmental stresses becomes slower.
7. Fluid volume deficit may result from abnormal fluid loss associated with gastroenteritis with vomiting or diarrhea, uncontrolled diabetes mellitus, diabetes insipidus, fever, infection, diuretic therapy, or copious mucus production related to chronic pulmonary disease.
8. Fluid volume deficit may be a consequence of inadequate fluid intake related to difficulty in swallowing, a diminished sense of thirst, difficulty in obtaining and handling fluids, or communication disorders that interfere with the ability to request fluids.
9. A fluid intake of 1500 to 2000 ml per day is desirable.
10. Older persons may voluntarily restrict fluid intake to prevent urinary incontinence.
11. Many older people do not tolerate both foods and fluids at mealtime.

ASSESSMENT CRITERIA
Physical

Poor skin turgor over sternum or forehead
Furrowed, thin, dry tongue, dry oral mucosa
Weight loss
Increased pulse rate
Decreased venous filling

Orthostatic hypotension
Diaphoresis
Vomiting, diarrhea
Dry, flaking skin
Cough with excessive sputum production
Swallowing difficulties
Diminished sensation of thirst
Immobility and dexterity problems
Decreased fluid intake
Increased or decreased urine output
Clinical evidence of body fluid or blood loss via wounds, tubes, lumens

History of diseases causing excess fluid loss, such as diabetes mellitus, diabetes insipidus, gastroenteritis with vomiting or diarrhea, pulmonary disease with excessive sputum production, overzealous diuretic therapy, hemorrhage

Psychosocial

Decreased sensorium
Depression or fatigue resulting in decreased motivation to drink liquids
Altered thought processes

Spiritual

Fasting related to religious practices

 ## NURSING CARE PLAN: FLUID VOLUME DEFICIT

Common contributing factors	Expected client outcomes	Nursing strategies
Vomiting, diarrhea, fever, infection, copious mucus production of chronic obstructive pulmonary disease	Client will have adequate fluid intake (as evidenced by intake greater than output) and relief of symptoms Client will experience relief of nausea, vomiting, and diarrhea Client will verbalize rationale for treatment plan	Assess skin turgor, tongue, and mucous membranes Monitor intake and output and record every 8 hours Daily weight (same scale, same clothes, same time) Report to physician changes greater than 3 pounds Administer antiemetics, intravenous fluids as ordered Offer preferred fluids every 30 minutes Monitor and record stools Monitor temperature every 4 hours while elevated Check blood pressure, pulse rate, respiratory rate, and level of consciousness every 4 hours Assess mucous membranes and skin turgor (over forehead or sternum) every 8 hours
Chronic obstructive lung disease, uncontrolled diabetes mellitus, diuretic therapy	Client will be able to discuss the relationship between the disease and fluid volume deficit Client's electrolytes will be within normal limits	Administer antibiotics as ordered for respiratory infections Monitor blood glucose as ordered, reporting values greater than 300 mg/100 ml or less than 80; check urine ketones if glucose is greater than 300 Diabetic diet as ordered Antidiabetic medications as ordered Teach client about fluid loss and fluid intake Monitor electrolytes as ordered Report symptoms of low potassium (weakness, muscle cramping, twitching)
Diminished sense of thirst, difficulty swallowing fluids	Client will have adequate fluid intake Client will be able to swallow sources of fluid available	Monitor fluid intake, setting goals for fluid intake greater than output Teach client about amount of desired intake Offer fluids every 2 hours Assess preferences for easy-to-swallow food with high fluid content, such as fruit, gelatin Assist client in drinking See also care plan for impaired swallowing, p. 87
Difficulty obtaining and handling fluids; voluntary restriction of fluid to prevent urinary incontinence; communication disorders that interfere with ability to request fluids	Client will obtain adequate fluids as evidenced by intake-output record Client will participate in developing bladder control program Client will receive fluids on a routine basis	Assess barriers to intake of fluids Place attractive fluids within reach of client; assist as needed Encourage client to ask for assistance with fluids; consult occupational therapist for assistive devices Place client on schedule for bladder emptying every 2 hours during day, every 4 hours at night; reevaluate in 72 hours Teach client that increased fluid decreases bladder irritability Assess communication deficit Identify system for client to indicate need if possible Offer fluids between meals, with meals, at bedtime, and one time during night if awake

EVALUATION

1. The client experiences relief of fluid volume deficit as evidenced by intake greater than output; weight returns to the client's baseline, with daily changes less than 3 pounds.
2. The client receives prompt treatment of the underlying cause of the fluid loss.
3. The client is able to identify foods that are high in water content.
4. The client participates in a plan to prevent fluid volume deficit in the future.

NURSING ALERTS

1. Decreased appetite, nausea, and discomfort related to eating may result from food and drug interactions or from drug toxicity, such as toxic digitalis levels. The refusal of the older individual to consume fluids with meals should alert the nurse that an evaluation of the client's medications with an eye to possible interactions is needed.

2. Age-related progressive increases in fat and decreases in lean body mass and total body water may result in a decreased volume of water for distributing water-soluble drugs and an increased distribution volume for fat-soluble drugs.

Bibliography

Carpenito LJ: Handbook of nursing diagnosis, Philadelphia, 1989, JB Lippincott Co.

Carpenito LJ: Nursing diagnosis: application to clinical practice, Philadelphia, 1983, JB Lippincott Co.

Esberger KK and Hughes ST Jr: Nursing care of the aged, Norwalk, Conn, 1989, Appleton & Lange.

Long B and Phipps W, editors: Medical-surgical nursing, St Louis, 1989, The CV Mosby Co.

Matteson, MA and McConnell ES: Gerontological nursing: concepts and practice, Philadelphia, 1988, WB Saunders Co.

Matz R: Diabetes mellitus in the elderly, Hospital Practice 21(3):195, 1986.

Thompson JM et al: Mosby's manual of clinical nursing, St Louis, 1989, The CV Mosby Co.

Fluid Volume Excess

Christine Clarkin

KNOWLEDGE BASE

1. Fluid volume excess is the state in which an individual experiences increased fluid retention and edema.
2. Decreased cardiac output contributes to depedent edema related to venostasis.
3. The elderly have a decreased ability to concentrate their urine, because of a reduction in glomerular filtration rate.
4. Fluid volume excess may be a consequence of abnormally high secretion of antidiuretic hormone (ADH), which may occur in pneumonia, meningitis, stroke, subdural hematoma, tuberculosis, central nervous system disorders, and pulmonary disorders.
5. Laboratory findings that are consistent with an oversecretion of ADH include low serum sodium level, low blood urea nitrogen concentration, low serum osmolality, and decreased hematocrit.
6. Congestive heart failure that has progressed to right-sided failure may result in congestion throughout the circulatory system, leading to increased pressure in the renal tubules.

7. The resulting increased pressure in renal tubules causes increased reabsorption of sodium, further contributing to edema and congestive heart failure.
8. Decreased excretion of sodium causes retention of potassium, which increases the risk of cardiac arrhythmias.
9. Laboratory findings consistent with fluid excess related to congestive heart failure and decreased cardiac output might include elevated serum sodium and potassium levels; decreased red blood cell count, hematocrit, and hemoglobin; and urine specific gravity less than 1.010.
10. A mentally ill client with compulsive traits who is on psychotropic drug therapy (which causes dry mouth) may ingest large volumes of water, resulting in water intoxication.
11. Other conditions that may cause hyposmolar states and fluid excess include renal disease, cerebral injury, alcoholism, and excessive intravenous hydration with hypotonic or isotonic solutions.
12. An individual who is vomiting and has intake limited to ice chips will also be at risk for water intoxication.

13. An elderly diabetic client who has decreased cardiac output with poor renal clearance may be at risk for the syndrome of inappropriate ADH secretion (SIADH) if he or she is taking chlorpropamide (Diabinese).
14. Many problems causing fluid excess will require collaboration of the registered nurse with the physician and other members of the health care team.

ASSESSMENT CRITERIA
Physical

Edema; noted on sacrum, feet, over sternum
Shiny, taut skin
Sudden weight gain
Increased pulse volume or blood pressure
Full neck veins
Tachycardia or arrhythmia
Puffiness of face
Third heart sound
Wet cough, rales, rhonchi
Increased respiratory rate
Muscle weakness, fatigue, or twitching
Dyspnea on exertion; orthopnea
Fluid intake greater than output

Decreased urinary output
Decreased reflexes, seizures, hemiplegia, coma
Low-protein diet
Very low sodium intake
Complaints of abdominal cramping, diarrhea
Low hemoglobin, low hematocrit
Low urine specific gravity
Low serum sodium, potassium, osmolality
Frequent use of tap water enemas
Gastric suction
Severe burns
Current medications

Psychosocial

Change in mental state
Lethargy or confusion
Restlessness, anxiety, irritability, hallucinations
Stressful occurrences, such as death of a loved one
History of psychotropic therapy that causes dry mouth or impaired water secretion, combined with compulsive behavior patterns causing excessive water ingestion

Spiritual

Fear of death

 ## NURSING CARE PLAN: FLUID VOLUME EXCESS

Common contributing factors	Expected client outcomes	Nursing strategies
Failure of renal regulatory mechanism related to decreased cardiac output	Client will regain fluid balance as evidenced by a return of vital signs to premorbid levels	Assess vital signs for evidence of fluid overload every 4 to 8 hours: Pulse rate, quality Heart sounds, presence of murmur Respiratory rate, depth, presence of adventitious sounds, dyspnea and orthopnea Blood pressure every 4 hours Weigh daily on same scale, same clothes, same time of day; report changes greater than 3 pounds Administer diuretics, digitalis as ordered Utilize measures to promote comfort and to reduce anxiety of client, including quiet room, Fowler's position, oxygen as ordered
Improper diet: high salt intake or low protein intake (low-calorie liquid diets are an example)	Client will identify appropriate diet, including reduced salt and adequate consumption of protein	Monitor diet, including use of salt and convenience foods Interview client and family to determine food preference, adequacy of resources to obtain food Develop teaching plan for client/family
Renal failure, acute or chronic	Client and/or family will verbalize rationale for monitoring and treatment	Monitor all output, including urine, emesis, stools, and gastric suction
Excessive fluid intake associated with mental illness, compulsive behaviors, psychotropic medication, SIADH	Client will take in appropriate volume of fluid	Restrict fluids as ordered; monitor fluid intake, including intravenous, oral, tube feedings, irrigations, fluids given with meals and with medications Collaborate with mental health professional for modifying behavior

NURSING CARE PLAN: FLUID VOLUME EXCESS—cont'd

Common contributing factors	Expected client outcomes	Nursing strategies
Dependent venous pooling, venous stasis	Client will experience relief from dependent edema	Assess limbs, sacrum for signs of venous pooling and skin integrity Assess for constricting clothing Encourage alternate periods of rest and activity Encourage client to elevate feet when sitting Inquire about use of elastic stockings Discourage ankle crossing and knee locking See also care plan for skin integrity, p. 75
Immobility	Client will move or change position (with assistance if necessary)	Turn or change position every 2 hours; develop exercise program (see care plan for altered mobility, p. 50, for additional specific strategies)
Stressful situations, surgery, acute infections	Client's temperature, vital signs, and level of consciousness will be within usual parameters	Monitor temperature every 8 hours; if elevated, every 4 hours Observe appearance of wounds, lesions Evaluate level of consciousness every 4 to 8 hours; if altered, report immediately and monitor more frequently Hourly intake and output Lung sounds every 2 hours Assess for dependent edema

EVALUATION

1. The client regains fluid balance, as evidenced by a pulse rate of 70 to 95 beats/min and blood pressure in the usual range for this individual, preferably under 100 mm Hg diastolic and 165 systolic. The respiratory rate should be 16 to 20 breaths per minute, with breathing not labored and no adventitious breath sounds. The client will have no third heart sound when fluid balance is restored. The client should have lost weight as compared with baseline, with daily fluctuations of less than 3 pounds.
2. The client will be able to describe an appropriate diet, including reduced salt and sodium along with adequate protein consumption. The client and/or family should be able to select meals that are consistent with the client's dietary restrictions.
3. The client will have urinary output of at least 30 ml per hour.
4. The client will take in an appropriate volume of fluid, as determined by his or her individual needs and the medical treatment plan.
5. The client will have decreased evidence of dependent edema.
6. The client will change position to relieve pressure and promote circulation every 2 hours.
7. The client's temperature, vital signs, and level of consciousness will be within the usual parameters for him or her.

NURSING ALERTS

1. Diuretics and medications that increase ADH secretion should be avoided in the client experiencing water intoxication. These drugs include vasopressin, aspirin, acetaminophen, haloperidol, narcotics, and barbiturates.
2. In the client with reduced renal flow, therapy should be aimed at correcting the problem causing congestive heart failure, correcting fluid volume, and returning blood pressure to normal levels.

Bibliography

Caine RM and Bufalino MK, editor: Nursing care planning guides for adults, Baltimore, 1987, The Williams & Wilkins Co.

Carpenito LJ: Handbook of nursing diagnosis, Philadelphia, 1989, JB Lippincott Co.

Carpenito LJ: Nursing diagnosis: application to clinical practice, Philadelphia, 1983, JB Lippincott Co.

Esberger KK and Hughes ST Jr: Nursing care of the aged, Norwalk, Conn, 1989, Appleton & Lange

Holloway NM: Medical-surgical care plans, Springhouse, Pa, 1988, Springhouse Corp.

Puderbaugh Ulrich S, Canale SW, and Wendell SA: Nursing care planning guides, Philadelphia, 1986, WB Saunders Co.

Thompson JM et al: Mosby's manual of clinical nursing, ed 2, St Louis, 1989, The CV Mosby Co.

Grieving, Dysfunctional

Sue E. Meiner

KNOWLEDGE BASE

1. Dysfunctional grieving is the state in which an actual or perceived loss is not resolved or accepted through a grieving process. Losses can include people, possessions, a job, status, home, ideals, and parts and processes of the body.
2. Grief is the emotional response to loss. Mourning is an attempt to adapt to the loss.
3. An elderly person's grief and adaptation are affected by many factors, such as personality, past experiences of loss, health status, relationships, support systems, and resources.
4. As aging occurs, the number of losses felt by an individual increases. However, in the years after age 60, a greater number occur and faster than ever before. This rapidly increasing number of losses requires better and more frequent use of coping skills and social relationships.
5. Coping mechanisms used by older people vary greatly. Common coping mechanisms include denial or minimizing the seriousness of a loss, requesting reassurance and emotional support, setting new goals when a loss necessitates dramatic change, rehearsing alternative outcomes before acting, and finding a general purpose or pattern of meaning in the course of events. The person's past experience with a particular coping style can influence the outcome of the handling of loss.
6. When a person is unable to cope, unresolved grief may result in a variety of responses: hopelessness, loneliness (a subjective sense of being alone), inability to maintain an independent level of functioning, depression (which may lead to suicide attempts), isolation, phobias, and somatic symptoms.
7. When losses occur in clusters, a person is less likely to be able to adapt and bereavement overload occurs, resulting in confusion, lethargy, lack of appetite, and withdrawal from social contact.
8. Depression in the elderly is a great imitator; other diseases are frequently diagnosed when depression is the underlying problem. Sluggishness and lethargy are prevalent signs of depression.
9. Multiple role losses and feelings of uselessness can have a significant impact on self-esteem and the elderly person's place in society.
10. A sense of loss may be experienced when organ removal or amputation has been necessary. When the loss involves a visible body part (e.g., a breast), the loss may have more importance to the person.
11. In an assessment of losses of roles, the importance of each role can be determined by assigning a percent of committment at the time that the role was a part of activities. Allow sufficient time for discussion of the various roles experienced throughout life.
12. Be cautious concerning your own value system and possible judgmental attitudes toward another person's spiritual practices.

ASSESSMENT CRITERIA
Physical

Physical losses such as:
    Organ removal
    Amputation
    Vision/hearing loss
    Muscle strength/coordination
General appearance
Alterations in eating habits
Abnormal sleep patterns
Lethargy
Decreased activity level
Decreased libido
Chronic pain
Degree of dependence/independence

Psychosocial

Inability to concentrate
Anger
Sadness/crying
Past experiences with loss
Coping strategies/skills
Denial of loss
Feelings of guilt
Ability to discuss the loss
Expressions of unresolved issues
Developmental regression
Relationships with others

Level of self-esteem
Need for community/financial support
Significance of a loss
Roles/purpose
Changes in life-style
Predictability of daily routine
Support systems

Productivity
Losses of significant others (spouse, family, friends)
Loss of financial or social status

Spiritual

Religious practices and beliefs
Feelings of hopelessness/helplessness

NURSING CARE PLAN: DYSFUNCTIONAL GRIEVING

Common contributing factors	Expected client outcomes	Nursing strategies
Grieving over a loss or losses	Client will demonstrate adaptive grieving behaviors	Assess for factors that may block adaptation Accept any behavior that is not self-destructive—i.e., screaming, crying, pacing, or talking to self Encourage ventilation of feelings; allow client to direct the conversation When the loss is an alteration in body form, recognize the response to the loss, the meaning of the loss, previous experiences with loss, and present support systems; provide emotional support as required
Insufficient knowledge about the process of loss resolution	Client will express understanding of a typical grief response to loss	Assess awareness of common grief responses Identify others' normal reactions to losses Give positive reinforcement to all attempts to adapt to losses Discuss that restitution will occur and negative feelings will diminish over time
Feelings of powerlessness, hopelessness, or loneliness	Client will verbalize a sense of control and adjustment to and/or acceptance of the loss.	Promote a trust relationship with a staff member or chaplain Intervene immediately with frequent visits to assess current state of mind Use communication techniques of listening, reflection Telephone reassurance when daily visits are not made Promote family/friend support Help client to seek spiritual resources Provide pet therapy if acceptable Allow time for ventilation of feelings related to losses Identify with the client the coping skills being used or planned
Fear over role changes caused by losses	Client will effectively cope with current situation with a minimum level of anxiety Client will assume other social and family roles	Acknowledge grief Assist the client to identify remaining roles Allow free expression of feelings about current situation Refer to other health care professionals as necessary Reinforce use of adaptive defenses Provide counseling for financial and spiritual needs/requests Encourage involvement in community activities to provide purpose Identify persons who would be a resource for intimacy, challenge, support, and acceptance

EVALUATION

1. The client verbalizes the feelings of loss (positive and negative) and identifies them as part of the normal grieving process.
2. The client utilizes significant others and situational support to cope with life-style changes related to losses.
3. The client participates in the situation as a sign of adaptation to the grieving process.
4. The client participates in decision making for the future.
5. The client resumes pre-loss roles and functions or modifies them as necessary.

NURSING ALERTS

1. Losses related to body image may require a period of time during which mirror viewing should be avoided.
2. After a new loss, an older person is at risk for abuse of sedative drugs if sleep interruption or insomnia is being treated with prescription medication. The added decline in appetite and poor nutritional intake compound the downward spiral of health.
3. Additional stressors need to be reduced to a minimum. Fully inform the client of all procedures in advance and at the time they are done. Reassurance is essential if stress is to be minimized.

Bibliography

Eliopoulos C: Gerontological nursing, ed 2, Philadelphia, 1987, JB Lippincott Co.
Eliopoulos C, editor: Health assessment of the older adult, Menlo Park, Calif, 1984, Addison-Wesley Publishing Co. Inc.
Kermis M: The psychology of human aging: theory, research and practice, Boston, 1984, Allyn & Bacon, Inc.
Miller J: Coping with chronic illness: overcoming powerlessness, Philadelphia, 1983, FA Davis Co.

Tools suggested for use

Zung Self-Rating Depression Scale, Copyright, American Medical Association

Zung W: A self-rating depression scale, Archives of General Psychiatry, 12:63, 1965.

OARS Social Resource Scale

Multidimensional functional assessment: the OARS methodology, Durham, NC, 1978, Duke University Center for the Study of Aging and Human Development, Duke University Press.

Mini-Mental State Examination, copyright, Pergamon Press, Ltd

Folstein S et al: Mini-Mental State: a practical method for grading the cognitive state of patients for the clinician, Journal of Psychiatric Research, 12:189, 1975.

Revised Philadelphia Geriatric Center Morale Scale

Lawton M: The Philadelphia Geriatric Center Morale Scale: a revision, Journal of Gerontology, 30:85, 1975.

Life Satisfaction Indices

Neugarten B, Havighurst R, and Tobin S: The measurement of life satisfaction, Journal of Gerontology, 16:134, 1961.

Self Esteem Scale

Goldberg W and Fitzpatrick J: Movement therapy with the aged, Nursing Research 29:339, 1980.

Health Maintenance, Altered

Christine Clarkin

KNOWLEDGE BASE

1. Altered health maintenance is the inability to identify or manage health problems or to seek out help in maintaining health.
2. An individual in such a situation is at risk of experiencing a disruption in his or her present state of wellness because of inadequate preventive measures or because of unhealthy life-style. This may apply to an asymptomatic person, or to an individual with chronic disease.
3. Aging is not synonymous with disease, but the fact remains that many of the elderly have physical disabilities that increase in frequency with age.
4. The ability of an older individual to function effectively in his or her environment is often a function of the person's ability to maintain wellness and prevent illness and injury.
5. Impairment of an individual's ability to make thoughtful and deliberate judgments will interfere with health maintenance.

6. Memory loss, toxic dosages of medication, adverse reactions to medications, and depression are found frequently in persons over 75. All of these factors may impair judgment and functioning.
7. An older person's access to health care may be compromised by financial constraints.
8. Communication impairments such as hearing loss may limit the success of older people in obtaining information about disease process and treatment regimens.
9. Elders may have difficulty recognizing and reporting signs of illness.
10. Health care management strategies will be more effective if they take into consideration a client's overall health status, life expectancy, life-style, and food preferences. A nurse's personal attention to these factors makes a positive outcome more likely.

ASSESSMENT CRITERIA
Physical

Unkempt, dirty hair
Inappropriately applied makeup
Unshaven
Poor oral hygiene
Missing dentures
Cuts, scrapes, bruises suggesting falls
Sores in various stages of healing
Long, dirty nails
Dirty, wrinkled, mismatched clothing
Food particles on clothing or self

Weight loss
Body odor

Psychosocial

Inappropriate speech
Disoriented talking
Repetition of words or phrases
Flight of ideas
Difficulty following simple commands
Difficulty following health maintenance practices
Lack of understanding of health maintenance practices
Lack of necessary resources
Lack of motivation
Absence of support system of family or friends
Difficulty accepting advancing age and/or physical disability
Bland affect
Monotone voice

Spiritual

Feelings of hopelessness or hopefulness
Ability to maintain religious practices
Belief in a supernatural power
Concerns about death, disability

General

Appearance of home:
  Unkempt or dirty
  Windows and doors tightly closed
  Inadequate resources for maintaining a clean environment
  Furniture in disarray
Lack of access to health care

 NURSING CARE PLAN: ALTERED HEALTH MAINTENANCE

Common contributing factors	Expected client outcomes	Nursing strategies
Impaired ability to make deliberate and thoughtful judgments	Client will seek help needed to maintain health	Assist client in identifying health maintenance needs: what help is needed; what resources can be utilized
Impaired ability to communicate	Client will relay health needs and concerns as well as plans to satisfy them	Identify source of communication difficulty; then develop strategies to overcome barriers
Insufficient material resources	Client will receive counseling on available assistance and will have access to these sources	Utilize social worker (if available) to determine needs and match them with available resources
Religious beliefs that discourage medical intervention	Client will discuss beliefs that prohibit health maintenance behaviors with a spiritual counselor or with nurse	Encourage client to discuss beliefs with competent counselor, family, nurse Contract explicitly with patient and family, if appropriate, to provide limited health maintenance care that is consistent with beliefs

Continued.

NURSING CARE PLAN: ALTERED HEALTH MAINTENANCE—cont'd

Common contributing factors	Expected client outcomes	Nursing strategies
Inadequate family/social supports	Client will use family and community resources appropriately to maintain health	Assist client in identifying family and community members who can be called on for assistance Encourage/assist client in contacting these resources and in specifying help that is needed Identify a resource for monitoring success of attempts to involve family and community in meeting health maintenance needs
Physical barriers to health maintenance such as poor vision, hearing impairment, declining energy	Client will utilize vision aids, hearing devices to simplify work to accomplish health maintenance	Explore aids client currently has and extent to which they have been used Assist client in contacting necessary providers to obtain needed devices Encourage and assist client in using devices
Feelings of discouragement, disappointment	Client will verbalize feelings and seek assistance in coping with such emotions	Encourage client to discuss feelings openly Assist client in realistic appraisal of opportunities available for support, counseling Encourage client to "reframe" negative thoughts, practice positive "self talk" Advise physician of client's feelings (antidepressant medications may be indicated)

EVALUATION

1. The client secures needed help in identifying and correcting health maintenance deficits.
2. The client develops a system for alerting others to his or her health maintenance needs (such as hearing aid, sign language, translator).
3. The client utilizes available resources to meet material needs (food stamps, medical assistance, family assistance with budgeting, shopping).
4. The client and family explores religious beliefs and contract with health care providers and family members for health maintenance care that is consistent with their beliefs.
5. The client obtains needed family or community support to maintain health.
6. The client obtains and effectively uses devices that can enable him or her to accomplish self-care.
7. The client experiences relief from feelings of discouragement.

NURSING ALERTS

1. Coexisting medical problems, poverty, social isolation, and poor access to medical services will compound a client's difficulties in managing health care needs.
2. Clients having difficulty with medication regimens should be evaluated for memory loss. Special accessories such as calendars and watches with alarms may help them remember to take their medications on time.

Bibliography

Carpenito, LJ: Nursing diagnosis: application to clinical practice, Philadelphia, 1983, JB Lippincott Co.

Feeney ET, Williams MP, and Coyle GC: Meeting the needs of the hospitalized elderly, Nursing Management, 17(9):24, 1986.

Matteson, MA and McConnell ES: Gerontological nursing, Philadelphia, 1988, WB Saunders Co.

Mion L, Frengley JD, and Adams M: Nursing patients 75 years and older, Nursing Management 17(9):24, 1986.

Kim MJ, McFarland GK, and McLane AM: Pocket guide to nursing diagnoses, ed 3, St Louis, 1989, The CV Mosby Co.

Yura H and Walsh MB: The nursing process, ed 5, Norwalk, Conn, 1988, Appleton & Lange.

Injury, Potential for: Falls

Sue E. Meiner

KNOWLEDGE BASE

1. Potential for injury is the state in which an individual is at risk for injury as a result of environmental conditions interacting with the individual's adaptive and defensive resources.
2. Maintaining one's balance depends on receiving and integrating information from many sources: the vestibular system, the eyes, and proprioceptors in the joints, muscles, and tendons. The brain's pyramidal tract, extrapyrymidal system, and cerebellum have balance functions.
3. Once an older person has fallen, he or she is at greater risk for additional falls.
4. Falls account for two thirds of the accidents among elderly people and are the second leading cause of accidental death.
5. The morbidity and mortality connected with falls increase with age.
6. Hip fractures that result from falls are the most common injury in elders.
7. Repeated falls are a major factor in the decision to admit an elderly person to a nursing facility.
8. Among hospitalized older people, falls usually occur during the first 2 weeks of hospitalization.
9. Multiple-system illness, depressants, and unfamiliar environment increase the likelihood of falls and injury.
10. Age-related changes of the sensory system increase the risk for falls:
    a. Presbyopia decreases the ability to see near objects clearly.
    b. Increased accommodation time causes an older person to be unable to see when first entering a dark room.
    c. Sclerosis of the pupil causes less light to enter the eye, resulting in decreased visual acuity.
    d. Opacities in the lens create a blinding glare in bright light.
    e. Inability to distinguish among blues, blue-greens, violets, and monotones creates hazards on steps and doorways.
    f. Alteration in depth perception causes an elderly person to misjudge distances, possibly resulting in a fall on stairs or street curbs.

11. Musculoskeletal problems are a major factor in falls and often result in injury. Decreased muscle strength, joint stiffness, and poor coordination create a high-risk situation.
12. Gait changes indicate a risk for falls. When an older person shuffles instead of stepping, tripping and falling are more likely.
13. Loss of neurons and slowed response time result in the inability to regain balance.
14. Minimal or slowed movement is a neurological indicator for imbalance and potential falls.
15. Postural sway and a wide base of support indicate an attempt to compensate for decreased balance.
16. Foot problems such as bunions, corns, or neuropathies may affect stability.
17. Cardiac and vascular problems increase an elderly person's risk for falls and injury:
    a. Orthostatic hypotension caused by age-related vascular changes or antihypertensive medication
    b. Transient ischemic attacks
    c. Vertigo, syncope, dizziness
    d. Drop attacks
    e. Arrhythmias
18. Premonitory falls are those that occur at the onset of a severe illness such as pneumonia.
19. Urinary incontinence, urgency, and frequency create a hazard. Many falls occur as an older person attempts to get to the toilet.
20. Disorientation and memory loss may cause an older person to leave a safe environment, resulting in a fall.
21. Environmental hazards include inadequate lighting, loose rugs, electrical cords, slick floor surfaces, clutter, unstable furniture, pets, and changes in furniture arrangement.
22. Loose-fitting footwear or long nightwear can precipitate a fall.
23. Improper use of canes, crutches, or wheelchairs creates a risk for injury.
24. Medications that cause or have side effects of hypokalemia, hypotension, or sedation increase the risk for falls.

25. Physical restraints are often used to prevent falls by institutionalized elderly people. However, restraints cause emotional trauma and increase disuse complications. In addition, it has been found that older people who have been restrained are actually much more likely to be injured.

ASSESSMENT CRITERIA
Physical

History of falls
Mobility
Postural stability
Muscle strength and control
Ability to recover from trip
Endurance
Activity tolerance
Assistive devices
Gait
Sensory
   Vision (including accommodation)
   Hearing
   Ear infections or disorders
Vital signs, including blood pressure (lying, sitting, standing)
Cardiac arrhythmias
Urinary alteration
   Urgency
   Frequency
   Nocturia

Vertigo
Medications

Psychosocial

Memory
Safety practices
   Footware
   Clothing
   Environment (throw rugs, cords)
   Lighting
Living arrangements
Supportive relationships; assistance with activities of daily living
Financial status/ability to maintain safe environment
Communication
Stressors

Spiritual

Source of strength and hope
Relationship between health, illness, disability, and spirituality
Participation in faith community in the past
Present limitations in participating in religious services
Relationships with others
Support systems

 # NURSING CARE PLAN: POTENTIAL FOR INJURY—FALLS

Common contributing factors	Expected client outcomes	Nursing strategies
Poor vision/cataracts	Client will have vision corrected to the extent possible Client will demonstrate prevention behaviors	Assess vision deficits Identify community services for vision testing and assist with arrangements as requested or required Teach client and family about cataracts and other visual problems Provide night-lights and easy accessibility to other lights Provide adequate nonglaring light Instruct client to avoid surfaces that have a high degree of shine Instruct client to avoid looking directly at bright lights Instruct client to use dark glasses to reduce glare Encourage client to use contrasting colors or black and white in environment for better discrimination of doors, stairs, light switches Instruct client to keep glasses clean and nearby when not being worn
Decreased darkness adaptation	Client will identify and correct areas of poor lighting in home Client will avoid movement until adaptation occurs	Suggest ways of correcting areas of poor lighting in the home Suggest turning head away from light when turning it on

NURSING CARE PLAN: POTENTIAL FOR INJURY—FALLS—cont'd

Common contributing factors	Expected client outcomes	Nursing strategies
Weakness or balance problems caused by medications or diagnostic procedures	Client will verbalize relationship between side effects of medications and the risk for falls	Assess for previous falls Identify medications and assess client's response and any side effects Establish schedule for blood pressure and pulse assessment Teach importance of taking medications as prescribed Monitor fluid intake and offer liquids Instruct client and family regarding medication side effcts Evaluate time of administration (i.e., diuretics, hypnotics) Evaluate need for assistive devices and instruct client in the use of the devices Consider bedside commode if urinary urgency and frequency are a problem Instruct client in bed exercises Instruct client to sit on side of bed before standing after any rest period Instruct client to avoid stooping
Unstable gait	Client will maintain mobility without decreasing physical safety	Assess client's ambulation and awareness of safety concerns Request consultation from physical therapist for evaluation and treatment In collaboration with physical therapist, assist with balance exercises, exercise program, range-of-motion exercises Provide degree of assistance needed and any assistive devices needed Communicate need, type, and degree of assistance to all other staff and family Teach client use of assistive devices, transfer and ambulation techniques, and method of getting assistance Remove barriers and clutter from the environment Instruct client to wear sturdy footwear with nonskid soles

Lack of safety awareness	Client will demonstrate safety measures	Instruct client/family in personal safety measures:
		    Avoid improperly fitted shoes or slippers
		    Wipe up spills promptly
		    Keep floors free of clutter
		    Secure extension and appliance cords
		    Remove items that block exits or hallways
		    Anchor area rugs
		    Avoid long robes
		    Do not enter unlighted rooms
		Teach hospitalized clients to keep bed in low position, use bed rails and call lights, use showers with rails or have assistance when entering or leaving a wet area (tub)
		Teach clients in wheelchairs to lock the brakes when transferring from wheelchair to bed, etc.

Unfamiliar surroundings or altered mental status	Client will use measures to remain safe to the extent of his or her ability	Assess history of falls Assess client's ability to understand information and his or her sensory abilities Orient client to surroundings, explain call system, evaluate client's ability to use the system Allow participation in decision making Visit at frequent intervals; provide orienting information Provide environmental safety measures (i.e., lights, signs, familiar objects) Explain provision for physical needs such as toileting, calling for assistance, bathing Plan schedule to assist client with toileting Avoid physical restraints Continue to evaluate risk for falls and modify plan if needed

EVALUATION

1. The client states the importance of optimal vision.
2. The client identifies intrinsic and extrinsic factors that increase the risk for falls.
3. The client demonstrates safety measures in activities of daily living.
4. The client follows medication schedules and reports side effects that may contribute to a fall.
5. The client maintains mobility in a safe manner.
6. The client states the importance of maintaining a safe environment.
7. The client identifies and removes environmental hazards in the home.

NURSING ALERTS

1. Careful monitoring is very important when an older person is first admitted to an institution, since most falls occur in the first 2 weeks.
2. Always monitor clients being placed on new medications. Side effects of dizziness or hypotension are common and can lead to falls.

3. Be alert to clients who have a history of falls. There is a high probability that they will continue to fall unless corrective measures have been taken.

Bibliography

Blumenthal J et al: Psychological and physiological effects of physical conditioning on the elderly, Journal of Psychosomatic Research, 26:505, 1982.

Botwinick J: Aging and behavior, ed 2, New York, 1978, Springer Publishing Co, Inc, p 262.

Burggraf V and Stanley M: Nursing the elderly: a care plan approach, Philadelphia, 1989, JB Lippincott Co.

Eliopoulos C: Gerontological nursing, ed 2, Philadelphia, 1987, JB Lippincott Co.

Kim K and Grier M: Pacing effects of medication instruction for the elderly, Journal of Gerontological Nursing 7:464, 1981.

Kim MJ, McFarland GK, and McLane AM: Pocket guide to nursing diagnoses, ed 3, St Louis, 1989, The CV Mosby Co.

Schow R et al: Communication disorders of the aged: a guide for health professionals, Baltimore, 1978, University Park Press, pp 138-146. (This book contains the Nursing Home Hearing Handicap Index.)

Knowledge Deficit

Christine Clarkin

KNOWLEDGE BASE

1. A knowledge deficit exists when an individual is unable to express understanding of concepts that pertain to his or her disease, disorder, or developmental needs.
2. An individual who is unable to perform certain psychomotor tasks may or may not have a lack of knowledge related to the task.
3. Older people are more likely to have knowledge deficits if they have chronic diseases that require new information for management.
4. Older clients may not have had formal health education about body functions and the effects of aging on these body functions.
5. Health education materials usually are not adapted to account for the sensory impairments of older individuals, making learning less likely to happen.
6. The physiological changes of aging may result in less effective adaptation to stress or overload.
7. Although there is no decline in intelligence, an older individual may need more time for the learning process to occur.

8. Thought processing, information receiving, and response time slow in advancing age.
9. Because recent memory will be less efficient than long-term memory, teaching needs to be offered at a slower pace for the elderly.
10. New information should be offered in short messages and in a context meaningful to the client. Helping him or her form associations will aid in retention of new material.
11. Utilization of the senses of sight, sound, touch, taste, and smell will also assist in retention of new information.
12. Clients who are experiencing a loss and demonstrating grief may not be able to retain information. The phase of grief response dictates specific teaching techniques.
13. The goal of client education is to alter the client's perceptions and encourage new behavior.
14. Helping the older person tie ideas together and link thoughts improves his or her ability to form concepts. Conceptualization is a necessary part of the process that places new information into one's memory bank for later recall.

15. Loss of visual acuity may make it difficult for older individuals to read certain types of print or to utilize audiovisual aids.
16. Talking louder to the hearing impaired does not help. Speaking slowly and distinctly and facing the individual is more effective in relaying a message.

ASSESSMENT CRITERIA
Physical

Barriers to learning
Signs of acute illness (e.g., elevated temperature, increased pulse rate, elevated blood pressure)
Shortness of breath
Easy fatiguability
Pain
Tremors
Loss of hearing, vision, tactile sense
Signs of anxiety:
  Restlessness
  Higher pitch to voice
  Constant motion of hands and feet

Psychosocial

Desire and willingness to learn
Current level of knowledge
Ability to process thoughts
Ability to receive information and follow instructions
Delayed response to touch or verbal instructions
Difficulties staying focused on a topic
Grief responses
Family or social support
Expression of need for information
Memory
Ability to perform health care practices safely
Responses to previous learning experiences

Spiritual

Religious beliefs
Values placed on life that affect responses to illness
Feelings of hopelessness or helplessness

 ## NURSING CARE PLAN: KNOWLEDGE DEFICIT

Common contributing factors	Expected client outcomes	Nursing strategies
Distrust of health care providers	Client will develop trusting/helping relationship with nurse	Allow sufficient time for one-to-one interaction Sit quietly, listen actively to client's concerns Give client your name and title
Delayed readiness to learn	Client will demonstrate readiness to learn	Assess interest and present knowledge base
Physical barriers to learning, such as acute illness, vision loss, hearing loss	Client will obtain necessary resources/aids enable him or her to learn	Assess barriers to learning (vision, hearing, acute illness, etc.) Initiate activities to lessen effect of these barriers through environmental control Identify family or community resource to support client's effort to accomplish self-care, or to perform care for him or her when support is not enough
Negative feelings about therapeutic regimen or organized learning	Client will identify his or her need/focus for information (what he or she wants to know)	Assist client in identifying what he or she wants to know—how illness is creating problems for him or her Form teaching plan beginning with need identified by client, then covering what you have identified as critical information
Slowed thought processing	Client will receive information in a manner appropriate to his or her needs and learning capabilities	Implement teaching plan in environment free of distraction Limit teaching to three to five points each session Utilize large-print materials, colorful charts, and slides or tapes that are available
Unsafe level of skill in health maintenance practices	Patient will demonstrate safe level of skills, appropriate to identified need	Evaluate effectiveness of teaching plan via return demonstrations, appropriate responses to questions that test knowledge
Lack of support systems in home environment	Client will identify one or more individuals who can support him or her in making needed changes in life-style	Include family members/close friends who can be available to client as he or she implements teaching If no family or friends are available to participate in learning, find community resources that may be of assistance

EVALUATION

1. The client discusses with the nurse fears and concerns about his or her health, previous experiences with health care systems, and the treatment regimen.
2. The client seeks assistance with financial concerns.
3. The client asks questions of the nurse.
4. The client states his or her most immediate concern with current health state, identifying the information they want first.
5. The client is able to read (using large-print materials if necessary). The client is able to repeat back simple sentence when spoken in normal voice. The client is able to utilize glasses/hearing aids to facilitate learning.
6. The client identifies plans to implement new information (e.g., to incorporate aerobic exercise into his or her activities by walking in a local shopping mall from 7 to 8 AM on Mondays, Wednesdays, and Fridays.
7. The client's response to specific teaching methods indicates mastery of the subject matter.
8. The client or care partner demonstrates a safe level of skill or knowledge appropriate to the identified problem.
9. The client's family or friends participate in the teaching process, indicating their commitment to support the client.

NURSING ALERTS

1. Lack of follow-through with developing new perceptions or behaviors may be related to factors such as anxiety or ineffective individual and family coping. The nurse should be alert to behavioral cues, and respond to them with appropriate interventions. Application of more information may not be an appropriate intervention.
2. There are practical limits to the amount of new information an elderly individual can remember. The amount forgotten, mistakes, and confusion increase with the volume of information given. A maximum of three to five points should be made during an instructional session.
3. People without adequate income, social support, and coping skills are going to require more assistance from health and community resources.

Bibliography

Doak CC: Communication with the elderly, The Diabetes Educator, 8(special issue):45, 1983.

Kim MJ, McFarland GK, and McLane AM: Pocket guide to nursing diagnoses, ed 3, St Louis, 1989, The CV Mosby Co.

Levin RF et al: Diagnostic content validity of nursing diagnoses, Image: Journal of Nursing Scholarship, 21(1):40, Spring 1988.

Matteson MA and McConnel ES: Gerontological nursing: concepts and practice, Philadelphia, 1988, WB Saunders Co.

Papatheodoro NH: The psychosocial aspects of aging in diabetics, The diabetes educator, 9(special issue):49, 1983.

Puderbaugh Ulrich, Canole SW, and Wendell SA: Nursing care planning guides: a nursing diagnoses approach, Philadelphia, 1986, WB Saunders Co.

Mobility, Impaired Physical

Jo Eva Ziegler Blair

KNOWLEDGE BASE

1. Impaired physical mobility is the state in which an individual experiences a limitation of ability for independent physical movement.
2. Impaired mobility is the most frequent problem experienced by institutionalized elders.
3. Some causes of impaired mobility are drug reactions, pain, malnutrition and weakness, depression (lack of motivation), sensory impairment, fear of falling, deconditioning after prolonged bed rest, and forced immobility because of restraints.

4. Some specific conditions forcing impaired mobility are fractures, chronic obstructive pulmonary disease, peripheral vascular disease, coronary artery disease, congestive heart failure, cerebrovascular accident, multiple sclerosis, Parkinson's disease, arthritis, osteoporosis, malignancies, spinal cord injuries, and surgery.
5. The effects of prolonged impaired mobility in the elderly can be irreversible, resulting in permanent loss of function.
6. To maintain strength, a muscle must actively contract; to increase strength, there must be an increased number of contractions or increased resistance.
7. The muscles most affected by impaired mobility are those necessary for locomotion and maintenance of an upright position.
8. Muscle endurance requires adequate nutrition and adequate respiratory and circulatory function so that muscle cells receive oxygen and nutrients and have waste products removed.
9. Joint tissues will remain elastic only with continued movement. Without movement, joint fluid becomes thick and tenacious, connective tissue becomes fibrotic, and ligaments, tendons, and muscles shorten to their maximum amount of stretch, resulting in contractures.
10. Early joint stiffness may be reversible with therapy; later, only surgical intervention can free the joint.
11. Lack of a planned exercise program will result in a prolonged recovery time for muscle strength.
12. Achieving sitting balance is the first step in relearning dressing, position transfers, ambulation, and other activities of daily living.
13. Fear of falling must be recognized and overcome.
14. Regaining mobility must be a health team collaborative project. Consistent directions, stepwise progression, patience, and praise are important factors in the client's success.
15. Inadequate nutrition, especially in protein intake, jeopardizes rehabilitative programs for elderly people.
16. As mobility becomes impaired, an older person may experience many psychological reactions, such as anger, withdrawal, depression, changes in self-concept, and dependence.
17. The measurable nursing outcome in caring for a client with impaired mobility is the prevention of any further decline in abilities, and thus the prevention of further dependence.
18. Periodic dismissal planning is necessary for clients. With adequate support services and a planned rehabilitative program, a client may be able to return home.

ASSESSMENT CRITERIA
Physical

Ability to move in bed
Balance: sitting and standing
Transfer ability
Walking ability
Gait and stability
Toileting ability
Feeding ability
Grooming ability
Ability to flex and extend extremities
Weakness or paralysis of extremities
Muscle strength in extremities
Pain in joints, with and without movement
Joint mobility/contractures/deformities
Amputations
Fine and gross motor coordination
Bradykinesia, cogwheel rigidity
Prothestic and adaptive devices being used
Restrictive devices medically prescribed (casts, traction)
Generalized pain
Endurance (tolerance for activity)
Edema
Respiratory status (rest and exertion)
Circulatory competence; postural hypotension
History of disease, trauma, or surgery
Drug therapy

Psychosocial

Apprehension, fear
Ability to comprehend
Ability to follow instructions/commands
Depression
Degree of motivation
History of falls
Mental status (alert to comatose)
Memory
Degree of cooperation
Self-concept

Spiritual

Feelings about ability to cope with the situation
Sense of hopefulness or despair
Source of strength and hope

NURSING CARE PLAN: IMPAIRED PHYSICAL MOBILITY

Common contributing factors	Expected client outcomes	Nursing strategies
Decreased muscle strength and endurance	Client will demonstrate measures to increase muscle strength and endurance Client will describe the rationale for exercise and self-care Client will report intolerance to activity, if experienced Client will discuss importance of nutrition in increasing mobility	Assess muscle strength of upper and lower extremities Assess activity tolerance by evaluating heart rate and respiration and report of fatigue and weakness Develop a program of progressive range-of-motion exercises and self-care activities in conjunction with occupational and physical therapists or physician Encourage client to maintain good body alignment while in bed; use foot boards and pillows Assist client in bed exercises; when ambulation is possible, limit time and distance, and progress as tolerated Assess nutritional status; collaborate with dietitian to provide nutrients necessary for energy needs Consider group exercises Assist client in evaluating progress; encourage client to assume responsibility for the exercise and mobility program

Neuromuscular, musculoskeletal impairment	Client will increase movement within the limitations of the disease/condition
	Client will be able to perform self-care activities with less difficulty
	Client will be able to discuss causative disease process, treatment plans, and activity limitations
	Client will have a safe environment
		Assess current status (see assessment criteria)
		Develop mobility goals in collaboration with physician, rehabilitative therapist, client, and family
		Develop program of exercise for joints and muscles within treatment plan designed by physician and therapist
		Encourage self-care
		Promote comfort through measures such as positioning and heat; develop pain management, including medications
		Encourage client to maintain good posture when up and good alignment when in bed
		For inflammatory joint disorders:
		  Teach energy conservation, such as sliding objects rather than lifting
		  Avoid positions of possible deformities (sitting for long periods of time, flexion deformities)
		  Avoid using the same muscle and joints for long periods of time; vary activities
		  Use good body mechanics
		Encourage correct use of assistive devices during self-care activities and ambulation
		Evaluate home environment for safety, such as grab bars, raised toilet seats, hand rails, nonskid floors, nonskid bath mat
		Refer to community support groups and services for home care

Pain during movement	Client will increase activity Client will report greater comfort with movement Client will experience increased joint function	Assess pain characteristics, location, events that increase the pain, relief factors Develop plan for pain management; schedule exercise or movement during peak comfort periods Balance rest and activity Collaborate with rehabilitative therapist to plan program of joint movement, exercise, and activities Collaborate with physical therapist and occupational therapist for assistive devices Teach client and family about comfort measures and analagesic medication Encourage client to direct care; encourage self-care Teach client about medications, side effects, and adverse reactions

NURSING CARE PLAN: IMPAIRED PHYSICAL MOBILITY—cont'd

Common contributing factors	Expected client outcomes	Nursing strategies
Mental/emotional impairments	Client will display less anxiety during exercise Client will participate in an activity program to his or her maximum potential	Assess events that increase anxiety and/or pain Assess for past history of falls Assign staff or family member to be exercise "buddy"; use games such as "Simon Says" to get the client to exercise If client is unable to follow instructions, use assistive-active range-of-motion exercises on all joints at least daily Reassure client of his or her safety; when mobilizing, use transfer belt and adequate assistants; use slow, confident movements; demonstrate movements before client move Evaluate safety of client's use of assistive devices such as walkers, wheelchairs

EVALUATION

1. The client experiences no further mobility impairment or dependence and meets specific goals (e.g., able to transfer, able to use walker).
2. The client is able to be more physically active.
3. The client balances rest and activity.
4. The client is able to explain prescribed activity limitations, treatment measures, and self-care goals.

NURSING ALERTS

1. Because of decreased motor ability, muscle weakness, depression, and disease, the elderly are at risk for experiencing limitations in physical movement.
2. If an elderly client loses muscle strength because restricted activity is medically necessary, it is possible that the strength will not be regained, making the client prone to more morbidity (pressure wounds, pneumonia, confusion, falls).

3. Immobility may be a direct result of pain or depression.
4. Pain management is an important adjunct to rehabilitative therapies. Careful development of a plan for pain relief in conjunction with exercises may determine the success or failure of rehabilitative therapy.

Bibliography

Caliandro G and Judkins B: Primary nursing practice: Glenview, Ill, 1988, Scott, Foresman/Little, Brown College Division.

Carpenito L J: Nursing diagnosis: application to clinical practice, Philadelphia, 1987, JB Lippincott Co.

Kim MJ, McFarland GK, and McLane AM: Pocket guide to nursing diagnoses, ed 3, St. Louis, 1989, The CV Mosby Co.

Long BC and Phipps WJ: Medical-surgical nursing: a nursing process approach, ed 2, St. Louis, 1989, The CV Mosby Co.

Potter PA and Perry AG: Basic nursing: theory and practice, St. Louis, 1987, The CV Mosby Co.

Nutrition, Altered: Less Than Body Requirements

Lisa Logan
Frances F. Rogers-Seidl

KNOWLEDGE BASE

1. Nutrition is a critical factor in health. For elderly people, nutrition becomes even more important for physical and emotional health.
2. A minimum amount of nutrients must be consumed to meet the metabolic requirements of the body.
3. Caloric requirements for older adults may be less than, more than, or the same as those of younger adults, depending upon activity, absorption of nutrients, and metabolic needs.
4. If metabolic needs are not met, loss of weight, poor health, and inability to repair tissue result.
5. Metabolic needs are increased when an older person has surgery, trauma, infection, or cancer.
6. Aging poses particular problems in nutritional health because of age-related physiological and life-style changes, increased incidence of chronic disease, psychosocial problems, medications/treatments, and functional disabilities.
7. The food patterns of an elderly person have been developed over many years. Food choices and eating habits are shaped by the interaction of early family experiences, cultural and financial factors, health status, knowledge, and environment.
8. Laboratory assessment is critical to the identification of malnourishment. The biochemical signposts of malnutrition are serum albumin level (normal value, 3.5 g/dl), serum transferrin level (180 to 260 mg/dl), and total lymphocyte count (1500-4000/mm³).
9. The planning of effective strategies for correction of malnourishment is based on the individual's profile.
10. Risk factors for nutritional deficits include anorexia, impaired memory or cognition, inability or difficulty in self-feeding, difficulty in chewing or swallowing, inadequate hydration, neurological disorders, poor dentition, shortness of breath, extreme fatigue, activity intolerance, loneliness, depression or death wish, use of depressants or multiple medications, alcohol abuse, lack of transportation, inability to prepare food, and inadequate finances.
11. Studies show that as age increases, mean caloric and nutrient intake decreases.
12. Nutrient deficits most often identified include iron, vitamin A, and vitamin C.
13. Early signs of malnourishment in older people are nonspecific and may be caused by other conditions. Examples of symptoms include lethargy, irritability, reduced appetite, depression, and cognitive impairment.
14. The use of anthropometric measurements for elderly people, such as skinfold thickness, is controversial. Norms for skinfold thickness have not been established for persons over age 75.
15. Drugs may cause nutrient losses.

ASSESSMENT CRITERIA
Physical

Food intake (past/present)
Usual weight
Anthropometric measurements
   Height/weight
   Midarm circumference
   Subscapular skinfold
Laboratory values
   Blood chemistry profile
   Complete blood count
   Serum albumin level
   Serum transferrin level
Skin turgor and integrity
Condition of hair, nails, mouth, teeth
Ability to chew, swallow, feed self
Ability to prepare food
Activity patterns
Exercise habits
Strength, endurance, fatigue
Chronic illness
Recent surgery
Presence of infection
Medications (prescription and over-the-counter)
Hydration status
Food intolerances/allergies
Presence of nausea, vomiting, anorexia
Presence of pain

Psychosocial

Knowledge of nutrition and healthy nutritional practices

Short-term memory status

Mood swings, indications of depression

Coping patterns

Meaning of food

Sense of control over own life

Motivation for change

Ability to obtain food

Transportation

Physical mobility

Vision

Finances

Intact memory

Socialization, especially at mealtimes

Long-established or cultural food habits

Spiritual

Concern about spirituality/religious activity

Meaning of suffering, life, death

Strength to cope with the situation

Sense of hopefulness or despair

 ## NURSING CARE PLAN: ALTERED NUTRITION—LESS THAN BODY REQUIREMENTS

Common contributing factors	Expected client outcomes	Nursing strategies

Difficulty in chewing and swallowing	Client will consume adequate nutrients	Assess caloric and nutrient intake, including liquids
		Identify factors in the eating problem
		Request consultation from dietitian, speech therapist
		If client has dentures, assess fit and request consultation with dentist if needed
		Position as upright as possible; flex neck, tuck chin
		Chewing helps:
		  Place a 1-inch portion of soft food in the strongest side of the mouth
		  Instruct client to chew, lip closure should be maintained if possible
		  If client can follow instructions, instruct him or her to swallow, if client is apraxic, distract and stroke throat to stimulate reflex (see care plan on swallowing, p. 87)
		  Wait until each bite is completely chewed and swallowed before presenting the next bite
		  Increase caloric density of foods and thicken liquids for easier swallowing
		  Blot client's mouth; do not wipe
		  Schedule small, frequent meals
		  Have suction equipment at feeding site; staff should be knowledgeable of Heimlich's maneuver

Difficulty in self-feeding related to functional impairments, inability to sit upright, or activity intolerance	Client will participate in the eating/feeding process Client will consume adequate calories and nutrients Client will be able to eat adequate amount of nutrients without extreme fatigue	Assess specific deficit contributing to problem Request consultation from occupational therapist for plate guard, material to anchor plate, spoons, cups, and orthotics Monitor intake of nutrient groups and collaborate with dietician to provide supplemental feeding Identify what the client can do for himself or herself; if client is unable to feed, allow him or her to direct the feeding Provide easily chewed calorie-dense food in small frequent feedings Allow a rest period before meal Do not require the client to sit more than 10 minutes before the meal Position in an upright or functional posture at a table if possible; stabilize head and trunk, tuck chin Pace feeding/eating to allow adequate time for chewing, swallowing, and breathing Identify the food before introducing the food into the mouth Stay in the client's intact field of vision when feeding Provide servings of finger foods Request evaluation for restorative feeding program

Continued.

NURSING CARE PLAN: ALTERED NUTRITION—LESS THAN BODY REQUIREMENTS—cont'd

Common contributing factors	Expected client outcomes	Nursing strategies
Reluctance to eat related to anorexia, nausea, pain, medications	Client will accept increasing amounts and variety of foods Client will verbalize enjoyment of favorite foods Client will verbalize increased comfort at mealtime Client will express an increased sense of well-being Client will maintain socialization skills and personality integration	Monitor and record intake of food and fluids; weigh weekly Monitor laboratory values Assess for contributing factors to the eating problem Identify food preferences (including ethnic/cultural) and provide foods if possible Identify time of day client most willing to eat; provide nutrient-dense foods Assess need for medication for pain or nausea and give 45 minutes before eating Give oral care, including cleansing of tongue; avoid strong mouthwash Do not give medications at mealtime; do not mix medications with food; consider suppositories when possible Establish an exercise program to client's tolerance Encourage client to eat with others; have social atmosphere Provide food that looks, smells, tastes good; season with allowed herbs and spices; serve hot food hot and cold food cold Divide total nutrients into more frequent meals, smaller portions Increase nutrient density of foods served Give supplemental feedings as indicated Instruct client to avoid lying down flat for at least 1 hour after meals

Altered mental status, memory loss, depression, distractibility during meal	Client will express verbally or nonverbally an increase in self-esteem
	Client will consume adequate quantity of food
	Client will consume a greater quantity of food within his or her usual eating time
		Assess client's level of understanding and perception of eating and adjust communication
		For distractibility/memory loss:
		    Limit directions to one or two words, short phrases
		    Select eating site according to best results; reduce stimuli
		    Do not allow other people to converse with one another
		    Music may be tried; low and soothing
		    Keep client focused on eating
		    Introduce food items one at a time
		    Sit with client during meal
		    Consistent time schedule and seating arrangements
		For depression:
		    Establish schedule for meals and supplemental feedings
		    Small, frequent feedings
		    Sit with client during meals
		    Distinguish between lack of appetite and depression
		    Request consultation for depression

Increased need for nutrients because of burns, infection, cancer, impaired digestion and absorption of nutrients	Client will meet his or her energy requirements
	Client will receive ample nutrients and vitamins to sustain bodily functions
	Intolerance of feeding will be minimized
	Client will receive prompt treatment for any infection
	Client will have less potential for aspiration pneumonia
		Request consultation from dietitian for an in-depth evaluation
		When enteral nutrition support is ordered, request consultation from a dietitian knowledgeable in enteral nutrition for correct formula prescription
		    Monitor fluid and electrolytes
		    Assess skin integrity
		    Maintain accurate intake and output record
		    Assess bowel sounds every 4 hours
		    Administer correct volume and concentration for tube feedings; initial feeding should be started at half-strength at 40 m/hr; the rate may be increased by 25 m/ every 12-24 hours if the client tolerates the feeding

NURSING CARE PLAN: ALTERED NUTRITION—LESS THAN BODY REQUIREMENTS—cont'd

Common contributing factors	Expected client outcomes	Nursing strategies
Increased need for nutrients because of burns, infection, cancer, impaired digestion and absorption of nutrients—cont'd		When final rate is achieved, the strength can be increased as tolerated; avoid altering rate and strength at the same time
		Infuse feeding at room temperature
		Maintain a closed system for infusing; change every 24 hours; use aseptic technique
		Record tube feeding intake separately
		Flush with 30-50 ml water every 6 hours; maintain adequate hydration
		Monitor for infection related to aspiration pneumonia and insertion-path necrosis
		Check correct tube placement before each intermittant feeding or every 8 hours
		Elevate head of bed 30-45 degrees
		Monitor respiratory status during feedings
Decreased quality of food intake related to difficulty in obtaining or preparing food because of economics, transportation, or knowledge	Client will develop a self-support system for independent living	Assess the situational problems and plan accordingly
		Identify service alternatives (both formal community services and informal resources)
		Assist the client in developing a plan of adequate food intake
		Negotiate a commitment for adequate nutrition

EVALUATION

1. The client consumes adequate nutrients as evidenced by body weight, laboratory data, and clinical signs.
2. The client has adequate hydration.
3. The client demonstrates decreased incidence of choking and aspiration pneumonia.
4. The client has optimal independence in eating and drinking.
5. The client verbalizes that eating is a positive experience.
6. The client maintains dignity and self-esteem.

NURSING ALERTS

1. The critical role of nutrition in the well-being of older people makes it imperative for the nurse to diagnose and intervene in nutritional problems.
2. High-quality patient care requires assessment of nutritional status, planning of interventions, and monitoring of progress.
3. Assessment of elderly persons' nutritional status encompasses many complex factors—physical, psychological, social, and spiritual.

4. The nutritional status of an older person is sometimes ignored during the initial contact with the client, allowing problems such as delayed wound healing, longer recovery time, pressure ulcers, and depression to develop.
5. Collaboration with other disciplines, such as dietetics, speech therapy, occupational therapy, and physical therapy, is important in solving nutritional problems of elders.

Bibliography

Butterfield G: Impact of aging on nutritional status, Geriatric Consultant, March-April, 1988, p 13.

Collingsworth R and Boyle K: Nutritional assessment of the elderly, Journal of Gerontological Nursing, 15(12):17, 1989.

Hunter A and Rogers F.: Assessment in long-term care: a co-operative venture, Topics in Clinical Nutrition, Oct 1988, p 40.

Iverson-Carpenter M et al: Fulfilling nutritional requirements, Journal of Gerontological Nursing, April 1988, p 16.

Kim MJ, McFarland, GK, and McLane AM: Pocket guide to nursing diagnoses, ed 3, St Louis, 1989, The CV Mosby Co.

Schlenker E: Nutrition in aging, St Louis, 1984, The CV Mosby Co.

Williams S: Nutrition and diet therapy, ed 6, St Louis, 1989, The CV Mosby Co.

Nutrition, Altered: More Than Body Requirements

Ann Pendlebury Hunter
Frances F. Rogers-Seidl

KNOWLEDGE BASE

1. Altered nutrition resulting in more than body requirements can be defined as the condition in which body weight exceeds ideal weight by more than 20%.
2. The incidence of obesity in the elderly not living in institutions is from 15% to 50%.
3. Food is an integral part of social function, religious ritual, and creative expression. It becomes symbolic, with the meaning being derived from each person's perception.
4. Many older people use food "to feel better"— that is, as a coping mechanism for increased anxiety, boredom, depression, or grief.
5. Common factors contributing to obesity in older people include social isolation, lifelong patterns of obesity, poor dentition, reduced mobility, decreased metabolic rate, and appetite-stimulating drugs.
6. Increased food intake without energy expenditure will result in weight gain. Activity (exercise) causes calories to be burned and raises the basal metabolic rate (BMR). Engaging in aerobic exercise for 20 minutes increases the BMR for 24 hours.
7. Increased quantity of nutrients does not ensure increased quality of nutrients. Therefore, even though a person is obese, he or she may be malnourished.
8. A deficit (intake vs expenditure) of 3500 calories is required to allow an elderly person to lose 1 pound.
9. The method used to arrive at ideal weight must be consistent with recent tables.
10. The BMR decreases approximately 5% per decade after 20 years of age, which necessitates a decrease in caloric intake and maintenance of activity.
11. Weight will not decrease unless the caloric level is significantly below the basal metabolic requirement. Caloric intake should be set 200 to 300 calories below this requirement.
12. Obesity leads to increased incidence of impaired mobility, diabetes, congestive heart disease, joint disease, hypertension, increased cholesterol and triglyceride levels, gallbladder disease, and some forms of cancer.
13. An obese elderly person who has mobility problems often suffers from negative feedback from caregivers and significant others.
14. The negative self-image associated with obesity can lead to unacceptable behaviors.
15. The three nutrients providing calories (energy) are carbohydrates, protein, and fats. A high fat intake appears to cause increased obesity.
16. The elderly are particularly susceptible to fad diets. Most fad diets lead to malnourishment and are injurious to general health.
17. Medications that stimulate appetite include tranquilizers, lithium carbonate, and vitamins.

ASSESSMENT CRITERIA
Physical

Food intake (past/present)
Usual weight
Anthropometric measurements
   Height/weight
   Midarm circumference
   Subscapular skinfold
Laboratory values
   Blood chemistry profile
   Complete blood count
   Serum albumin
   Serum transferrin
Skin turgor and integrity
Condition of hair, nails, mouth, teeth
Ability to chew, swallow, feed self
Ability to prepare food
Activity patterns
Exercise habits
Strength, endurance, fatigue
Chronic illness
Recent surgery

Presence of infection
Medications (prescription and over-the-counter)
Hydration status
Food intolerances/allergies
Presence of pain

Psychosocial

Knowledge of nutrition and healthy nutritional practices
Past attempts at dieting
Short-term memory status
Mood swings, indications of depression
Coping patterns
Meaning of food
Sense of control over own life

Motivation for change
Ability to obtain quality food
    Transportation
    Physical mobility
    Vision
    Finances
    Intact memory
Socialization, especially at mealtimes
Long-established or cultural food habits

Spiritual

Concern about spirituality/religious activity
Meaning of suffering, life, death
Strength to cope with the situation
Sense of hopefulness or despair

 NURSING CARE PLAN: ALTERED NUTRITION—MORE THAN BODY REQUIREMENTS

Common contributing factors	Expected client outcomes	Nursing strategies
Excessive intake of high-calorie foods	Client will consume adequate nutrients within the caloric limits Client will experience weight reduction of 1-2 pounds per week	Establish acceptable calorie intake Monitor intake of nutrients and calories, and record Request consultation with dietitian Monitor weight on a weekly basis Limit intake of simple sugars and fats; provide foods with complex carbohydrates and adequate protein Provide for food holiday for special occasions Teach family and friends acceptable foods to bring to the client Allow the client choices within the established limits
Anxiety, depression, boredom, or grief	Client will verbalize adaptive mechanisms not involving food	Assess psychosocial status and factors contributing to food intake Assess meaning of food; cultural influences Listen to expressions of hopelessness, anger, grief Allow and encourage client to participate in meal planning Encourage family and significant others to plan activity not involving food; if food is involved, allow the food and alter the next meal Consider referral to counseling or support group (Overeaters Anonymous) Help client to increase control over other areas of care Provide recreational and productive activity
Decreased activity related to habit, disease, psychological status	Client will increase activity within prescribed limitations Client will verbalize the rationale for increased activity	Assess activity tolerance and prescribed limitations Increase activity as allowed Include exercise in the client's daily schedule Teach the client exercises within his or her limitations—e.g., bed exercises, chair or floor exercises Include the client in development of the plan for activity Schedule other activities of daily living to support the exercise program Gradually increase activity; avoid overfatigue

EVALUATION

1. The client consumes adequate nutrients within the caloric limits.
2. The client experiences weight reduction of 1 to 2 pounds a week.
3. The client utilizes adaptive mechanisms not involving food.
4. The client verbalizes an understanding of the need for increased activity.
5. General health and stamina remain good.
6. Hemoglobin and hematocrit are in normal ranges, as are other chosen laboratory values.

NURSING ALERTS

1. Severe dietary restrictions often make an elderly client less compliant, while a more liberal approach (small pieces of dessert) allows him or her to feel happier and still achieve the goal.
2. Correction of boredom and depression and a willingness and desire to comply on the part of the client are essential if the treatment plan is to be effective.
3. Medications must be carefully chosen to avoid appetite stimulation.
4. Family and friends must help the client by not providing forbidden items.
5. In addition to improved diet, increased activity is essential.
6. A holiday meal or some regular relief from the prescribed diet helps.
7. A reward for decreased weight should be nonfood but something the client wants.

Bibliography

Alford BB and Bogle ML: Nutrition during the life cycle, Englewood Cliffs, NJ, 1982, Prentice-Hall, Inc.

Hunter AP and Rogers FF: Assessment in long-term care: a cooperative venture, Topics in clinical nutrition, 3(4):40.

Kim MJ, McFarland GK, and McLane AM: Pocket guide to nursing diagnoses, ed 3, St Louis, 1989, The CV Mosby Co.

Roe DA: Geriatric nutrition, ed 2, Englewood Cliffs, NJ, 1987, Prentice-Hall, Inc.

Ross Laboratories: Nutritional support in the long-term care institution, Columbus, Ohio, 1984, Ross Laboratories.

Ross Medical Nutritional System: Nutritional assessment of the elderly through anthropometry, Columbus, Ohio, 1984, Ross Laboratories.

Simko MD, Cowell C, and Gilbride JA: Nutrition assessment, Rockville, Md, 1984, Aspen Publishers, Inc.

Pain

Sue E. Meiner

KNOWLEDGE BASE

1. Pain refers to the state in which an individual experiences and reports the presence of severe discomfort or an uncomfortable sensation. Chronic pain refers to pain that continues more than 6 months.
2. The experience of pain is influenced by personality, developmental state, and cultural background.
3. Pain can be adaptive, warning the person of an abnormal situation, or maladaptive, causing additional emotional and physical stress.
4. Anxiety and fear augment the pain perception and thus intensify the response to pain.
5. The pain experience cannot be generalized on the basis of age, sex, or cause. It is unique to the person, a subjective experience, thus it is whatever the person reports.
6. The elderly are at high risk for pain-inducing situations because they often have several chronic diseases or conditions at one time. A single pain-producing condition may be overlooked in the complexity of the overall health status.
7. Muscle and joint pains are the most common complaints of elders. Pain as a symptom of infection is usually absent in the elderly. Rather they display apathy, loss of appetite, lethargy, and decreased mental acuity.
8. Older people may or may not display decreased sensitivity to pain. The variability may be due to degenerative changes in nerve receptors, decreased numbers of neurons both in the brain and in the periphery, and decreased velocity of impulse transmission. Older people have a decreased ability to localize painful stimuli.
9. Absence of pain where pain should be present is significant. In elderly people pain cannot be used as the early warning symptom for injury or infection; for example, in appendicitis, urinary tract infections, or myocardial infarctions, pain may not be present.
10. Nonverbal behaviors may be the only assessment parameters in elderly people who are confused.
11. Older people and health professionals themselves often consider pain an expected part of the aging process. Because of this myth, many reversible conditions go untreated.
12. For elderly people, pain weakens and interrupts the sense of wholeness of self, others, and the environment. It may have meanings of loss of independence or even death.

13. Effective pain management is necessary for physical and emotional functioning. Pain control has important implications for maintaining independence and enhancing the quality of life. A holistic approach must be taken. A variety of theories and models have been researched and can be used in developing strategies.

ASSESSMENT
Physical

Quality of pain
Severity of pain (use scale of 0 to 10)
Location of pain
Onset, duration, and conclusion of pain
Precipitating and alleviating factors
Nausea or syncope
Signs/symptoms of pain
    Guarding behavior
    Grimacing
    Withdrawal from social activities and contacts
    Impaired thought processes
    Rigidity or listlessness of body posture
    Self-focus
    Narrowed focus
    Altered time perception
    Crying/moaning
    Sweating
    Pupillary dilatation
    Changes in vital signs
    Disorientation
    Restlessness, pacing
Current medications (over-the-counter and prescription)
Effectiveness of pain relief measures

Psychosocial

Level of anxiety/fear
Attitude toward and perception of pain
Energy level/reserve
Diagnosis and prognosis
Coping strategies
Previous experience and meaning of pain

Spiritual

Influence of religion on pain
Cultural beliefs

 NURSING CARE PLAN: PAIN

Common contributing factors	Expected patient outcomes	Nursing strategies
Injury, infection, or surgery resulting in acute pain	Client will verbalize a reduction in pain	Use active listening to acknowledge pain Assess descriptors of pain and pain behavior Use a pain rating scale for consistency of understanding and managing pain Develop a plan for pain management with the client, using a combined approach of medication and noninvasive strategies With the client, initiate noninvasive pain-relief measures such as distraction, relaxation, cutaneous stimulation, and music therapy Monitor effectiveness of pain management, using a flow sheet for pain intensity, duration, medication, and comfort measures Eliminate or minimize additional stressors and sources of discomfort Provide for uninterrupted rest following medication Instruct client to request medication as needed before pain is severe Instruct family in comfort measures such as back rubs and positioning
Altered body function resulting in chronic pain	Client will perform without preoccupation with pain; level of pain will be controlled	Plan activities that will minimize painful effects Plan rest and activity at intervals during the day Plan diversional activities as appropriate Ask client to record intensity and duration of pain, activities in daily routine, and pain medication taken; use the pain diary to evaluate present therapy and to consider changes Instruct family by explaining the causes of the pain and the client's responses Monitor for impaired balance and cognitive functioning Give oral medications with food Begin a bowel regimen early to prevent constipation Listen to the client and assist in assigning meaning to the pain experience Teach effective use of analgesics aimed at control of pain

Continued.

NURSING CARE PLAN: PAIN—cont'd

Common contributing factors	Expected patient outcomes	Nursing strategies
Fear of pain	Client's pain will be lessened by use of adaptive coping mechanisms and a reduction in anxiety	Assess anxiety level and depression behaviors Use pain-relieving measures before pain becomes severe Provide accurate information about medications, condition Encourage verbalization of feelings about the pain and its relief Plan diversional activities Reassure the client about addiction possibility when necessary Remain supportive and teach family about the fear-pain cycle Support the client in regaining control over the pain through self-medication, establishing a plan, etc.

EVALUATION

1. The client verbalizes comfort and pain relief after medication has had time to become effective.
2. The client demonstrates only mild levels of anxiety.
3. The client establishes a schedule for rest periods, with activities at tolerance levels but not exceeding them.
4. The client describes measures that have been successful in relieving pain.
5. The client uses diversional measures such as audiotapes, television, and progressive relaxation techniques at appropriate times.
6. The client performs activities of daily living within the limitations of his or her abilities.
7. The client sets realistic goals for daily activities.
8. The client collaborates with the nurse and includes the family in planning actions.
9. The client allows family members to share in this life experience through touch, physical care, and emotional and spiritual support.
10. The client makes fewer statements about fear of pain or fear of addiction to prescribed medications but openly discusses these issues at intervals.

NURSING ALERTS

1. Special attention must be exercised in regard to dosages of all medications for the elderly. The diminished liver and kidney function and metabolism can lead to higher concentrations and longer-lasting drug effects.
2. Drug overload is a frequent concern when multiple medications are being prescribed and taken, and the dosages are the same as the recommended adult dosages. Dosages may need to be adjusted downward if signs and symptoms of prolonged action are present.
3. Side effects common in the elderly, such as nausea, dyspepsia, and constipation, should be anticipated and prevented.

4. Cognitive impairment may be exacerbated by pain and its treatment.
5. Frequently the elderly cannot accurately localize pain.
6. An older person may not report pain. He or she may fear the meaning of the pain, diagnostic workups, or the cost of diagnosis and treatment, or may assume that the pain is to be expected with age.
7. An elderly client in obvious pain should not be interviewed.
8. Pain consumes much of the energy of an older client. Conservation of energy is very important in his or her care.
9. In the postsurgical elderly client, restlessness may result from either hypoxia or pain. The cause must be carefully evaluated before analgesics are given. Respiratory arrest may occur if a hypoxic client is given a narcotic analgesic.
10. Caution must be exercised in attributing pain exclusively to a psychological cause. Failure to investigate physiological sources can result in needless suffering.

Bibliography

Eliopoulos C: Gerontological Nursing, ed 2, Philadelphia, 1987, JB Lippincott Co.

Eliopoulos, C, editor: Health assessment of the older adult, Menlo Park, Calif, 1984, Addison-Wesley Publishing Co., Inc.

Kermis M: The psychology of human aging: theory, research and practice, Boston, 1984, Allyn & Bacon, Inc.

Kim K and Grier M: Pacing effects of medication instruction for the elderly, Journal of Gerontological Nursing, 7:464, 1981.

Kim MJ, McFarland, GK, and McLane AM: Pocket guide to nursing diagnoses. ed 3, St. Louis, 1989, The CV Mosby Co.

McCaffery M. and Beebe A: Pain: clinical manual for nursing practice, St Louis, 1989, The CV Mosby Co.

Simonson W: Medications and the elderly, Rockville, Md; 1985, Aspen Publishers, Inc.

Self-Care Deficit

Jo Eva Ziegler Blair

KNOWLEDGE BASE

1. A self-care deficit is a state in which an individual experiences an impaired ability to perform or complete the following activities: bathing and hygiene; dressing and grooming; feeding; toileting.
2. Self-care is valued by individuals and society.
3. The ability to complete self-care functions depends on circulatory, musculoskeletal, respiratory, and nervous system competence.
4. Self-care is threatened by any of the following factors, alone or in combination: poor motivation, poor self-esteem, depression, environmental barriers, cognitive impairment, activity intolerance, pain, musculoskeletal conditions, restricted joint motion, paralysis.
5. The ability to perform self-care functions is important to the comfort, dignity, and self-esteem of an elder.
6. Self-care deficits may contribute to a loss of autonomy and foster dependence.
7. Assisting another person in self-care involves intimate contact. Both client and caregiver may have feelings of shame and guilt. The client's privacy must be respected and measures taken to decrease anxiety.
8. Threatening situations, stress, or illness may cause regression in self-care activities.
9. The likelihood of institutionalization increases as functional dependence increases.
10. Rehabilitation requires analysis of the client's deficits in knowledge, skill, motivation, and orientation in regard to a self-care activity.
11. An individual's performance may be recorded on a scale:
    0 = Completely independent
    1 = Requires use of equipment or assistive device
    2 = Requires help of another person; supervision or assistance
    3 = Requires assistance and assistive devices
    4 = Dependent in activity; unable to participate
12. Rehabilitation goals must be realistic and consider all aspects of the client's status, including other health problems, physiological status, resources, strengths, and willingness to participate in the treatment plan.
13. The total health care team, including client and family, must be involved in setting goals.
14. Goals are established for regaining function, adapting to lost function, preventing further disabilities, and maintaining psychological and physical integrity.
15. A consistent approach by all team members is critical to the client's relearning of self-care.
16. The purpose of care is to help the elderly client move from dependence to independence to the extent possible.
17. Teaching strategies for the older client must consider what the client perceives as important needs, as well as motivating factors, learning abilities, sensory losses, environment, and optimal time frame.
18. An older person's grief resulting from the loss of function may inhibit relearning.
19. Activity intolerance necessitates inclusion of principles of energy conservation and task simplification in helping the client relearn self-care.
20. Adaptations in utensils, clothing, environment, and methods may afford the elderly client independence in self-care.

ASSESSMENT CRITERIA
General

Past medical and surgical history
Present conditions and illness
Nutritional status
Medications

Physical

Mobility
Extremity function and strength
Gait
Posture; control of position
Balance; sitting and standing
Neurological status
Ambulation ability
Transfer ability
Joint movement
Joint deformity; contractures
Pain on movement
Tremor
Amputation
Motor skills/coordination
Activity tolerance
   Respiratory status
   Angina

Leg cramps
Extreme fatigue
Sensory deficits: vision, touch, hearing
Self-feeding ability
    Bringing food to mouth
    Using utensils
    Chewing, swallowing, drinking
    Cutting food; adding seasoning
    Wiping mouth
Self-bathing ability
    Getting to bathroom
    Getting into shower/tub
    Washing body
    Regulating water temperature or flow
    Brushing teeth/caring for dentures
    Shampooing hair/shaving
Self-dressing/grooming ability
    Putting on or removing clothing
    Zipping or buttoning
    Tying shoes
    Hair care

Toileting ability
    Control of bowel and bladder
    Getting to and/or rising from toilet
    Cleaning self
    Removing and replacing clothing

Psychosocial

Cognitive status
Anxiety level
Independence/dependence needs
Depression
Self-esteem
Motivation
Potential for learning
Adaptability
Economic resources
Support from others

Spiritual

Sense of hopefulness/hopelessness
Anger toward God, self, others related to condition
Meaning of condition in relationship to God

 ## NURSING CARE PLAN: SELF-CARE DEFICIT

Common contributing factors	Expected client outcomes	Nursing strategies
Inability to feed self	Client will be able to consume adequate nutrients	Assess and analyze specific causative factors contributing to deficit
		Request consultation from dietitian, speech therapist, occupational therapist, and social worker
		Provide preferred foods in balanced diet
	Client will be able to participate in the eating experience	Help client to assume position most conducive to self-feeding
		Provide assistive devices such as rocker knife, large-handled spoon, plate guard, etc.
		Schedule other activities to avoid fatigue at mealtime
		Consider small, frequent feedings if client has poor energy levels
	Client will maintain control over the eating process	Provide assistance to the extent needed, from feeding to only providing verbal or physical prompting
		Allow client to direct pace, sequence of food eaten, fluids taken, and amount of food eaten
		Avoid mixing foods on plate, such as scrambled eggs in oatmeal
	Client will be able to express satisfaction with eating	Maintain a social atmosphere with conversation and a pleasant environment
	Client will demonstrate self-esteem	Consider privacy needs; avoid embarrassing situations for the client, especially with drooling or food spillage
		Modify diet consistency to increase ease of handling, consider finger foods
		Assist in placing dentures, glasses, and/or hearing aids
		See care plan for alteration in swallowing, p. 87
Inability to provide for own hygiene	Client will use remaining abilities to his or her maximum	Assess and analyze barriers to self-care in hygiene
		Request consultations from physical and occupational therapists

NURSING CARE PLAN: SELF-CARE DEFICIT—cont'd

Common contributing factors	Expected client outcomes	Nursing strategies
	Client will express satisfaction with the bathing activity	Identify type of bath setting desired by the client and most conducive to abilities
		Use contractual style in setting hygiene schedule
		With clients having activity intolerance, consider energy conservation measures
		Provide adaptive equipment such as long-handled brushes, shower stools, and hand-held shower heads
	Client will identify safe practices in bathing	Assess and teach client about safety hazards
		Encourage client to direct the bathing procedure if he or she is unable to perform the activity
	Client will demonstrate only mild levels of anxiety	Provide privacy
		Identify client's level of anxiety and encourage verbalization of feelings
	Client will verbalize feelings about being bathed (if able)	Adopt matter-of-fact attitude when cleansing intimate areas of the body, but be sensitive to the client's feelings
		Convey caring through tender and unhurried touch
		If pain prevents self-care, give medication 45 minutes before client performs task
Inability to dress or groom self	Client will use strengths while participating in dressing/grooming	Assess and analyze components of dressing and grooming in relation to specific client deficits
		Request consultation from physical and occupational therapists
	Client will dress and groom to his or her maximum ability	Allow adequate time for the client to dress or groom at his or her own pace
		Provide assistance only to the extent needed; from verbal or physical prompting to direct assistance with the task
		Encourage the client/family to have clothing that is conducive to a positive self-image
		Use a consistent approach when teaching dressing sequences; simplify tasks; use clothing that is easy to put on (larger sizes, Velcro fastners, elastic waists, large buttons, elastic shoelaces, etc.)
		Divide tasks into parts; continue on one part until mastered then proceed to next task
	Client will demonstrate safe practices while grooming and dressing	Identify the most functional position for the client; provide safety devices such as side rails, grab bars, sturdy chair
		Be sensitive to anger and frustration if client is unable to complete a task; employ previously identified stress-relief actions and avoid any additional stress; the task may need to be completed for the client
		To the extent possible, allow the client to make decisions about the selection of clothing or the time frame for grooming
		Schedule activities to maximize self-care; avoid over-fatigue; provide adequate pain relief
Inability in toileting	Client will demonstrate increased ability to toilet in a timely manner	Assess and analyze components of self-toileting and identify deficits
		Record present toileting patterns for both bowel and bladder
		Identify present methods of getting assistance
	Client will verbalize feelings about dependence in toileting	Identify meaning of the toileting deficit to the client
		Provide privacy to the extent possible
		Assess skin integrity
	Client will not experience secondary problems related to toileting deficit	Assess for urinary tract infection, retention, urgency, frequency, and incontinence
		Assess for constipation and bowel incontinence
		Provide for adequate fluid intake
		See care plan for constipation, p. 23
		Provide cleansing with soap and water if incontinence occurs
		Remove barriers to toilet

Continued.

NURSING CARE PLAN: SELF-CARE DEFICIT—cont'd

Common contributing factors	Expected client outcomes	Nursing strategies
Inability in toileting—cont'd	Client will identify safety practices	Assess safety hazards to the client in self-toileting
		For activity intolerance or when energy expenditure negates other activities, provide bedside commode
		For cognitive impairment establish schedule of toileting based on recorded data
		Provide the degree of assistance necessary, from removing clothing to verbal cues
	Client will have increased ability to eliminate when on the toilet	For an apraxic client, distraction during toileting allows reflex voiding and defecation

EVALUATION

1. The client is clean, well groomed, and appropriately dressed.
2. The client is well nourished.
3. The client maintains skin integrity.
4. The client is able to use the toilet for bowel and bladder elimination.
5. The client verbalizes feelings about self-care deficits.
6. The client maintains independence and self-esteem.

NURSING ALERTS

1. A complete daily bath may not be necessary for each client. As a person grows older, there is decreased function of sweat and oil glands, resulting in less waste on the skin. Excessive bathing may dry the skin.
2. Nurses should set reasonable long term goals— is it possible for the client to become more independent with self-care?
3. Because of decreased motor ability, muscle weakness, depression, activity intolerance, and disease, the elderly are at risk for experiencing limitations in self-care.
4. The shared expertise of all health team members is needed in rehabilitation for self-care deficits.

Bibliography

Caliandro G and Judkins B: Primary nursing practice, Glenview, Ill, 1988, Scott, Foresman/Little, Brown College Division.

Carpenito LJ: Nursing diagnosis: application to clinical practice, Philadelphia, 1987, JB Lippincott Co.

Kim MJ, McFarland GK, and McLane AM: Pocket guide to nursing diagnoses, ed 3, St Louis, 1989, The CV Mosby Co.

Long BC and Phipps W: Medical-surgical Nursing: a nursing process approach, ed 2, St Louis, 1989, The CV Mosby Co.

Potter PA and Perry AG: Basic nursing: theory and practice, St Louis, 1987, The CV Mosby Co.

Sensory-Perceptual Alterations

Tally N. Bell

KNOWLEDGE BASE

1. Sensory-perceptual alteration is a state in which an individual experiences a change in the amount or patterning of incoming stimuli, accompanied by a diminished, exaggerated, distorted, or impaired response to such stimuli.
2. Age-related changes in the special senses can profoundly affect the elderly's ability to perceive and respond to their environment. Sensory-perceptual alterations can occur whenever sensory reception, conduction, and/or interpretation are compromised. An accurate nursing history and an accurate assessment are essential in order to examine the amount and type of sensory stimuli an elderly client receives, as well as his or her interpretation and recognition of the stimuli.
3. Sensory deprivation results in feelings of isolation, frustration, anxiety, fear, and anger. The reaction of many older people to sensory deprivation is to withdraw socially and to limit their interactions with others, resulting in further deprivation.
4. Elderly people who receive an excess of sensory stimuli can experience exaggerated emotional responses, suspicion, paranoia, and fear.
5. A significant nursing challenge is to provide the elderly with a proper balance of appropriate sensory input and to ensure that the sensory input received is accurately interpreted.
6. The integration of sensory function and motor function declines with age.
7. Pathophysiological changes such as altered circulation, oxygenation, and cerebral perfusion can cause sensory-perceptual alterations, resulting in dizziness, lightheadedness, and vertigo.
8. Age-related changes cause slower processing of information and slower reaction time. Multiple commands can lead to confusion.
9. The sensory receptors become less efficient with aging, so fewer stimuli reach them.
10. Inability to interpret sensory stimuli can cause anxiety and fear of the unknown, both of which can contribute to sensory overload.
11. Absence of rapid-eye-movement (REM) sleep aggravates sensory-perceptual deficits and can lead to sensory overload or sensory deprivation.
12. An older person's response to stimuli varies with his or her ability to adapt. Increased anxiety, misperceptions, distortion of time, and altered thought processes can occur if the person is unable to adapt.
13. Unfamiliar sounds and objects may have no relevance for sensory stimulation.
14. Steady, firm touch provides more sensory stimulation to the elderly, and it is perceived as more calming.
15. Reminiscence is a useful strategy to stimulate the elderly. Long-term memory usually remains intact even when short-term memory declines.
16. Private rooms, isolation, immobility, and confinement can decrease the amount and type of sensory stimulation that a person receives.
17. Sensory deprivation occurs when special senses are impaired and compensatory aids such as glasses and hearing aids are not used.
18. When a person is deprived of one sense, the other senses become keener, thus providing some compensation for the sensory impairment.
19. Medication interactions, side effects, overdosage or underdosage, and toxicity can cause sensory impairment.
20. Sensory-perceptual alterations can cause a person to be unable to interpret correctly stimuli indicating hunger, thirst, pain, or position.
21. Uncompensated sensory impairments put the client at high risk for injury.
22. Consistency and familiarity with the environment facilitate safety for the client with sensory-perceptual alterations.
23. Age-related visual changes can add to sensory-perceptual alterations.
24. Severe hearing impairment can necessitate alternate means of communication to prevent sensory deprivation.
25. A person's response to vestibular and kinesthetic stimulation declines with age, leading to impairment in equilibrium, coordination, and proprioception.
26. The sensory threshold is increased with aging, so more intense stimulation is required to produce a response.
27. Common physical stressors include sense organ alteration, neurological disease, neurological in-

jury, metabolic imbalance, impaired gas exchange, paralysis, amputation, medications, surgical procedures, substance abuse, and altered sleep/rest pattern.
28. Common psychological stressors include social isolation, physical isolation, immobility, pain, stress, and unfamiliar environment.

ASSESSMENT CRITERIA
General

History (may need family/significant other to assist)
  Onset, pattern, duration, and site of symptoms
  Changes in behavior and personality
  Past and present medical problems
  Use of corrective devices, such as glasses, hearing aids, prostheses
  Nutritional intake pattern and status
  Pattern of activities of daily living (ADL)
  Medication history

Physical

Neurological examination
  Level of consciousness
  Pupil size and reaction
  Accommodation reflex
  Motor deficits
  Sensory deficits
  Orientation to time, place, person
Presence of altered thought processes

Reported and/or measured changes in:
  Special sense organ function: visual, auditory, kinesthetic, gustatory, tactile, olfactory
  Recognition of sensory input
  Response to sensory stimulation
  Coordination, posture, proprioception, mobility
  Effects of sensory-perceptual alterations on client's functioning
Vital signs
Review of other body systems
Self-care deficits

Psychosocial

Coping strategies and support systems, adaptive or maladaptive
Communication patterns (verbal and nonverbal) and adaptive responses
Current behavior (note restlessness, irritability, apathy, anxiety)
Intellectual function
  Conceptual thinking
  Abstract thinking
  Reasoning
  Problem-solving
  Memory
  Judgment
  Insight
  Concentration

Spiritual

Religious beliefs and practices

 NURSING CARE PLAN: SENSORY/PERCEPTUAL ALTERATIONS

Common contributing factors	Expected client outcomes	Nursing strategies
Sensory overload	Client will attain optimal level of sensory stimulation without experiencing sensory overload Client will maintain usual orientation and level of mentation	Assess neurologic/mental status, intellectual functioning, behavior, interpretation of stimuli on admission and on an ongoing basis; report changes immediately Reduce unnecessary noise, light, activity, clutter, and furniture in client's environment Maintain good room lighting (i.e., lights on/off to denote day/night, curtains open during day, and lighting that prevents shadows) Explain unusual sounds, smells, equipment, and procedures Cluster treatments, activities, and nursing care as tolerated; provide a consistent, structured outline Encourage uninterrupted sleep/rest periods Speak in a calm, quiet voice and maintain good eye contact with client while speaking (however, be sensitive to cultural preferences regarding eye contact) Reorient client to environment and give verbal clues as needed Place clock and calendar within client's field of vision Avoid belittling the client when stimuli are misinterpreted Avoid supporting inaccurate interpretations of the environment, and help client to interpret accurately Document altered thought processes and exaggerated responses to the environment Encourage the client to validate perceptions

NURSING CARE PLAN: SENSORY/PERCEPTUAL ALTERATIONS—cont'd

Common contributing factors	Expected client outcomes	Nursing strategies
Sensory deprivation	Client will attain optimal level of sensory stimulation Client will maintain orientation and usual level of mentation	Identify elements of the therapeutic regimen that restrict the client's sensory stimulation, and plan further nursing strategies Determine communication deficits and establish alternative systems Monitor and document client's response to stimuli Determine effects of sensory deprivation on client's self-care activities, and intervene as appropriate Engage in frequent, meaningful conversation with client Provide opportunities for client to interact with others, as appropriate Touch client at frequent intervals using firm, steady pressure, and encourage significant others to do the same Provide clock, television, radio, and/or music in client's environment; place in client's field of vision Encourage wearing of glasses, hearing aids, prostheses, and other adaptive devices; if necessary, help client to put them in place Modify environment to compensate for sensory impairments Provide meaningful sensory stimulation to all special senses through conversation, touch, music, and/or pleasant smells Assess neurologic/mental status, intellectual functioning, and behavior on an ongoing basis; report changes immediately Reorient client to environment and give verbal cues as needed Provide a consistent, structured routine Ensure adequate, uninterrupted sleep/rest periods Evaluate client's ability to adapt to decreased stimulation level Encourage diversional activities
Altered visual and/or auditory reception, conduction, and/or interpretation	Client will attain optimal level of sensory stimulation Client will become aware of visual impairment and ways to compensate	Assess gross hearing deficits by noting client's response to conversational tones or through use of an audioscope; recommend further consultation, if indicated Examine the auditory canal with an otoscope to detect the presence of excessive cerumen Assess visual acuity and visual fields bilaterally and report deficits Encourage wearing of glasses, hearing aids, prostheses and other adaptive devices; if necessary, help client to put them in place; check equipment for functioning Utilize bright, contrasting colors in the environment Patch eyes alternately every 2 hours if diplopia present Provide large-print reading materials, such as books, clocks, calendars, and educational materials Maintain room lighting that distinguishes day from night and that is free of shadows and glare Teach client to scan the environment to locate objects Help client to locate food on the plate using "clock" system, and describe food if client is unable to visualize; assist with feeding, as needed Arrange physical environment to maximize functional vision Place personal items, call light, etc., within client's field of vision Coordinate the health care team's effort to reinforce compensatory mechanisms Encourage involvement of significant others in treatment plan

Continued.

NURSING CARE PLAN: SENSORY/PERCEPTUAL ALTERATIONS—cont'd

Common contributing factors	Expected client outcomes	Nursing strategies
Altered visual and/or auditory reception, conduction, and/or interpretation—cont'd	Client will become aware of visual impairment and ways to compensate—cont'd	Modify education plan to maximize intact senses, such as utilizing demonstration/return demonstration, written and/or verbal instructions, as appropriate Explore means to make adaptive equipment available, if needed Encourage client to express feelings about sensory loss/impairment Identify previous adaptive coping strategies, and encourage client to use them
	Client will become aware of auditory impairment and ways to compensate	Encourage client to ask questions to clarify his or her perception of what has been said Teach the client to watch the speaker Have adequate, nonglare lighting Reinforce wearing of hearing aid; if client does not have an aid, use a communication device Communicate clearly, distinctly, and slowly, using a low-pitched voice and facing client; avoid overarticulation Remove as much unnecessary background noise as possible Do not use slang or extraneous words Position yourself at eye level and no farther than 6 feet away Get the client's attention before speaking Avoid speaking directly into the client's ear If the client does not understand what is being said, rephrase the statement rather than repeating
	Client will demonstrate ability to perform activities of daily living, with assistance if necessary	Provide a consistent ADL routine that includes placing toiletry items in specific locations and a verbal explanation of the items and their locations Break activities into small, clear, simple, one-step commands, and allow client adequate time to complete activity Reorient client to environment as needed Avoid moving furniture in room; keep bedside objects in same places Institute safety measures such as bed in low position, side rails up, no smoking while alone, and call light within reach Provide adequate room lighting Teach client to increase use of unimpaired senses Encourage client to ask for assistance, when necessary

EVALUATION

1. The client demonstrates absence of sensory overload or deprivation, as evidenced by appropriate verbal and/or nonverbal behavior.
2. The client remains oriented to time, place, and person, to the extent that his or her condition allows.
3. The client demonstrates accurate interpretation of internal and external stimuli as evidenced by appropriate verbal or nonverbal behavior.
4. The client demonstrates compensatory mechanisms for each sensory impairment or deficit.
5. The client utilizes adaptive equipment.
6. The client causes no injury to self or others as a result of sensory-perceptual alterations.
7. The client assists with activities of daily living, as far as he or she is able.

NURSING ALERTS

1. To maximize the client's functioning when sensory-perceptual alterations are present, use a multisensory approach to his or her activities of daily living.
2. Age-related changes in color discrimination can cause the elderly difficulty in differentiating between medications, reading dipsticks for glucose levels, and clarifying color-illustrated patient education materials.
3. Sensory changes experienced by the elderly pose a distinct safety risk as they perform their normal activities. It is imperative that all sensory alterations be noted on the nursing care plan so that nursing strategies are implemented in a consistent manner by all caregivers.

Bibliography

Carpenito J: Nursing diagnosis: application to clinical practice, ed 3, Philadelphia, 1987, JB Lippincott Co.

Doenges M, Moorhouse M, and Geissler A: Nursing care plans: guidelines for planning care, ed 2, Philadelphia, 1989, FA Davis Co.

Eliopoulos C: Gerontological nursing, ed 2, Philadelphia, 1987, JB Lippincott Co.

Eliopoulos C: A guide to the nursing of the aged, Baltimore, 1987, Williams & Wilkins.

Esberger K and Hughes S Jr: Nursing care of the aged, Norwalk, Conn, 1989, Appleton & Lange.

Kim MJ, McFarland GK, and McLane AM: Pocket guide to nursing diagnoses, ed 3, St Louis, 1989. The CV Mosby Co.

Long B and Phipps W: Medical-surgical nursing: a nursing process approach, St Louis, 1989, The CV Mosby Co.

Matteson M and McConnell E: Gerontological nursing: concepts and practice, Philadelphia, 1988, WB Saunders Co.

Murray R and Zentner J: Nursing assessment and health promotion strategies through the life span, ed 4, Norwalk, Conn, 1989, Appleton & Lange.

Rudy E: Advanced neurological and neurosurgical nursing, St Louis, 1984, The CV Mosby Co.

Taylor C and Cress S: Nursing diagnosis cards, Springhouse, PA, 1987, Springhouse Corp.

Wyness M: Perceptual dysfunction: nursing assessment and management, Journal of Neuroscience Nursing, 17(2):105, 1985.

Sexuality Patterns, Altered

Elaine E. Steinke

KNOWLEDGE BASE

1. Altered sexuality patterns is the state in which an individual expresses concern regarding his or her sexuality.
2. Psychological responses, misperceptions, and insufficient knowledge of physical changes that occur with aging are often the greatest barriers to sexual satisfaction.
3. Sexuality is individually defined, which may or may not include coitus. Therefore the changes occurring with age may not be a concern for some older adults.
4. A client may express concerns about changes in sexual patterns. These changes could be related to psychosocial factors, normal physical changes with age, and/or pathological mechanisms.
5. Lack of partner availability is one of the major causes of diminished sexual activity in older women. There are more available older women than older men.
6. An older adult may withdraw from social interaction, which inhibits the development of meaningful relationships. Reasons for such social isolation include lack of transportation, fear of leaving home or of crime, and physical health problems, or the isolation may occur by choice.
7. Psychological variables may prove to be inhibiting factors for sexual expression. The older adult may show diminished interest in sexual activity, exhibit signs of depression, or find monotony in a long-term sexual relationship.
8. Negative attitudes and conflicting religious beliefs may preclude sexual expression. For example, an older adult might believe that sexual activity should be reserved for marriage; however, the person might be interested in another older adult but does not want to remarry.
9. A lack of privacy may preclude sexual activity. A person in a retirement center, nursing home, or other group living arrangement may have little opportunity for sexual expression. However, privacy for the purpose of enhancing sexual satisfaction may or may not be a need for an older adult.
10. Resolution of sexual tension and venous engorgement of sex organs are of longer duration for both men and women.
11. Slowed sexual response occurs in both men and women.
12. There is less venous engorgement of sex organs.
13. Vaginal lubrication and wall expansion are decreased in women. Problems with vaginal lubrication can be alleviated with the use of a water-soluble jelly. Estrogen therapy might also be prescribed.
14. Erection in older males takes two to three times longer as compared with younger males.
15. Once erection is achieved, it can be maintained longer before ejaculation. Prolonged erection in males can be a benefit, with longer time to stimulate the partner to orgasm.
16. There may be a single-stage rather than a two-stage ejaculation. The older male may report diminished sensation of ejaculation because of this normal physical change.

17. Ejaculation may be a seepage of semen rather than a forceful emission. The older male may believe that this represents an end of sexuality rather than a normal result of aging.

For women:
  Difficulty with arousal
  Changes in vaginal lubrication
  Difficulty achieving orgasm

ASSESSMENT CRITERIA
Physical

Underlying physical health problems
Effect of health problems and treatment on sexual function
Degree of sexual activity:
  Active or not active
  Times per month
  Sexual practices
Pain with intercourse
For men:
  Ability to attain/maintain erection
  Changes in ejaculation

Psychosocial

Concerns about sexuality/sexual function
Knowledge of sexuality and aging
Degree of sexual interest
Relationship patterns
Partner availability
Sexual satisfaction
Mood changes (e.g., depression, guilt)
Need for privacy

Spiritual

Conflicting values or religious beliefs

 # NURSING CARE PLAN: ALTERED SEXUALITY PATTERNS

Common contributing factors	Expected client outcomes	Nursing strategies
Reported changes in usual sexual patterns related to physical health problems	Client will return to usual sexual patterns or adapt to new sexual patterns	Assess usual sexual patterns and behaviors and changes in physical health Provide teaching about sexual response with physical health problems; individualize teaching to specific problem Allow client to discuss problems freely in nonjudgmental atmosphere
Insufficient knowledge and/or negative attitudes about sexual changes with age	Client will describe normal changes in sexual function with age Client will have increased knowledge of sexuality and aging Client will exhibit positive attitudes about sexuality and aging	Assess knowledge of sexuality and aging Explore attitudes with client in a nonjudgmental manner Discuss the impact of societal attitudes about sexuality and aging on the older adult Provide teaching that corrects misinformation about sexuality and aging Expose the client to older adults with positive attitudes about sexuality and aging Evaluate client's understanding of teaching content
Diminished sexual interest, monotony	Client will verbalize reasons for psychosocial changes in sexuality Client will incorporate strategies into sexual relationships	Assess degree of sexual interest and interaction Explore reasons for changes in sexual interest (e.g., depression or monotony, sexual patterns that are unchanged after years of marriage) Discuss approaches and develop strategies with the client to enhance sexual satisfaction (creating romantic mood, allowing plenty of time for sexual activity, planning sexual activity at a time when well rested, creating a mood of excitement, positioning, etc) Evaluate utilization of strategies by the client and achievement of satisfaction
Lack of partner availability, withdrawal from interaction related to loss of spouse	Client will express ways to reopen social world Client will attempt to develop meaningful relationships	Assess client's desire for social interactions and meaningful relationships Develop with the client strategies to increase meaningful relationships (interaction with other older adults at senior centers, church activities, etc.)
Lack of privacy	Client will have time periods available for privacy	Assess the need for privacy Provide an environment free from distraction Allow time periods for privacy
Conflicting values or religious beliefs	Client will express feelings about values or beliefs	Explore feelings about sexuality and aging in reference to religious beliefs and values Encourage the older adult to discuss his or her views with others in the same age group Support the client in his or her decisions about sexuality

EVALUATION

1. The client is able to identify and discuss problems that are contributing to his or her altered sexual patterns.
2. The client demonstrates understanding of sexuality and aging.
3. The client expresses more positive attitudes about sexuality and aging.
4. The client states that he or she will increase social interactions and attempt to develop meaningful relationships.
5. The client uses strategies to enhance sexual satisfaction and privacy.
6. The client openly discusses his concerns about values and religious beliefs.

NURSING ALERTS

1. The nurse should be aware of his or her own attitudes about sexuality and aging and should take care not to impose them on the client.

2. A broad understanding of normal and abnormal changes in sexuality with age is paramount. This knowledge provides a sound basis for client teaching.

Bibliography

Carpenito LJ: Handbook of nursing diagnosis, ed 2, Philadelphia, 1987, JB Lippincott Co.

Carpenito LJ: Nursing diagnosis: application to clinical practice, ed 2, Philadelphia, 1987, JB Lippincott Co.

Kim MJ, McFarland GK, and McLane AM: Pocket guide to nursing diagnoses, ed 3, 1989, St. Louis, The CV Mosby Co.

Roberts SL: Nursing diagnosis and the critically ill patient, Norwalk, Conn, 1987, Appleton & Lange.

Steinke EE: Older adults' knowledge and attitudes about sexuality and aging, Image: Journal of Nursing Scholarship, 20(2):93, 1988.

Steinke EE and Bergen MB: Sexuality and aging: a review of the literature from a nursing perspective, Journal of Gerontological Nursing, 12(6):6, 1986.

Taylor CM and Cress SS: Nursing Diagnosis Cards, Springhouse, Pa, 1987, Springhouse Corp.

Sexual Dysfunction

Elaine E. Steinke

KNOWLEDGE BASE

1. Sexual dysfunction is the state in which an individual experiences a change in sexual function that is viewed as unsatisfying, unrewarding, or inadequate.
2. Slowed sexual response is often attributed by the older adult to a medical condition rather than seen as a normal change with age. Hence, some older adults with medical conditions mistakenly believe that the capability for sexual response has ended.
3. Performance anxiety is compounded by the stereotype that impotence necessarily occurs with age. Physical versus psychological impotence is an important distinction that should be made.
4. Performance anxiety is often related to unrealistic expectations or inadequate knowledge of sexual changes with age and/or medical problems. Anxiety reduction should be targeted to addressing concerns arising from the underlying cause.
5. Approaches to deal with sexual dysfunction will vary depending on the underlying problem.

6. Clients may express dissatisfaction with sex roles. Problems such as illness often cause changes in previously assumed roles. The older adult may need to acquire different roles to adapt to a given situation.
7. The older adult may experience changes in both sexual and social relationships. Problems may arise that have not been experienced in the past. In general, improvement in general areas of a relationship should have a positive effect on a sexual relationship.
8. Knowledge of the normal sexual changes that occur with age (see Appendix C or the nursing care plan for altered sexuality patterns, p. 71) may in itself alleviate the problem of sexual dysfunction.

ASSESSMENT CRITERIA

For assessment criteria in addition to those listed here, see the nursing care plan for altered sexuality patterns, p. 71.

Physical

Effect of physical health problem/treatment on sexual function (see the accompanying box)

Comparison of usual sexual patterns to current patterns

Onset of sexual dysfunction

Psychosocial

Concerns about sexual function

Sex roles and relationship patterns

Knowledge of:

    Sexual changes with aging

    Effect of physical health problems on sexuality

    Alternative methods for achieving sexual satisfaction

Anxiety about sexual performance

Common Etiologies for Sexual Dysfunction in the Older Adult

Diabetes mellitus	Colostomy
Decreased hormone production	Fear
	Fatigue
Chronic renal failure	Absence of sexual teaching
Arthritis	
Myocardial infarction	Anxiety
Congestive heart failure	Pain
Peripheral vascular disorders	Lack of partner availability
Chronic lung disease	Low self-concept
Cerebrovascular accident	Altered body image
Cancer	Alcohol
Liver disease	Radiation therapy
Ileostomy	Medications

 ## NURSING CARE PLAN: SEXUAL DYSFUNCTION

Common contributing factors	Expected outcomes	Strategies
Medical condition or its treatment	Client will have improved sexual function and/or will adapt to changes in function	Perform a complete physical, sexual, and psychosocial assessment Explore the client's perception of the problem Determine if sexual dysfunction existed before the onset of the medical problem Discuss ways to achieve sexual satisfaction that take into consideration the effects of the medical problem on sexual function (e.g., other sexual pleasuring behaviors, timing of sexual activity)
Dissatisfaction with sex roles	Client will express satisfaction with and/or make adaptations in sex roles	Assess the older adult's expectations in regard to sex roles as compared with his or her perception of the present roles Explore alternative methods of sex role development (e.g., a spouse may take a more initiatory role in sexual activity than was assumed previously, referral to support group)
Changes in relationship with significant other	Client's social and sexual relationship with significant other will be improved	Assess present communication and relationship patterns
	Client will openly discuss changes in sexual relationship	Encourage open communication between client and significant other
	Client will note an alleviation of problems in the sexual relationship	Encourage the client to utilize strengths of the relationship to mutually develop strategies for improvement in problem areas; strategies should be individualized to the specific problem Allow client and significant other to role-play difficult situations within the relationship
Performance anxiety	Client will experience a reduction in anxiety	Determine reasons for performance anxiety Develop strategies to decrease anxiety (e.g., patient teaching to correct misinformation, relaxation techniques as needed)
Insufficient knowledge of sexual changes with age and/or physical health problems	Client will have increased knowledge of the normal changes in sexual function that occur with age and the effects of physical health problems on sexuality	Assess knowledge of sexuality and aging Provide teaching that corrects misinformation about sexuality and aging or about sexual responses in persons with physical health problems

EVALUATION

1. The client expresses satisfaction with sex role development.
2. The client demonstrates increased knowledge of normal sexual changes that occur with age.
3. The client reports a decrease in performance anxiety.
4. Client and significant other are able to discuss sexual problems and develop acceptable approaches to resolve them.

NURSING ALERTS

1. The nurse will need to investigate further the impact of specific medical conditions on sexual function and provide teaching as appropriate.
2. The nurse should be aware of medications that can cause impotence as a side effect.

3. Physical versus psychological impotence is an important distinction that influences intervention.

Bibliography

Carpenito LJ: Handbook of nursing diagnosis, ed 2, Philadelphia, 1987, JB Lippincott Co.
Carpenito LJ: Nursing diagnosis: application to clinical practice, ed 2, Philadelphia, 1987, JB Lippincott Co.
Kim MJ, McFarland GK, and McLane AM: Pocket guide to nursing diagnoses, ed 3, St. Louis, 1989, The CV Mosby Co.
Roberts SL: Nursing diagnosis and the critically ill patient, Norwalk, Conn, 1987, Appleton & Lange.
Steinke EE: Older adults' knowledge and attitudes about sexuality and aging, Image: Journal of Nursing Scholarship, 20(2):93, 1988.
Steinke EE and Bergen MB: Sexuality and aging: a review of the literature from a nursing perspective, Journal of Gerontological Nursing, 12(6):6, 1986.
Taylor CM and Cress SS: Nursing diagnosis cards, Springhouse, Pa, 1987, Springhouse Corp.

Skin Integrity, Impaired

Marilee Kuhrik
Nancy Kuhrik

KNOWLEDGE BASE

1. Impaired skin integrity is a state in which there is a potential for damage to the skin or in which damage has already occurred.
2. Assessment of risk factors on first contact with the client is critical to prevention.
3. Factors that jeopardize skin integrity include the following:
   a. Impaired oxygen transport
   b. Nutritional and fluid deficits
   c. Neurological disorders
   d. Difficulty/inability in movement
   e. Severe depression
   f. Altered mental state
   g. Mechanical pressure or trauma
   h. Continued presence of moisture
   i. Radiation therapy
   j. Friction or shearing force
   k. Systemic disorders and elevated body temperature
   l. Overexposure to sun, wind, heat, cold
   m. Age
4. The process of aging results in changes in the epidermis, the dermis, and subcutaneous tissue.

Each layer loses its former number of cells, causing each layer to thin and become less functional.
5. Epidermal cells lose their ability to retain moisture, resulting in dry, less supple skin. The skin surface becomes more fragile and more easily injured.
6. Changes in the dermis result in loss of fluid and decreased elasticity. A decrease in the number of neurons in the dermis causes a decrease in the ability to sense pressure and injury. The small blood vessels become increasingly fragile and easier to compress.
7. The thinning of the subcutaneous layer causes it to lose its cushioning properties for blood vessels and nerves. Thermoregulatory ability decreases, predisposing the elder to hypothermia and hyperthermia.
8. Tissue necrosis occurs when external pressure exceeds the intracapillary blood pressure, resulting in hypoxia. The area is termed a pressure ulcer.

9. The injury may involve one or more layers of the skin and extend to muscle and bone. One system describing ulcer depth or layers of tissue involved follows:

Stage 1: reddening of the skin that does not disappear within 30 minutes after the pressure is relieved. The skin is not broken.

Stage 2: the top layer of skin may be broken or blistered. The skin around it is red. This stage is very painful.

Stage 3: the ulcer goes through all layers of the skin and looks like a crater. It contains thick yellow, green, or gray secretions. If the secretions are not removed, they will become a "leather-like" black crust (eschar).

Stage 4: skin and muscle are involved, exposing the bone or joint. Eschar is present. The wound may be infected and usually has drainage.

10. Management of pressure ulcers focuses on principles of moist wound healing, prevention of pressure, and enhancement of the client's nutritional and circulatory status.

ASSESSMENT CRITERIA
Physical

Examination of the skin
 Color
 Moisture
 Texture
 Turgor
 Edema
Medical history
Impaired oxygen transport/tissue perfusion
Activity
Ability to turn or move
Body temperature
Sensory perception
Trauma, injuries, spasticity, tremors, shearing force
External pressure caused by casts, traction, braces
Incontinence
Medications
Treatments such as chemotherapy or radiation therapy
Nutritional status/hydration
Hygiene
Laboratory data
 Serum albumin
 Total protein

Psychosocial

Cognitive impairment
Stress level
Environmental factors: exposure to sun, wind, heat, cold

Spiritual

Sense of hope/hopelessness
Values

 NURSING CARE PLAN: IMPAIRED SKIN INTEGRITY

Common contributing factors	Expected client outcomes	Nursing strategies
Decreased vascularity	Client will be free of skin breakdown Client will participate in activities to enhance circulation Client will request changes in position	Relieve all areas from pressure Check whether erythema subsides within 30 minutes after turning; test for capillary refilling Schedule and assist with ambulation and bed exercises; teach lifting exercises; limit sitting time If client is immobile, turn every 1-2 hours; inspect for reddened areas Palpate tissue firmness over bony prominences after each turning; note tissue edema Cleanse skin gently; apply lotion to skin with slow, smooth stroking motions; avoid aggressive massage Utilize pressure-relief bed surfaces (RoHo, Clinitron bed, etc.) Ensure adequate warmth; avoid chilling Use warmed blankets in immediate postoperative period Evaluate effectiveness of turning schedule by inspecting skin 30 and 60 minutes after turnings
Reduced sensation	Client will be free of injury to skin Client will be aware of dangers of excessive heat and cold Client will direct position-change schedule Client will inspect skin on a scheduled basis	Assess sensory nerve function (pain, tactile, temperature) Avoid extreme temperatures (bath water, heating pads) Teach client the hazards of using heat and cold on skin Advise client to avoid overexposure to sun, to decrease the chance of skin cancer Instruct client/family in skin inspection methods Establish position-change schedule

NURSING CARE PLAN: IMPAIRED SKIN INTEGRITY—cont'd

Common contributing factors	Expected client outcomes	Nursing strategies
Inadequate nutrition and/or hydration	Client will consume adequate nutrients and fluids	Assess nutrition/hydration Assess knowledge of good nutrition and readiness to learn Instruct client to consume a diet high in protein, carbohydrates, and vitamins Request consultation with dietitian Explore community resources (e.g., senior citizens centers, Meals on Wheels) Assist client in individualizing meal plans (e.g., frequent feedings, ethnic preferences) Modify diet as necessary (e.g., soft or pureed foods)
Lack of bowel or bladder control	Client will establish a bowel and bladder routine if possible; client will be kept clean and dry	Establish a bowel and bladder rehabilitation program Toilet client every 1-2 hours If client is incontinent, clean promptly with mild soap; rinse well; avoid vigorous scrubbing; use a gloved hand or very soft cloth. Perineal area may be cleansed with peri-bottle filled with warm soapy water, followed by clear warm water; pat dry If soiling is constant, consider pouching
Decreased moisture	Client will have increased moisture and resilience of skin	Assess for dry, flaky, rough skin Assess hydration Encourage client to gently rub, not to scratch itchy skin Use soap only on soiled areas Use super-fatted soaps (Basis Soap, Lowila Soap) Avoid perfumed bath oils Put a small amount of mineral or baby oil in water for tub baths; caution must be taken to avoid falls Have client apply mineral or baby oil directly to the moist skin when showering Apply lotion or emolients several times a day Maintain an environment with adequate humidity Discourage hot baths and showers Limit the number of baths and showers
Trauma/friction	Client will be free from injury	Eliminate friction and irritation to the skin (e.g., wrinkled sheets or food crumbs) Avoid shearing force when moving or positioning the client If client is unable to assist with turning, use a turn sheet for transfers to a cart or repositioning in bed; lift client off the bed when turning; avoid dragging the client on the bed Limit time for semi-Fowler's position (30-40 degrees) to 30 minutes Encourage client to sit upright Use footboard to maintain position in bed Use linen with low surface resistance Assess skin surfaces exposed to external devices (cast, restraints, braces) If external device can be removed, do so on scheduled basis; if nonremovable, pad and position to change pressure points Carefully evaluate any client report of discomfort, especially a burning sensation under a cast or brace or with traction devices Protect the skin with padding if tremors are a potential source of injury

EVALUATION

1. The client maintains skin integrity.
2. The client voices understanding of the danger of exposing skin to extreme temperatures.
3. The client's daily routine includes measures to increase the resilience of the skin.

4. The client's diet is high in protein, carbohydrates, and vitamins and includes adequate fluids.
5. The client's skin is free from continued exposure to moisture.

NURSING ALERTS

1. Preventive measures should be initiated when a client is immobile or incontinent or suffers from poor nutrition.
2. Exercise caution when applying hot and/or cold devices.
3. Be alert for the first signs of skin breakdown, and institute therapeutic measures at once.
4. Elderly people are at risk for skin cancers. Preventive measures should be followed in the sun and the client taught to seek medical advice for any skin lesions.
5. Do not use circular "doughnut" devices. Pressure decreases the circulation within the ring.
6. Caution must be exercised in moving a client in bed, to avoid sliding the layers of skin (shear).

Bibliography

Berliner H: Aging skin, American Journal of Nursing. 86(10):1138, 1986.

Burggraf V and Donlon B: Assessing the elderly, American Journal of Nursing 85(9):974, 1985.

Calkins E, Davis P, and Ford A: The practice of geriatrics, Philadelphia, 1986, WB Saunders Co.

Ebersole P and Hess P: Toward healthy aging, St Louis, 1981, The CV Mosby Co.

Kim MJ, McFarland GK, and McLane AM: Pocket guide to nursing diagnoses, ed 3, 1989, St Louis, The CV Mosby Co.

Malasanos L: Health assessment, St Louis, 1986, The CV Mosby Co.

Potter PA and Perry AG: Fundamentals of nursing: concepts, process, and practice, ed 2, St Louis, 1989, The CV Mosby Co.

Sleep Pattern Disturbance

Mary E. Allen

KNOWLEDGE BASE

1. Sleep pattern disturbance refers to the state in which a disruption of sleep causes discomfort or interferes with desired life-style.
2. Levels of deep sleep are less prominent and brief arousals are more frequent with aging. However, the total sleep time is reduced only slightly from that of younger persons.
3. Sleep deprivation may result in a variety of symptoms, including short-term memory loss, decreased attention span, decreased motor coordination, decreased coping ability, irritability, and neurological symptoms.
4. Any disease that causes problems with adequate oxygenation or comfort will result in sleep disturbance.
5. Sleep disturbance is a common symptom of anxiety, fear, depression, delirium, or dementia.
6. Inadequate nutrient intake, especially in regard to proteins, contributes to sleep disturbance.
7. The presence of physical illness, anxiety, and/or depression may cause pain or discomfort resulting in an inability to sleep.
8. Inadequate exercise or activity during the waking hours will result in an imbalance in the sleep/wake cycle.
9. Elderly persons may need more time to get adequate sleep in the presence of degenerative diseases.
10. Being required to sleep in unfamiliar surroundings can initiate or contribute to sleep pattern disturbance.
11. Elderly persons may experience nocturnal cardiac arrhythmias and/or nocturnal shortness of breath.
12. There is an increased incidence of sleep apnea in the elderly population.
13. For some elderly people, falling asleep may be correlated with a fear of death, thereby resulting in sleep pattern disturbance. The meaning of sleep to an elderly person will influence the extent to which goal setting between the nurse and client will be mutual.
14. Increased use of prescribed and over-the-counter medications, with subsequent drug-drug and drug-food interactions, coupled with less efficient use of drugs by the aging body, can contribute to disturbances in sleep pattern.
15. Sedative-hypnotics can reduce the time before the onset of sleep and decrease the number of arousals, but only temporarily.
16. When an elderly person with a sleep pattern disturbance is being cared for, the midlife parameters of normal sleep patterns must be reexamined.
17. The long-term goal for a plan of care would be the establishment and maintenance of a sleep pattern that would promote an optimal balance of activity, rest, and sleep.

18. Baseline data on what is considered a "normal" sleep pattern for a particular elderly person should be collected and compared to current disturbances in that person's sleep. A thorough medical history, a current physical examination, and a complete drug profile should be part of the assessment data analyzed in order to formulate realistic and age-appropriate nursing strategies and expected outcomes.

ASSESSMENT CRITERIA
Physical

Medical, surgical history
Symptoms that interfere with uninterrupted sleep
    Angina
    Paroxymal nocturnal dyspnea
    Leg cramps
    Incontinence of bowel or bladder
    Nocturia
    Gastric reflux
    Discomfort or pain
    Sleep apnea
    Orthopnea
Medications
Alcohol use
Daytime activity; degree of mobility
Activity before sleep time
Nutritional status; intake of caffeine
Time of retirement; time of awakening

Overt physical signs of fatigue
    Yawning
    Flat affect
    Frequent falls or accidents
Difficulty falling asleep
Awakening earlier than desired
Difficulty in awakening
Interrupted sleep
Not feeling rested
Amount of sleep obtained

Psychosocial

Early morning awakening
Dreams, nightmares
Environmental factors
    Temperature
    Noise
    Familiar room
    Comfortable mattress
Presence or absence of roommate or bed partner
Change in rituals before sleep
Importance of sleep to the individual
Flexibility; ability to adjust to change
Anxiety levels; history of stressors
Changes in behavior and performance during waking hours as a result of sleep deprivation
Changes in speech patterns resulting in communication difficulties during waking hours
Misuse/abuse of sedative-hypnotic drugs

Spiritual

Fear of dying while asleep

 ## NURSING CARE PLAN: SLEEP PATTERN DISTURBANCE

Common contributing factors	Expected client outcomes	Nursing strategies
Internal sensory alterations related to physical illness, psychological stress, altered nutritional status	Client will verbalize being able to sleep adequately by his or her own definition (specify length of time) Client will be able to identify factors that facilitate or inhibit sleep Client will exhibit no overt behavioral signs of excessive fatigue	Identify specific cause(s) of internal sensory alteration Provide client education on sleep Identify with client factors or substances that promote sleep (e.g., warm milk) or interfere with sleep (e.g., ingestion of substances containing caffeine) Evaluate the diet for adequate nutrients (e.g., protein, niacin, vitamin B_{12}, water) Request consultation with dietitian to provide adequate diet Provide comfort measures to induce rest and sleep (e.g., back rub, pain medications, positioning) Position to enhance breathing Schedule diuretic therapy early in day to avoid nocturia Avoid extreme fatigue but discourage lengthy daytime naps Identify with client sleep-inducing relaxation techniques or use of imagery Avoid rigorous activity during late evening Give medications for sleep as prescribed, but only as a last resort, with ongoing monitoring of their effectiveness and side effects Refer to appropriate agency or person in cases of severe psychological stress (e.g., overwhelming feelings associated with fear of dying)

Continued.

NURSING CARE PLAN: SLEEP PATTERN DISTURBANCE—cont'd

Common contributing factors	Expected client outcomes	Nursing strategies
External sensory alterations related to changes in environment, social cues	Client will verbalize that the environment is conducive to sleep Client will verbalize adequate balance between level of activity and pattern of sleep	Identify specific causes of external sensory alteration Modify the environment to produce comfort and induce rest and sleep (e.g., cool, well-ventilated room, clean linens, light-weight blankets, restful lighting) Play selected tapes of soft music, sound of water, or a monotonous lecture Reduce the number of interruptions by staff just before and during hours of sleep Maintain ritual for getting ready for sleep; discourage vigorous mental activity before bedtime Identify with client an appropriate activity level during waking hours; gradually increase activity to this level Reduce the potential for injury during sleep (e.g., use of bed rails as needed, call light within easy reach)

EVALUATION

1. The client states that he or she is able to sleep adequately according to his or her own definition.
2. The client identifies factors that facilitate or inhibit sleep.
3. The client states that his or her environment is conducive to sleep.
4. The client is able to verbalize having an adequate balance between level of activity and pattern of sleep.

NURSING ALERTS

1. Withdrawal of sedatives may cause rebound rapid-eye movement (REM) sleep.
2. Early morning awakening may indicate depression.
3. With some debilitating long-term illnesses or in the case of terminal illness, palliative nursing strategies may need to be ongoing, with limited probability of achieving the expected outcomes.
4. Recovering alcoholics may not reestablish a normal sleep pattern for 6 to 12 months.

Bibliography

Budden F: Adverse drug reactions in long-term care facility residents Journal of the American Geriatric Society 33(6): 449, 1985.

Butler RN and Lewis MI: Aging and mental health, St. Louis, 1982, The CV Mosby Co.

Foxall MJ: Elderly patients at risk of potential drug interactions in long-term care facilities, Western Journal of Nursing Research 4(2):134, 1982.

Goebel G and Boech B: Ego integrity and fear of death: a comparison of institutionalized and independently living older adults, Death Studies 11:193, 1987.

Goldman R: Aging changes in structure and function. In Carnevali DL and Patrick M, editors: Nursing management for the elderly, New York, 1986, JB Lippincott Co, pp 73-101.

Haley WE and Dolce JJ: Assessment and management of chronic pain in the elderly. In Brink TL, editor: Clinical gerontology: a guide to assessment and intervention, New York, 1986, Haworth, pp 435-455.

Hurley ME editor: Classification of nursing diagnosis: proceedings of the Sixth Conference, North American Nursing Diagnosis Association, St Louis, 1986, The CV Mosby Co, p 542.

Kao Lo C and Kim MJ: Construct validity of sleep pattern disturbance: a methodological approach. In Hurley ME, editor: Classification of nursing diagnoses: proceedings of the Sixth Conference, North American Nursing Diagnosis Association, St Louis, 1986, The CV Mosby Co, pp. 197-206.

Kim MJ: McFarland GK, and McLane AM: Pocket guide to nursing diagnoses, ed 3, 1989, St Louis, The CV Mosby Co.

Lamy PT: OTC drugs and the elderly, Journal of Gerontological Nursing 11(2):44, 1985.

McNairy SL, et al: Prescription medication dependence and neuropsychologic function Pain, 18:169, 1984.

Richardson K: Assessing communication, Geriatric Nursing 4:237, July/August 1983.

Rottenberg RF: Prescribing for the elderly—safely, Patient Care 16(12):13, 1982.

Spiegel R: Aspects of sleep, daytime vigilance, mental performance and psychotropic drug treatment in the elderly, Gerontology, 28 (suppl 1): 68, 1982.

Todd B: Drugs and the elderly: identifying drug toxicity, Geriatric Nursing 6(4):231, 1985.

Social Isolation

Rhonda W. Comrie

KNOWLEDGE BASE

1. Social isolation can be defined as aloneness experienced by an individual, who perceives the situation as imposed by others and as a negative or threatening state.
2. Loneliness and social isolation are two separate problems. Social isolation is a risk factor for loneliness, but some older people intentionally adopt an isolated life style, thereby experiencing loneliness.
3. Loneliness is perceived insufficient human contact and may be the result of social isolation.
4. Elders often have difficulty finding others who are of equal or similar age.
5. As persons age, various role changes occur. These may include changes from worker to retiree, spouse to widow, parent to grandparent. Role changes may cause an elderly person to question his or her worth to society.
6. Social isolation may cause further role changes.
7. Social isolation may occur as a result of an older person's dissatisfaction with his or her body because of loss of mobility or inability to function. Physical problems such as changes in appearance with aging, incontinence, disfiguring surgery, or loss of body parts affect an elderly person's ability to maintain a positive body image and self-concept.
8. Sensory deficits may create so many difficulties for an older person when he or she leaves his home environment that the person tends not to risk going out into the community and thus becomes isolated. Loss of sensory function may also negatively affect self-concept and self-esteem, causing the person to withdraw from interactions with others.
9. Self-concept is reinforced through other persons. Isolation may become a protective mechanism for self-concept if a person fears negative appraisal by others.
10. Behaviors associated with confusion, dementia, alcoholism, eccentricity, deviance, or egocentricity may alienate others and lead to social isolation of an elderly client.
11. Geographic isolation may occur as an elderly client becomes separated by distance from friends or family (e.g., newly widowed elderly person who moves to a new community). In urban areas a tendency toward anonymity exists, which can cause an elderly person to become isolated as a result of fear or lack of social contacts. Institutionalization is another form of geographic isolation.
12. Social isolation may lead to deterioration of interpersonal skills, resulting in further alienation.
13. Older people who are at risk for social isolation require assistance in planning preventive measures.

ASSESSMENT CRITERIA
Physical

Current health status
Presence of physical barriers
    Chronic illness
    Physical impairments
    Decreased mobility
Unacceptable body image change
    Disfiguring surgery
    Wrinkling of skin
    Fecal or urinary incontinence
    Skin burns
    Cancer
Sensory deficits (hearing/visual)
Nutritional status/appetite
Sleep patterns

Psychosocial

Mental status
Ability to communicate
Sensorium
Fears/sense of security
Sad/dull affect
Perceived feelings of loneliness; time of day these are felt most
Lack of interests
Withdrawal from others
Feelings of shame in regard to use of assistive devices
Feelings of uselessness or anomie
Income
Role changes
Extent of social network
Opportunities for social contact
Availability of supportive significant others
Living arrangements (alone or with others)
Environment/community (familiar or changed)
Ability and desire to interact meaningfully
Group memberships
Patterns of social activity/relationships
Means of transportation

Spiritual

Ethnic/cultural values
Belief systems
Involvement in a church or other religious community
Desire for visitation by religious leader at client's home

NURSING CARE PLAN: SOCIAL ISOLATION

Common contributing factors	Expected client outcomes	Nursing strategies
Decreased physical mobility	Client will decrease social isolation Client will express a willingness to participate in social activities	Assess function, mobility, activity tolerated, and sensory alterations Recommend correction or treatment for identified causes of decreased mobility Help client to consider canes or wheelchairs to enhance mobility and safety Refer client to community agencies for assistance in modifying dwelling or home for increased accessibility Assist client in exploring options for increased socialization both within and outside the home, considering his or her limitations Consider fluctuations in activity tolerance when planning activities
Reduced number of opportunities for social interaction	Client will express the desire to develop or maintain meaningful relationships Client will assume responsibility for developing or maintaining relationships Client will increase the number of contacts with others	Assess present relationships and preferences Consider lifelong patterns of relationships Assist client in identifying interesting activities involving other people Assist with selection of functions or activities within chosen religious community that the client finds interesting or that are accessible Encourage significant others to maintain telephone or physical contact with elderly client Identify available means of transportation and possible use by the client Assess for existing programs such as retirement communities, adult day care, foster grandparent programs, friendly visitor programs, or telephone contacts Assess environment to determine if location of home or nearby persons are felt to be threatening Consider the feasibility of pet therapy
Memory loss or behavioral changes	Client will verbalize that the interactions were positive Client will have interactions with others	Assess social interactions that increase anxiety or inappropriate behavior and those interactions that result in a positive experience Help client to participate in a small group of similar clients Help client to develop relationships with one or two other people Encourage adult-to-adult communication Provide environment most conducive to interactions Consider memory training, reminiscing, and music therapy for group activity See care plan for alteration in thought processes, p. 90
Decreased self-concept	Client will operationalize methods of enhancing self-esteem and body image	Encourage the elderly client to talk about feelings of loneliness or low self-esteem Use touch as a means of conveying acceptance if this is accepted as a means of communication by the client Focus on the values and interests of the elderly client Invite the client to participate in group work, such as reading or discussions Provide structure and expect participation in discussion group to allow expressions of fear, anger, loneliness, depression, and grief Demonstrate openness to assisting with aesthetic problems resulting from incontinence, surgery, etc. Use music therapy; familiar songs often stimulate communication about happier times and discussions of life experiences in the present Refer client to agencies for financial assistance for needed prostheses, wigs, dentures, clothing, etc. Use a form of life review designed to help client to analyze the past

EVALUATION

1. The client is able to move about home and other environments safely.
2. The client makes contact with one significant other or group at least one time each week.
3. The client expresses positive feelings about himself or herself.

NURSING ALERTS

1. Medications that depress the client's cortical functions, such as narcotics, psychotropic medications, or sedatives, may worsen confusional states and contribute to social isolation.
2. Elderly clients who are socially isolated may not have their health care needs met. A system for periodic assessment of needs should be established.
3. Social isolation of an elderly family member may be a symptom of abuse or neglect and should be assessed for this possibility. Appropriate social service resources need to be contacted if this is the case.

Bibliography

Bond CL and Miller MJ: Reading: the ageless activity, Geriatric Nursing 8(4):192, 1987.

Burnside I, editor: Nursing and the aged, ed 3, New York, 1988, McGraw-Hill Book Co.

Carpenito LJ: Nursing diagnosis: application to clinical practice. Philadelphia, 1989, JB Lippincott Co.

Decker SD and Kinzel SL: Learned helplessness and decreased social interaction in elderly disabled persons, Rehabilitative Nursing 10(2):31, 1985.

Ebersole P and Hess P: Toward healthy aging, human needs and nursing response, ed 2, St Louis, 1985, The CV Mosby Co.

Gioiella EC and Bevil CW: Nursing care of the aging client, Norwalk, Conn, 1985, Appleton-Century Crofts.

Guerin ME: Come sing along with me, Geriatric Nursing 3(3):170, 1982.

Kim MJ, McFarland, GK, McLane AM: Pocket guide to nursing diagnoses, ed 3, 1989, St Louis, The CV Mosby Co.

McFarland G and McFarlane L: Nursing diagnosis and intervention, St Louis, 1989, The CV Mosby Co.

Ochoco L and Shimamoto Y: Group work with the frail ethnic elderly, Geriatric Nursing 8(4):185, 1987.

Ravish T: Prevent social isolation before it starts, Journal of Gerontological Nursing 11(10):10, 1985.

Seaman L: Affective touch, Geriatric Nursing 3(3):162, 1982.

Spiritual Distress

Karen Osterman Fieser
Frances F. Rogers-Seidl

KNOWLEDGE BASE

1. Spiritual distress is defined as a disruption in one's relationship with God, or that person's concept of a higher power, which gives identity, values, and meaning to life.
2. The concept of a higher power allows for individual definitions and expression. Some would consider nature or universal truth to be their higher power.
3. Religiosity has been defined in recent studies as the giving of outward expression to life's meaning by affiliation with a faith community.
4. An elder's spirituality is distinguished not by age but by history (experience through life).
5. For an older person spirituality may have increased value, whereas religiosity may decrease.
6. A rich spiritual life is the single most important factor in one's perception of quality of life, regardless of age or socioeconomic status. It gives an older person a sense of value not for what is done or is owned but because "I am."
7. Older people become acutely aware of the unity of mind, body, and spirit. Spiritual interventions facilitate health in both the physical and psychosocial dimensions and reduce the use of health care resources.
8. An older person's acceptance of death may be related to the perceived nearness of death rather than chronological age. An elderly person may perceive each day to be lived either as a gift or simply as one day closer to death.
9. An elderly person's life journey with its joys and sorrows allows him or her to experience the nearness of God as well as the times when God is hidden.
10. Expressions of giving one's destiny into God's keeping may indicate spiritual peace rather than despair, depression, or lack of the will to live.
11. An older person's spiritual/religious state is shaped by his or her unique spiritual journeys and participation in faith communities. Figure 1 illustrates four spiritual/religious baseline patterns.

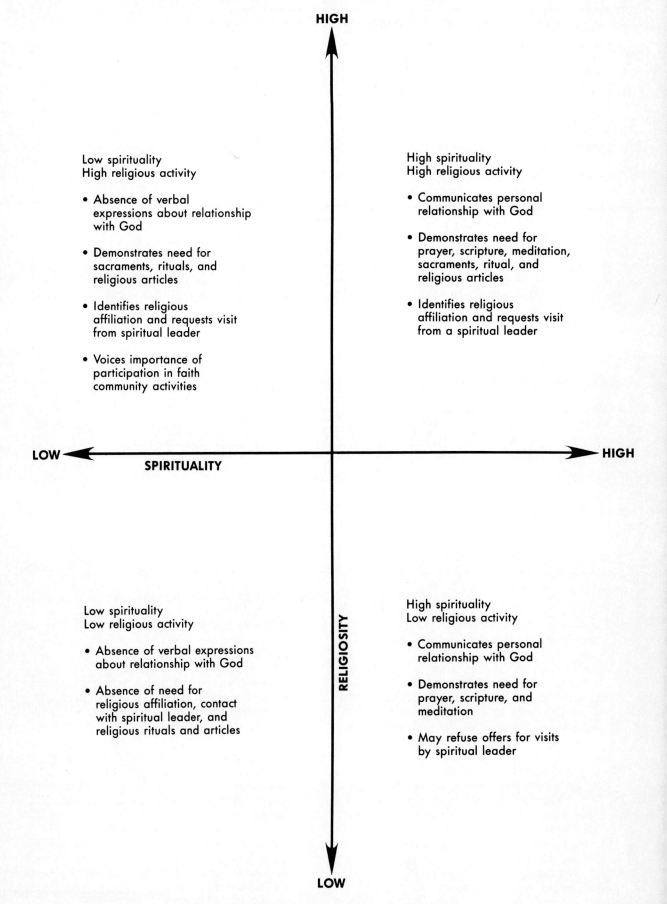

Fig. 1. Variability in the spiritual/religious dimension.

12. The overlay of a person's response to illness and loss can increase the variability in spirituality/ religious state and may produce spiritual distress. Equilibrium may be disturbed when a person is unable to integrate the experience of illness into a sense of a relationship with God. There may be one or more contributing factors to spiritual distress. Elements of spiritual distress center around God, self, others and/or a faith community. Spiritual distress may be caused or manifested by an inability to trust God, self, or others; maintain a sense of hopefulness; adjust to the situation; participate in a faith community and/or usual religious practices; or a combination of these factors.

13. To determine the nature of spiritual distress, not only must the spiritual/religious baseline pattern be identified but also the person's response to illness and loss. By assessing the baseline and the response, the nurse can formulate a plan for intervention. Assessment at one point in time does not provide permanent data because spirituality is always in process.

ASSESSMENT CRITERIA

General concerns about spirituality and religious activity

Comparison of spiritual/religious patterns before the health problem or loss with the patterns at present

Diminished sense of trust in God,* self, or others
  Questions meaning of suffering
  Unresolved feelings about the meaning of life and death
  Anger toward God or spiritual leader
  Verbalizes doubt about inner strength to cope with the situation
  Questions motives, competence, or caring of health care professionals and/or support network

Diminished sense of hopefulness
  Discouragement or despair
  Expressions of futility in living
  Sense of spiritual emptiness, abandonment, or loss of God's companionship
  Unable to identify source of strength and hope

Diminished adjustment to the situation
  Regrets choices made in past
  Excessive verbalization about the relationship between health, illness, and spirituality
  Expresses inability to control any outcomes in life
  Assumes disproportionate amount of blame for illness or situation

*"God" includes the concept of a higher power.

> ### *Guidelines for Assessing Spiritual Distress*
>
> 1. Do you have concerns about your spirituality or religious activity?
> 2. Have there been any changes in your relationship with God since the beginning of your problem?
> 3. Have there been any changes in your religious activities since the beginning of your problem?
>
> **Diminished Sense of Trust in God, Self, or Others**
> 4. How can I help you maintain your spiritual strength or spiritual base?
> 5. How will your illness, hospitalization, or loss affect your spiritual life?
> 6. Who or what helps you the most when you need it? Is that available to you?
>
> **Diminished Sense of Hopefulness**
> 7. Has being sick made any difference in how you see the future?
> 8. What is your source of strength and hope?
> 9. On a scale from 0 to 10, is life empty or full?
>
> **Diminished Acceptance of Self or Situation**
> 10. If you could change something in your past, what would that be?
> 11. Do you think you are doing as well as other people in the same situation?
>
> **Inability to Participate in a Faith Community**
> 12. To whom do you turn when you need help? Are they available?
> 13. Do you want your spiritual leader (pastor, priest, rabbi) notified?
> 14. Are there any religious practices or items that are especially important to you?
> 15. Is prayer helpful to you? Would you like to have someone pray with you?

Recreates the early events of the disease or illness with "if only I . . ." statements

Inability to share diagnosis with close family or friends

Inability to participate in a faith community and/or practice religious rituals
  Voices longing for faith community
  Unable to be independent in participating in faith community activities
  Limitations in practicing religious rituals

NURSING CARE PLAN: SPIRITUAL DISTRESS

Common contributing factors	Expected client outcomes	Nursing strategies
Inability to trust God, self, or others	Client will confide in at least one other person	Help identify one or two people who are trusted Assess ability to trust others prior to illness Be sensitive to increasing discomfort as a signal to terminate the visit Consider referral to mental health professional Keep promises and confidences Respect right to privacy Be cautious about a probing communication style Designate a primary nurse and a chaplain to provide care
	Client will express confidence in a loving God	Be attentive to client's expressions about his or her perceptions of God's part (causing, testing, supporting, caring) in the illness Help name the spoken and unspoken feelings Avoid premature reassurances and clichés (e.g., "Don't cry; everything will be OK." "It's God's will.")
	Client expresses ability to make decisions	Support decision making by the client
Inability to maintain hope	Client will talk about events or relationships that can be looked forward to	Assess pessimism versus optimism prior to illness/loss Assess whether life is now empty or full on a scale from 1 to 10 Encourage talk about source of strength and hope Be alert to the potential for self-destructive behavior Consider referral to mental health professional Assist through reminiscence in identifying positive events in past Refer to spiritual leader for assessment and intervention
	Client will consider new treatment plans	Educate client about treatment plans Help client assume maximum control in treatment plan
Inability to adjust to the situation	The client is able to limit anxiety or guilt to mild levels	Identify stressors in life Assist in planning stress reduction Identify personal means of coping (e.g., prayer, meditation, exercise)
	The client uses adaptive coping mechanisms	Use reminiscence to identify success in coping in the past Allow coping mechanisms Introduce problem solving
	Client assigns meaning to the situation	Listen actively, giving honest, open responses Refer to spiritual leader for assessment and intervention
Inability to participate in faith community and/or religious practices	Contact with the client's faith community is maintained	Identify the client's usual practices; determine if spiritual leader is to be notified; if so, call and document Assess need for religious items and provide Arrange for opportunity and privacy to practice rituals and/or prayer Refer to chaplain for assessment and intervention
	Client accepts the religious resources provided	Invite participation in individual and group activities for prayer or religious rituals Provide information about resources (e.g., local congregations, transportation, home-bound ministry) and facilitate contacts

EVALUATION

1. The client demonstrates an increased ability to trust and confide in others.
2. The client continues to express hope or future goals throughout the illness or trauma.
3. The client verbalizes a sense of meaning in terms of God, self, others, and life.
4. The client's relationship with God and the faith community is continued.

NURSING ALERTS

1. Differing religious values held by the nurse and the client do not negate the importance of providing spiritual care.
2. The nurse can plan and provide spiritual care by assessing the client's spiritual state.
3. Recovery may be blocked if spiritual distress is present and care is not provided.

Bibliography

Bowers, C: Spiritual dimensions of the rehabilitation journey, Rehabilitation Nursing 12:2, March-April, 1987.

Chatters L and Taylor R: Age differences in religious participation among black adults, Journal of Gerontology 44(5): S183, 1989.

Cowell V et al: Guidelines for pastoral care of older persons in long-term care settings, Washington, DC, 1989, American Association of Retired Persons.

Forbis P: Meeting patient's spiritual needs, Geriatric Nursing 9:158, May-June, 1988.

Jones W: Gerontheology: spirituality and aging, Quarterly Papers on Religion and Aging 1:1, Summer 1984.

Koenig, H et al: Religion and well-being in later life, The Gerontologist 28:18, Feb 1988.

Markides K et al: Religion, aging, and life satisfaction, The Gerontologist 27:660, Oct 1987.

McSherry E: The spiritual dimensions of elder health care, Generation, 8:18, Fall 1983.

Noreen D: Extending ministry with the aging, The Center Letter 17(3):1, 1987.

Stoll, R: Guidelines for spiritual assessment, American Journal of Nursing 9:1574, Sept 1979.

Swallowing, Impaired

Dixie M. Flynn
Sharyn L. Mills

KNOWLEDGE BASE

1. Dysphagia (difficult swallowing) commonly occurs as a result of a cerebrovascular accident or other catastrophic illness, such as tumors of the pharynx or progressive neurological disorders. The problem most often occurs after a left hemisphere or brainstem cerebrovascular accident.

2. The problem may be mild, or it may be severe enough that the client cannot take nourishment by mouth and must be fed by other means.

3. A great danger is aspiration, in which food or fluids enter the lungs, possibly causing pneumonia.

4. To understand the pathophysiology of swallowing, it is necessary to understand normal swallowing mechanisms. Swallowing is a combination of purposeful movement and reflexes that normally take no more than 3 seconds. This process can be divided into four stages:

   Stage 1 (preparatory phase): the food enters the mouth and is chewed. The combined efforts of the teeth, tongue, lips, and cheeks along with sensations of taste, temperature, and texture prepare food to be swallowed.

   Stage 2 (oral phase): the food, having been chewed to the proper consistency, is moved to the back of the throat by the tongue pressing against the roof of the mouth or palate, and actual swallowing begins.

   Stage 3 (pharyngeal phase): the swallowing reflex is triggered by the sensation of the food entering the pharynx. The coordinated muscle movements in the pharynx prevent food from being regurgitated through the nose, waves of tiny muscle contractions help the food descend into the esophagus, the vocal cords close tightly to protect the airway, and a muscular valve relaxes to allow the food to actually enter the esophagus.

   Stage 4 (esophageal phase): waves of tiny muscle contractions and gravity help move the food into the stomach.

5. A dysfunction in any of these areas can result in dysphagia.

6. The cranial nerves play a major role in the function of swallowing:

   Cranial nerve I (olfactory): responsible for sense of smell, which increases a person's desire to eat

   Cranial nerve V (trigeminal): motor function for the face and jaws; sensory function for face, particularly temperature

   Cranial nerve VII (facial): motor function of face, particularly around the mouth; sensory function of taste

   Cranial nerve IX (glossopharyngeal): sensory function of taste; motor function for gag reflex and swallowing

Table 2 **Example of a dysphagia diet**

Stage	Acceptable foods	Restricted foods
Stage 1	Yogurt, creamed or blended jello, pureed fruits, ice cream, sherbet, blended cottage cheese, thick soups	All others, especially foods that disperse in mouth or form lumps; water; thin liquids
Stage 2	All foods from stage 1; oatmeal; cottage cheese; soft-boiled, poached, or scrambled eggs; pureed foods; mashed potatoes; tomato juice; nectars	All others, especially thin liquids, stringy vegetables, dry foods
Stage 3	All foods from stages 1 and 2; pasta, rice, macaroni and cheese, ground meats, gravy, egg salad, crackers, toast (no crust), chopped canned fruits, cold cereal that easily disperses (e.g., Cheerios), thin liquids if tolerated	All others
Stage 4	Provide regular diet (or soft diet) with mechanical consistency; adjust menus according to tolerance	No restrictions

Cranial nerve X   (vagus): sensory function in the nasopharyngeal area; motor function for swallowing at the nasopharyngeal area

Cranial nerve XII (hypoglossal): motor function of tongue movement and strength

7. Few changes in the physiology of swallowing occur until individuals reach 80 years of age. At that time, there is a reduction in the strength of pharyngeal peristalsis and esophageal peristalsis.
8. Changes in swallowing are generally a result of pathophysiology.
9. Symptoms may be acute or insidious.
10. A speech pathologist is educated in the diagnosis and treatment of swallowing disorders and should always be consulted when a swallowing difficulty is suspected.
11. Diagnostic examinations are available to determine exactly where the swallowing pathology originates. The primary test is videofluoroscopy (barium swallow). This test provides information on transit time of food and liquids through the oral and pharyngeal phases, motility problems, and amount and etiology of aspiration.
12. Once the exact nature and location of the swallowing difficulty have been identified, treatment can begin.

13. Treatment must be achieved through a multidisciplinary approach, including physician, nurse, speech pathologist, and dietician.
14. Treatment must begin as soon as possible to prevent the complications of malnutrition, dehydration, and aspiration.
15. Clients may be retrained to swallow. The success of retraining depends on the severity of damage to the brain, the motivation of the client, the compliance of client and family with the plan of care, and prevention of complications as a result of the dysphagia.
16. If swallowing through normal means cannot occur, alternative feeding methods become necessary, i.e., nasogastric tube, gastrostomy tube, total parenteral nutrition. These may be temporary or permanent, depending on the severity of the injury and the client's recovery.
17. A diet progression is structured in stages. Each stage allows foods of a certain consistency, and individual tolerance and preference must be considered. Clear liquids are not easily tolerated. Therefore, thin liquids taken orally should usually not be given until stage 3. The speech pathologist, nurse, or dietitian may provide a substance called Thick-it to thicken liquids and some food, which may enable the client to swallow easier. Table 2 is an example of a dysphagia diet.

ASSESSMENT CRITERIA
Physical

Condition of teeth, tongue, cheeks, lips
Cranial nerves I, V, VII, IX, X, XII
Ability to swallow, including history of:
  Choking or need to clear airway during/after eating
  Ability to clear mouth totally after chewing
  Difficulty in initiating a swallow
  Need to swallow two or three times
  Excessive drooling, especially after eating
  "Gargled" sound in voice, especially after eating
Chest sounds
Weight (baseline and ongoing)
Fluid intake and urinary output
Body temperature
Level of consciousness
Ability to communicate verbally

Psychosocial

Changes in meal routine
Cognitive status
Social withdrawal
Motivational status
Coping techniques, individual and family
Support systems

General

Previous swallowing capability
Health history
Dietary habits
Recent health status changes

NURSING CARE PLAN: IMPAIRED SWALLOWING

Common contributing factors	Expected client outcomes	Nursing strategies
Inability to swallow (general)	Client will display adequate orientation, alertness, sequencing, and reasoning to participate in swallowing retraining Client will maintain clear, unobstructed airway Client will maintain adequate hydration and nutrition Client will demonstrate appropriate positioning and eating techniques during meals Client will maintain adequate oral hygiene Client will demonstrate ability to clear oral cavity/eradicate pockets of food Client will complete oral and pharyngeal phases in less than 10 seconds Client will experience minimal or no choking and/or aspiration while eating	Obtain order for evaluation by speech pathologist Document in chart observable behaviors concerning swallowing Position client's body in an upright position with the hips at a right angle to the body; use pillows to support clients who are too ill to sit upright Monitor client during meals in case food obstructs airway Follow instructions presented by speech pathologist, physician, and dietitian Provide dysphagia diet, as ordered Thicken liquids and foods as indicated Document amount of coughing, choking, spitting out of food, liquid Nutrient count if warranted Assist with feeding as needed Monitor weight
Problems in preparatory and oral phases of swallowing	Client will achieve adequate lip closure Client will have improved tongue movement Client will have awareness of reduced oral sensitivity	If recommended by speech therapist: 　Encourage use of straw 　Encourage client to perform tongue exercises 　Direct client to position food on the more sensitive side of his or her oral cavity
Problems in the pharyngeal phase of swallowing	Client will have improved swallowing reflex	If instructed by the speech therapist: 　Instruct client to tilt head forward while swallowing 　Alternate swallows of liquid and food 　Have client turn/tilt head toward affected side to close pyriform sinus on the affected side and direct material down the more normal side 　Instruct client to dry swallow after swallowing food/liquid 　May have client clear throat/cough 　Instruct client to hold breath before swallowing

EVALUATION

1. The client displays orientation, alertness, ability to sequence and reason, and ability to comprehend swallowing retraining.
2. The client maintains a clear, unobstructed airway.
3. The client reaches/maintains his ideal body weight (as determined by dietitian).
4. The client takes adequate hydration (as determined individually), as demonstrated by urine output of at least 30 ml/hr and moist buccal membranes.
5. The client demonstrates an ability to sit in an upright position, and he or she positions the head correctly to facilitate swallowing.
6. The client maintains oral hygiene.

7. The client demonstrates an ability to clear the oral cavity and eradicate pockets of food.
8. The client completes the oral and pharyngeal phases in less than 10 seconds.
9. The client demonstrates a decreased incidence of choking and no aspiration while eating.
10. The client achieves adequate lip closure, improved tongue movement, and awareness of oral sensitivity.
11. The client demonstrates improved swallowing.

NURSING ALERTS

1. Any client with a diagnosis of head injury or nasopharyngeal injury or disease should be observed for signs and symptoms of dysphagia.
2. If any symptoms of dysphagia occur, the client should be referred to a speech pathologist for evaluation and treatment as necessary.
3. Clients are at risk for malnutrition and dehydration, even after being diagnosed with dysphagia, because of their fear of choking on food or fluids.
4. Monitor temperature, and if the client becomes febrile, alert the physician.
5. These clients are also at risk for aspiration. Keep a suction machine at the bedside in the early phases of the dysphagia. Teach client and family the Heimlich maneuver for clearing the airway.

Bibliography

Carr E and Hawthorn PJ: Lip function and eating after a stroke: a nursing perspective, Journal of Advanced Nursing, vol 13, p 15 1988.

Dereiko M and Stout P: Swallowing safely, swallowing nutritiously: a manual for the swallowing impaired, Portland, Ore, 1986, Lincoln Tower.

Logemann J: Evaluation and treatment of swallowing disorders, San Diego, 1983, College-Hill Press, Inc.

Marriott Corporation, Health Care Division: Modified consistency diets—dysphagia diets. Diet manual, revised Jan 1986.

Rader T and Rende B: Swallowing disorder: what families should know, Tucson, Ariz, 1988, Communication Skill Builders, Inc.

Seidel HM, Ball JW, Dains JE and Benedict W: Mosby's guide to physical examination, St Louis, 1987, The CV Mosby Co.

Thought Processes, Altered

Tally N. Bell

KNOWLEDGE BASE

1. Altered thought processes is a state in which an individual experiences a disruption in such mental activities as conscious thought, reality orientation, problem solving, judgment, and comprehension.
2. Because of the relatedness of the nervous system to all the other body systems and its complexities of function, age-related changes in the nervous system are difficult to examine in isolation.
3. Marked cognitive declines should not be considered normal age-related changes and can, in fact, be early indicators of medical problems. It is important to rule out physical conditions that can affect the elderly's thought processes.
4. Decreased neuronal function arises from a variety of factors. One factor is a decreased availability of nutrients to the neurons because of a decreased volume of the extracellular fluid. If nutrients are unavailable to the neurons, neuronal death will ensue.
5. Although there is a consistent decline in the number of neurons, beginning with the age of physical maturity and continuing throughout the older years, the loss rate is not uniform throughout the brain's structure, nor is the rate steady. This loss may or may not affect an older person's functioning. It is believed that atrophy of dendrites may have more of an impact on neurological function in the elderly than neuron loss.
6. Slower synaptic transmission resulting from decreased neurotransmitter production causes the elderly's reaction time to be lengthened.
7. Since memory and acquisition of new information decrease with aging, the elderly's thought processes can be mistakenly interpreted as altered. The elderly take longer to learn new skills and to process new information. Increased distractibility, decreased concrete thinking, and difficulty in problem solving can all influence the elderly's learning and responses. Using verbal repetition and visual and verbal clues, as well as providing an older person with sufficient time to complete tasks, should be incorporated into a nursing care plan.

8. Age-related losses, such as death of a spouse, moving to a retirement home, and altered sensory integration, can lead to suspicious or paranoid behavior. Careful assessment of the client's stressors can give the nurse valuable data to guide the plan of care.
9. Many mental changes attributed to the aging process can be the result of other, potentially reversible physical problems and should not be considered normal age-related changes.
10. Sleep deprivation can cause alterations in thought processes and can affect the client's ability to cope with environmental stressors.
11. Unnecessary and excessive stimuli can contribute to altered thought processes through sensory overload and increased confusion.
12. Restraining a client may increase confusion and provide a distorted interpretation of the environment. However, external controls such as restraints may be necessary until the client regains control.
13. Physiological abnormalities such as electrolyte, acid-base, oxygenation, and fluid imbalances, can be manifested, in part, as altered thought processes.
14. A stable environment with consistent, nurturing caregivers assists an older client in maintaining contact with reality and decreasing confusion. Maintaining respect for the client promotes maintenance of integrity and provides a good foundation for reality-based thinking.
15. Reminiscence is a useful strategy to stimulate an elderly client and assists with reality orientation and normal thinking.
16. It is important to promote normal sensory input to assist in maintaining orientation and to compensate for age-related changes. Uncompensated sensory deficits can lead to altered thought processes.
17. Meaningful touch provides important sensory stimulation and denotes caring. However, clients with altered thought processes may misinterpret the purpose of the touch, leading to distorted thinking.
18. It is important to assist a client in decision making when his thought processes are altered.
19. Providing boundaries in regard to inappropriate behavior gives security to a client and avoids injury to self or others.
20. A fast, hurried approach to interaction may cause a confused client to feel threatened.
21. Communication patterns that neither support nor challenge non–reality-based thinking help the client to decrease altered thought processes, such as paranoia, confusion, and delusions.
22. Hallucinations, suicidal behavior, and/or delusions may be experienced by some clients with altered thought processes.
23. Altered thought processes can prevent a client from eating, drinking, and performing activities of daily living (ADL).
24. Drug interactions, side effects, underdosage or overdosage, and toxicity can cause alterations in thought processes.

25. A compromised neurological status resulting in disorientation, confusion, and altered thought processes increases the risk of injury.
26. Multiple commands can lead to confusion in an elderly client. In addition, brain pathologies can damage the communication centers and produce further difficulty in processing information.
27. Forcing a client's participation in the plan of care or activities can increase suspicion and the incidence of delusional thoughts.
28. It is important to involve the client's significant others in the treatment/discharge plan, particularly if the alteration in thought processes does not resolve. Educational opportunities provided for significant others permit them to learn how effectively to deal with the alteration in thought process and/or the disease process. This strategy also promotes transfer of useful nursing strategies during hospitalization into the home or health facility setting.

ASSESSMENT CRITERIA
Physical
Health history (may need family to assist)
  Onset and pattern of symptoms
  Previous confusional states
  Personality and behavior changes
  Sleep pattern
  Social behavior (e.g., withdrawn, isolated)
  Past/present surgical and medical problems
  Medication history
  Substance use/abuse
  Nutritional status
Neurological examination
  Level of consciousness
  Pupil size and reaction
  Motor function and deficits
  Sensory deficits
  Orientation to time, place, person
  Hypervigilance or hypovigilance
  Self-care deficits
  Vital signs
  Review of other body systems

Psychosocial
Conceptual/abstract thinking
Reasoning/problem solving
Judgment, insight
Concentration/attention span
Long- and short-term memory
Ability to interpret internal/external stimuli
Motor response to stimuli (e.g., combativeness, restlessness, agitation)
Presence of sensory overload or deprivation
Presence of anxiety, depression, or mood swings
Affect
Communication patterns, verbal and nonverbal
Coping strategies and support systems

Spiritual
Religious beliefs and practices

NURSING CARE PLAN: ALTERED THOUGHT PROCESSES

Common contributing factors	Expected patient outcomes	Nursing strategies
Physiological or psychological stressors; sensory-perceptual limitations	Client will experience optimal contact with reality, relative to condition	Provide client with consistent, nurturing caregivers and a consistent routine Maintain a respectful attitude and discuss appropriate subjects with the client Explain all procedures in a simple manner and introduce unfamiliar persons who interact with the client Provide opportunities for the client to interact with others, as appropriate Discuss current and past events with the client Use the client's name when speaking to him
	Client will experience appropriate and adequate sensory and motor stimuli	Maintain good room lighting (i.e., curtains open to denote day or night; prevention of shadows) Place familiar objects and personal possessions in the client's room Monitor sleep/wake patterns (see also care plan for sleep pattern disturbance, p. 78) Monitor noise and activity levels in the client's environment Assist or encourage the client to move about in bed at least every 2 hours and/or to be up in a chair or ambulate twice a day, as appropriate Ensure that hearing aids, glasses, prosthetic devices are worn Utilize meaningful touch while providing nursing care, and evaluate the client's response to touch
	Client will accurately interpret internal and/or external stimuli	Observe for distorted interpretations of internal or external stimuli Assist client with problem solving and differentiation between internal and external stimuli Evaluate verbal and nonverbal behavior in response to internal or external stimuli Avoid belittling the client when he or she misinterprets stimuli Validate the client's interpretation of internal or external stimuli Use a calm, slow approach when interacting with the client
	Client will differentiate reality from nonreality	Establish communication patterns that neither support nor challenge non–reality-based thinking and that divert non–reality-based thinking into reality Reorient the client to reality concisely and simply; when client has poor short-term memory, focus on feelings, not facts. Set limits on inappropriate behavior Implement measures to divert the client from inappropriate behaviors, such as distraction or removing the client from the situation Positively reinforce reality-based thinking and behaviors Observe for indications of hallucinations, suicidal behavior, and/or delusions
	Client will maintain usual level of orientation	Review client's medication history for potential drug-drug or drug-food interactions, side effects, underdosage or overdosage, and toxicity, and consult with physician and/or pharmacist, as appropriate Place clock and calendar within the client's line of vision, and call client's attention to these items often Assess neurological/mental status on admission and on an ongoing basis; report changes immediately
	Client will demonstrate attempts to maintain orientation and to reduce non–reality-based thoughts	Encourage the client to validate his or her thoughts and decisions

NURSING CARE PLAN: ALTERED THOUGHT PROCESSES—cont'd

Common contributing factors	Expected patient outcomes	Nursing strategies
	Client will not experience injuries	Institute safety measures, such as bed in low position, side rails up, no smoking while alone, call light within reach Judiciously evaluate the use of arm, leg, hand, and/or chest restraints Structure the environment to remove potential hazards and to demarcate areas in which the client may move around Stay with the client when he or she is frightened, anxious, agitated, restless, etc. Perform ongoing assessments according to appropriate assessment criteria, and intervene promptly when indicated Identify events that increase the client's anxiety, fear, confusion, and altered thought processes Monitor laboratory work and diagnostic studies to detect abnormalities Document therapeutic interventions and the client's response
	Client will demonstrate ability to perform activities of daily living, with assistance if necessary	Help client to identify self-care deficits Assist client in ADL routine to maximize functioning Encourage/monitor client's daily nutrition and fluid intake
	Client/significant other will participate in treatment/discharge plan	Break activities into small, clear, simple, one-command steps, and allow client adequate time to complete activity Do not force client's participation in care Involve significant others in the treatment/discharge plan, particularly if client's thought processes remain altered
	Client/significant other will demonstrate appropriate coping strategies	Help client/significant other to identify community support programs, such as support groups, home health agencies, church-based programs Provide educational opportunities for client/significant others to learn to deal effectively with altered thought processes and/or disease processes Encourage client and/or significant other to express feelings

EVALUATION

1. The client demonstrates optimal contact with reality, relative to his or her condition, as evidenced by appropriate verbal and nonverbal behaviors.
2. The client experiences no sensory overload or deprivation, as evidenced by verbal and nonverbal indicators.
3. The client verbalizes accurate interpretation of internal and external stimuli.
4. The client demonstrates an absence of or a decrease in non–reality-based thinking, relative to his or her condition.
5. The client remains oriented to time, place, person, and self, relative to his or her condition.
6. The client utilizes visual and verbal clues to maintain orientation.
7. The client validates thoughts and decisions with the nurse and/or significant other.
8. The client experiences no injury to self or others as a result of altered thought processes.
9. The client assists with activities of daily living, as far as he or she is able.
10. The client or significant other actively participates in the treatment/discharge planning.
11. The client or significant other verbally identifies the community support systems available.

NURSING ALERTS

1. Alterations in thought processes can often be the initial indication of a disease process. Careful multisystem assessments must be performed to attempt to discover causes of changes in mental status. Careful attention to the methods used to test the client's mental processes must be given, since the client's sociocultural and educational backgrounds can dictate that alternative methods of assessment be utilized.

2. The slow clearance of drugs in the elderly predisposes them to drug overdosage, which can be manifested, in part, as alterations in thought processes.
3. It is important to provide elderly clients with adequate time to perform tasks and to respond to requests, because of their slower reflexes and their slower response to multiple stimuli.
4. Thought processes in the elderly can become altered when they are unable to compensate for the physiological, psychological, and environmental stressors they encounter.
5. Alterations in thought processes can cause a client to become completely negligent in activities of daily living, as well as in meeting basic physiological needs, such as food and water.
6. Alterations in thought processes put a client at high risk of injury.
7. If a client's mental condition makes him or her an unreliable source of information, the client's history should be obtained from or validated by a significant other.

Bibliography

Carpenito L: Nursing diagnosis: application to clinical practice, ed 3, Philadelphia, 1989, JB Lippincott Co.

Eliopoulos C: Gerontological nursing, ed 2, Philadelphia, 1987, JB Lippincott Co.

Eliopoulos C: A guide to the nursing of the aged, Baltimore, 1987, Williams & Wilkins.

Esberger K and Hughes S Jr: Nursing care of the aged, Norwalk, Conn, 1989, Appleton & Lange.

Long BC and Phipps WJ: Medical-surgical nursing: a nursing process approach, ed 2, St Louis, 1989, The CV Mosby Co.

Matteson M and McConnell E: Gerontological nursing: concepts and practice, Philadelphia, 1988, WB Saunders Co.

Murray R and Zentner G: Nursing assessment and health promotion strategies through the life span, ed 4, Norwalk, Conn, 1989, Appleton & Lange.

Ozuna, J: Alterations in mentation: nursing assessment and intervention, Journal of Neuroscience Nursing 17(1):65, 1985.

Taylor C and Cress S: Nursing diagnosis cards, Springhouse, Pa, 1987, Springhouse Corp.

Ulrich S, Canale S, and Wendell S: Nursing care planning guides: a nursing diagnosis approach, Philadelphia, 1986, WB Saunders Co.

Urinary Elimination, Altered Patterns

Sue E. Meiner

KNOWLEDGE BASE

1. Altered urinary elimination is a state in which an individual experiences a disturbance in voluntary control over micturition.
2. Normal bladder function requires an intact brain and spinal cord and competent bladder and sphincters.
3. Loss of urine control is not a normal outcome of aging, but increasing age is a risk factor.
4. A variety of physical, psychosocial, and environmental factors may cause or contribute to incontinence.
5. Incontinence is the second leading cause of institutionalization.
6. Incontinence and mental confusion may be the first and only signs of urinary infection in older people.
7. The incidence of urinary incontinence in institutionalized elders has been found to be about 50%, contrasted with 15% to 30% for those not living in institutions.
8. The most common types of urinary incontinence in older people are stress incontinence, urge incontinence, and overflow incontinence. (For more information on types of incontinence, see the nursing care plan for urinary incontinence, p. 274).
9. Age-related changes that may predispose an older person to urinary problems include the following:
   a. Muscles associated with urinary function lose their elasticity, and supportive structures (pelvic floor) lose muscle tone.
   b. The bladder's elasticity is diminished, decreasing bladder capacity.

c. Symptoms of urinary tract infections are masked in older people; dysuria is not sensed; frequency and urgency are incorrectly assessed as incontinence.

d. The neurological system of an older person is not as efficient, which may cause lack of inhibition of the voiding reflex.

10. Arteriosclerotic changes may affect vessels that supply blood to the urinary system, resulting in less ability to resist infection and to recover from trauma.

11. Slowed mobility and manipulative difficulties associated with arthritis may hamper toileting functions and add to incontinence. Clothing adjustments using snaps or zippers and supportive devices such as elevated toilet seats with hand and arm rails may be useful.

12. Mental status changes may impair a client's ability to recognize stimuli for voiding, with resultant retention or incontinence.

13. Many prescription medications add to difficulties with abnormal urinary patterns. Antispasmodics and anticholinergics interfere with the action of acetylcholine at postganglionic neuroeffector sites. This can cause urinary retention. Antihistamines have anticholinergic effects that may cause frequency, dysuria, or retention. Antipsychotics may cause hesitancy or retention, as does levodopa (used to treat Parkinson's disease).

14. Elderly persons who have dependent edema during the day will have increased urine production when they elevate their legs at night or at rest.

15. Fear of incontinence is prevalent among older people. They may void frequently to prevent incontinence and thus may develop a low-capacity bladder.

16. Incontinence interferes with social interactions outside of the home setting. If fluids are restricted to reduce frequency, dehydration may occur. Concentrated urine becomes a bladder irritant, and the potential for incontinence increases.

17. Sleep disruption and potential for falls result when frequency or urgency occurs at night.

18. A complete history and physical examination must be made. Only when data are gathered about the problem can a logical treatment and care plan be developed.

19. There is a high rate of continence recovery when treatment and care are offered, even in the frail elderly population. When recovery is not possible, management of urine elimination is the major goal.

20. The assessment process must be sensitive to the client's emotional response to the problem. Privacy and comfort should be provided during the assessment.

21. Treatment and nursing measures are designed for the specific type of incontinence. Outcomes are either for cure or for minimizing the extent of the incontinence. An overriding aim is to maintain the client's self-esteem and dignity.

22. General measures include the following:
    a. A positive attitude should be maintained by client, family, caregiver, and physician.
    b. Evening fluid restrictions may aid in reduction of nighttime voiding; however, adequate fluids must be taken during the morning and daytime hours. Diuretics should be timed to peak during waking hours and not at night.
    c. Activity levels that are moderate to high, decrease urinary stasis with its potential for infection. Prolonged inactivity or immobility may result in stasis of urine and poor kidney output, leading to calculi or infection.
    d. Acidic urine assists in reducing infections of the bladder. Intake of cranberry juice increases acidity of the urine, as does ingestion of vitamin C, prunes, plums, grains, fish, and cheese.
    e. Institute behavioral programs such as a toileting schedule developed from baseline data and biofeedback.
    f. Teach Kegel exercises for pelvic floor strengthening.
    g. See that the client has access to toilets with assistive devices such as grab bars and raised toilet seats.
    h. For management of irreversible incontinence, protective clothing or urinary devices are needed.

ASSESSMENT CRITERIA
Physical
History/physical evidence of illnesses
Neurological disease or disorder
Diabetes
Prostatic hypertrophy
Genitourinary infections
Urinary tract or renal calculi
Strictures
Urologic tumors
Extrinsic obstructions
Menopausal status
Multiple births or grand multigravida
Status after use of indwelling catheter
Surgical procedures
Medications
  Sedatives and hypnotics
  Diuretics
  Antidiuretic hormone
  Phenothiazines
  Anticholinergics
  Tricyclic antidepressants
  Cholinergics
  Levodopa
  Nonprescription medications, especially sinus medications
Physical examination
  Bowel sounds
  Distended bladder
  Pelvic floor tone
  Retracted penis

Swelling, infection of penis
Cystocele
Rectocele
Uterine prolapse
Laboratory and diagnostic studies
  Analysis of urine elements (midstream specimen)
  pH urodynamic studies
  Renal, ureteral, bladder, urethral examination
History of symptoms
  Change in voiding patterns (e.g., frequency, nocturia)
  Specific complaints of retention, urgency, hesitancy, dribbling
  Incontinence; description and duration
Urine output data (three consecutive 24-hour periods)
  Fluid intake: time of intake, amount and type of fluid
  Time log of urine elimination
  Presence of sensation of need to void; time period from sensation to voiding
  Incontinence episodes, including volume, frequency, and surrounding events
  Difficulty stopping or starting urine stream
  Symptoms of burning, itching, pain, or pressure
  Character of urine; odor, color, sediment
  Residual volume studies

Accessibility; ability to toilet self
  Mobility/assistive devices
  Activity tolerance
  Ability to manipulate clothing
  Toilet aids such as grab bars, raised toilet seats; wheelchair accessibility
  Toilet substitutes

Psychosocial

Mental status
  Awareness of the need to void
  Ability to call for assistance
  Memory
  Orientation to surroundings
Ability to learn
Depression
Motivation
Meaning of problem
Changes in living arrangement and immediate environment
Level of social interaction and recent changes
Attitude of caregivers, family, and friends
Support systems
Financial resources/insurance coverage for remedial treatment

Spiritual

Degree to which participation in a faith community is limited by the problem
Beliefs and values in regard to excretory behaviors

 NURSING CARE PLAN: URINARY ELIMINATION—ALTERED PATTERNS

Common contributing factors	Expected client outcomes	Nursing strategies
Untimely elimination of urine related to urgency or physical stress	Client will verbalize the treatment schedule and rationale	Assess for pattern, concomitant events, amount, and frequency (see Knowledge Base)
	Client will experience fewer incontinent episodes	Develop a program for retraining if client is capable of participation
		Establish pattern for adequate fluid intake; avoid diuretic fluids late at night, such as coffee and tea; evening intake of fluids may be limited to avoid nocturia; provide fluids producing acid urine, such as cranberry juice
		Provide assistance to toilet if needed and provide methods for the client to remember toileting schedule
		Communicate an accepting attitude about incontinent episodes; be sensitive and allow client to verbalize feelings
		Give positive feedback for any degree of success
		Provide for easy accessibility to toilet or toilet substitutes
		Teach client to do Kegel exercises and help establish schedule
		Request consultation for biofeedback
		Assist to the extent needed with cleansing (warm soap and water) and skin protection with lubricant or ointment

NURSING CARE PLAN: URINARY ELIMINATION—ALTERED PATTERNS—cont'd

Common contributing factors	Expected client outcomes	Nursing strategies
Neurologic conditions that result in inability to perceive need to void	Client will have increased number of voidings on toilet or toilet substitute	Assess characteristics and time of the urine loss; intake of fluids; residual urine; and duration of problem For accuracy of baseline data, consider use of devices to signal wetting Identify any existing behaviors preceding the voiding, such as restlessness, sounding, or withdrawal Schedule toileting time; encourage postural emptying of bladder (rocking back and forth or bending forward) If client is apraxic, distract with conversation; voiding will be reflexive Schedule fluid intake in conjunction with the toileting schedule; specify amount and type of fluid, with suggestion on how to get the client to drink Cleanse client while on toilet with perineal care bottle filled with warm soap and water, and rinse with clear water; dry carefully Provide protective clothing and bed pads to the extent needed
Environmental impediments to normal bladder function	Client will adapt to the need to locate toilet facilities when away from familiar surroundings Client will adapt home environment to meet the needs of problems of mobility	Instruct client to locate toilet facilities when in unfamiliar surroundings in order to prevent putting off urination and overextending the bladder; voiding before leaving the home and at intervals of 2 to 3 hours may prevent incontinence related to an overly full bladder Assistive devices in the home bathroom may aid the elderly client in toileting; rails and/or elevated seat with rails may need to be installed
Inability to pass urine or empty the bladder fully when the need to void is felt	Client will be able to void and empty the bladder	Assess for causative factors; offer the client warm fluids to drink; ensure adequate hydration; let the client listen to running water or place the client's hand in warm water; a light brushing action on the inner thigh may produce urination To put pressure on a distended bladder, instruct client or assist in using a gentle downward pressure on the lower abdomen; avoid rushing; have the client rock back and forth on the toilet; instruct client to stay in an upright position even when using a bedpan; help the client to relax and provide privacy throughout
	Client will establish a normal pattern of urinary elimination	Collaborate with the client to establish a voiding schedule; a bladder training program can be initiated
Use of prescribed medications and/or bladder irritants	Client will adjust the daily use of diuretics to morning hours	Instruct client to take diuretics in the morning instead of later in the day, to avoid nocturia; sweetening agents and caffeine may need to be reduced or eliminated from the diet; if medications are suspected of causing urinary difficulties, consult the physician for an alternative medication If a history of frequent voiding has decreased bladder capacity, gradually increase time between voidings If client is incontinent before scheduled voiding time, readjust schedule and restart lengthening schedule Distinguish between frequency and overflow incontinence; measure residual urine after voiding

EVALUATION

1. The client identifies the amounts and types of fluid useful in urine control and in prevention of urinary infections.
2. The client takes fluids primarily in the morning and early afternoon as a way to prevent nighttime voiding patterns.
3. The client adheres to an established voiding schedule; preferably 300 to 400 ml of urine is voided every 3 hours while he or she is awake.
4. The client maintains hygiene and considers methods to control urine loss (e.g., absorbing pads).
5. The client identifies methods that can aid in urinary elimination if voiding does not begin following stimuli when a toilet facility is present.
6. The client assumes the responsibility of locating toilet facilities whenever the environment changes (e.g., social activity or relocation).
7. The client follows his or her medication schedule, which includes limiting the administration of any diuretics to the morning hours.
8. The client notifies his or her physician when medication side effects are present that interfere with normal urinary elimination.
9. The client experiences improvement in his or her urine control problem.

NURSING ALERTS

1. The subject of elimination may produce anxiety on the part of a client during an interview. Provide a positive environment and privacy throughout the assessment.
2. Be alert for changes in a client's mental status resulting from fluid and electrolyte imbalances caused by dehydration that occurs because fear of urinary control difficulties.

3. Review all medications that are prescribed for a client. If more than one physician's name appears on the medication bottles, ask the client if each physician knows that the others are prescribing drugs also.
4. To be effective, instructions to the elderly need to be given slowly or paced according to the client's ability to understand them. The client needs to feel that the instructions are relevant and meaningful.
5. The response time to questions may be lengthy, so the interviewer needs to be attentive.

Bibliography

Carotenuto R and Bullock J: Physical assessment of the gerontologic client, Philadelphia; 1981, FA Davis Co.

Eliopoulos C: Gerontological nursing, ed 2, Philadelphia, 1987, JB Lippincott Co.

Eliopoulos C, editor: Health assessment of the older adult, Menlo Park, Calif, 1984, Addison-Wesley Publishing Co., Inc.

Kim K and Grier M: Pacing effects of medication instruction for the elderly, Journal of Gerontological Nursing, 7:464, 1981.

Kim MJ, McFarland GK, and McLane AM: Pocket guide to nursing diagnoses, ed 3, St Louis, 1989, The CV Mosby Co.

Mandelstam D: Special techniques: strengthening pelvic floor muscles, Geriatric Nursing, 1:251, 1980.

McLane A and McShane R: Elimination. In Thompson JM et al, editors: Mosby's manual of clinical nursing, ed 2, St Louis, 1989, The CV Mosby Co.

Ouslander J: Urinary incontinence in the elderly, Western Journal of Medicine 135:482, 1981.

Simonson W: Medications and the elderly, Rockville, Md, 1985, Aspen Publishers, Inc.

Violence, Potential for

Mary E. Allen

KNOWLEDGE BASE

1. Potential for violence is a state in which risk factors for self-directed or other-directed physical trauma are present.
2. Violent behavior toward others has an underlying basis of either a sense of powerlessness or an inability to cope with the demands or stimuli of the environment.

3. Assaultive behavior by a client may be triggered by the following situations:
   a. A perceived threat to self-esteem or self-concept
   b. A demand that the client perform a specific task
   c. Restriction of movement or behavior

d. Lack of listening or attentiveness to the client
e. Environmental isolation or excessive stimuli (noise, number of people)
f. Unpredictability in routine or a change in the environment
g. Presence of unknown staff
h. Scolding from others

4. The potential for violent behavior increases in direct proportion to the client's level of anxiety and fear.
5. Fear, anxiety, or cognitive deficits may result in misinterpretation of motives, events, or environment, thus increasing the likelihood of violent behavior.
6. Substance abuse impairs judgment and decreases the ability to control behavior, thus increasing the potential for violent behavior.
7. Using violence as a coping response may be a lifelong behavior or may result from cognitive deficits.
8. Sensory-perceptual alterations related to the presence of organic or functional disorders can impair the ability to test reality and thus can lead to ineffective coping with multiple stressors.
9. Impaired ability to test reality and subsequent inability to control behavior can occur as a result of patterns of battering or abuse, organic mental disorders, affective disorders, substance-use disorders, paranoid disorders, and other psychotic disorders.
10. A catastrophic reaction is an overreaction to a minor stressor.
11. Staff response to violent behavior may either diminish or exacerbate the problem.
12. Staff education is critical to managing the environment and events that may trigger violent behavior.
13. Self-directed violence may have the following contributing factors:
a. Social or psychological isolation
b. Experience of multiple losses (bereavement overload) without adequate grief work
c. Uncontrolled pain as a part of terminal illness
d. Depression
e. Sense of hopelessness
f. Sense of failure related to past and present life
g. Increased dependence on caregivers and the loss of personal freedom, which can influence the severity, duration, and resolution of violence potential
14. Elderly people tend to give fewer warning signals or messages and are more "successful" in suicide attempts.
15. Any direct or indirect signal of suicide must be taken seriously and discussed with the client. A direct question may be desirable.
16. Cultural and religious beliefs influence a client's attitudes toward self-violence.

ASSESSMENT CRITERIA
Physical

Medical, surgical, and trauma history showing conditions that would result in neurological abnormalities
Head injury
Epilepsy
Stroke
Alzheimer's disease
Substance abuse
Psychiatric history: treatment modalities and medication therapies
History of family conflicts, violence
History of legal problems or criminal cases
Diagnostic studies
Drug levels
Glucose tolerance
CT scans, magnetic resonance imaging
Electroencephalogram
Blood gas levels
Blood alcohol level
Aggressive body language
Clenched fists
Tense facial expressions
Rigid posture
Increased motor activity
Pacing
Irritability
Agitation
Overt uncontrollable rage
Self-destructive, suicidal behavior
Chemical dependency withdrawal
Sensory impairment
Recent change or loss in functional abilities or health status

Psychosocial

Hostile, threatening verbalizations
Overt aggressive acts (e.g., destruction of objects in the environment)
Possession of weapons or destructive objects with intent to harm
Depression with no outlet for anger
Paranoid ideation, delusions and/or hallucinations
Relationships and behaviors within relationships
Coping styles, resources, and deficits
Cognitive abilities
Memory (long-term and short-term)
Problem-solving abilities
Recent losses and change in support system
Meaning of losses and changes in physical, psychological, and social realms
Environmental restrictions on autonomy, mobility, and privacy
Level of stimuli in the environment

Spiritual

Sense of loss of control over one's life; powerlessness
Guilt felt about own behavior
Belief about control over one's death

NURSING CARE PLAN: POTENTIAL FOR VIOLENCE

Common contributing factors	Expected client outcomes	Nursing strategies
Sensory-perceptual alterations	Client will be able to use the problem-solving process to cope with sensory-perceptual alterations	Identify specific cause(s) of sensory-perceptual alterations Encourage client to talk about how the alterations are affecting or contributing to the inability to cope with multiple stressors Identify with the client problem-solving approaches to minimize sensory-perceptual alterations Maintain client's personal space Be cautious about touching the client; only touch with permission Decrease stimuli in the environment or move the individual to a quiet room Use a neutral tone in giving messages, which should be worded concisely

Inability to control behavior; related to:
  Patterns of battering/abuse
  Organic mental disorders
  Affective disorders
  Substance-use disorders
  Paranoid disorders
  Other psychotic disorders
	Client will be able to verbalize feelings of anger (specify length of time)
	Client will be able to identify the source of anger
	Client will be able to use the problem-solving process to identify ways of overcoming the anger
	Client will learn to use constructive outlets for angry feelings
	Client will use assertive rather than aggressive behaviors to have needs met
		Decrease probability that the patient will harm self or others by creating a safe physical environment (e.g., remove potentially harmful objects)
		Create a safe psychological environment by approaching the client in a calm, reassuring manner
		Encourage client to talk about what he or she is experiencing and feeling
		Provide alternative, constructive outlets for the expression of angry feelings
		Decrease symptomatic behavior by giving prescribed medication and, when necessary, using physical restraint measures
		Evaluate lethality potential of suicidal/homicidal clients by identifying planned method, availability of weapons or destructive mechanisms, specificity of plan, and degree of weapon or mechanism lethality
		If needed, refer client to an appropriate agency or person for more intensive psychological care

Sense of hopelessness related to losses, chronic pain, fear of the future	Client will verbalize a purpose for the immediate future Client will explain rationale for planned interventions	Assess the feelings about and meanings of recent and past events Develop a trusting relationship Listen to the client's story; focus on his or her perceptions and feelings Provide opportunities for decision making and successful outcomes Assist in developing internal and external resources Develop plan for pain management Assist the client in setting achievable goals; establish a schedule for reevaluating goals and celebrating success Assist the client in assigning meaning and value to life events Create a safe environment Evaluate the need for visits or attendance

EVALUATION

1. The client is able to use the problem-solving process to cope with sensory-perceptual alterations.
2. The client is able to verbalize angry feelings.
3. The client is able to identify the source of anger.
4. The client is able to use the problem-solving process to identify ways of overcoming the anger.
5. The client is able to establish or reestablish constructive outlets for angry feelings.
6. The client is able to use assertive rather than aggressive behaviors to have his or her needs met.
7. The client verbalizes a sense of purpose.
8. The client experiences fewer episodes of aggressive behavior.
9. The client and others remain free from harm.

NURSE ALERTS

1. Be alert to the high potential for suicide among elderly males, especially those who are in poor health and alone.
2. After the nursing strategies have been implemented and evaluated, it is important to refer the client to an appropriate agency or person for long-term psychological care and follow-up if necessary.
3. Irreversible organic disorders or other psychopathology will require long-term medical management and follow-up.
4. Fear reactions of staff may lead to inappropriate use of chemical or physical restraints.

Bibliography

Addington J and Fry PS: Directions for clinical-psychosocial assessment of depression in the elderly. In Brink, TL, editor: Clinical gerontology: a guide to assessment and intervention, New York, 1986, Haworth, pp 97-118.

Butler RN and Lewis MI: Aging and mental health, St Louis, 1982, The CV Mosby Co.

Chaisson M et al: Treating the depressed elderly, Journal of Psychosocial Nursing 22(5):25, 1984.

Fry PS: Assessment of pessimism and despair in the elderly: a geriatric scale of hopelessness. In Brink TL, editor: Clinical gerontology: a guide to assessment and intervention, New York, 1986, John Wiley & Sons, Inc, pp. 193-201.

Goebel G and Boech B: Ego integrity and fear of death: a comparison of institutionalized and independently living older adults, Death Studies 11:193, 1987.

Hurley ME, editor: Classification of nursing diagnoses: proceedings of the Sixth Conference, North American Nursing Diagnosis Association, St Louis, 1986, The CV Mosby Co, pp 545-546.

Kim MJ, McFarland GK, and McLane AM: Pocket guide to nursing diagnoses, ed 3, St Louis, 1989, The CV Mosby Co.

Manfredi C and Pickett M: Perceived stressful situations and coping strategies utilized by the elderly, Journal of Community Health Nursing 4(2):99, 1987.

Newman MA and Gaudiano JK: Depression as an explanation for decreased subjective time in the elderly, Nursing Research 33(3):137, 1984.

Reed PG: Development resources and depression in the elderly, Nursing Research 35(2):368, 1986.

Whall A: Suicide in older adults, Journal of Gerontological Nursing 111(8):40, 1985.

Individualized Nursing Care Plans

CARDIOVASCULAR SYSTEM

Acute Myocardial Infarction, Dysrhythmias, and Temporary-Pacemaker Insertion

Sharon Bowles

KNOWLEDGE BASE

1. The elderly experience a higher rate of complications from acute illnesses than do younger adults.
2. Heart disease, cancer, and stroke are the leading causes of death for persons age 65 and over.
3. Heart rate slows, stroke volume decreases, and cardiac output is reduced by 30% to 40% as a result of aging.
4. The aged heart has relatively less blood in the coronary arteries because the venous vessels and sinusoids dominate, whereas the capillary network and coronary arteries dominate in childhood. At age 60, the maximum coronary blood flow is estimated to be 35% less than that of a younger adult.
5. Acute myocardial infarction occurs when there is lack of blood supply or increased oxygen demand without sufficient blood flow to the myocardium, resulting in tissue damage (necrosis). In an elderly person the diagnosis may be missed or delayed because of an atypical set of symptoms and the frequent absence of the pain that is usually present with younger adults.
6. Myocardial infarction is more frequently seen in elderly men with a history of hypertension and arteriosclerosis than in elderly women.
7. The mortality rate from acute myocardial infarction in the elderly is twice that of younger adults.
8. Measurements of creatine kinase-MB (CK-MB) isoenzyme levels and lactate dehydrogenase (LDH) isoenzymes levels are the most specific laboratory tests used to verify acute myocardial infarction. Normal ranges vary from laboratory to laboratory. The specific marker for damaged myocardial cells is the isoenzyme MB. CK-MB elevation and total CK elevation will occur within 2 to 5 hours after the onset of myocardial infarction, with peak elevation seen between 12 and 24 hours after onset. LDH isoenzymes separate into five bands. Levels of LDH-1 and LDH-2 are used to determine cardiac muscle damage. Normally, LDH-2 is greater than LDH-1. With myocardial damage, LDH-1 will be greater than LDH-2. LDH levels begin to rise about 12 hours after infarction and peak in 3 to 4 days.
9. Initial treatment for acute myocardial infarction is aimed at decreasing pain, increasing myocardial oxygen supply, and decreasing myocardial oxygen demand.
10. Medical and surgical interventions aimed at reperfusion to limit the size of infarction include thrombolytic therapy to lyse clots; percutaneous transluminal coronary angioplasty, laser therapy, and arthrectomy to improve blood flow through stenosed coronary arteries; and coronary artery bypass grafts to bypass obstructed portions of coronary arteries.

11. Guidelines are used to determine which initial treatment can or should be used. Thrombolytic therapy, for instance, may be contraindicated in persons over age 75 because of the increasing potential risk of intracranial bleeding. The benefit from thrombolytic therapy diminishes over time, with maximum benefits being achieved when therapy is initiated within 6 hours of the onset of chest pain. Bypass surgery may be contraindicated in an aged client who has advanced atherosclerosis, because the client's vessels (e.g., saphenous vein or internal mammary artery) would be used for the graft(s).

12. The majority of the elderly have normal sinus rhythm. Atrial or ventricular premature contractions and atrial fibrillation are the most common dysrhythmias in the aged. Atrial fibrillation is of particular notice because of the loss of atrial kick, which reduces cardiac output by 15% to 25%. The incidence of life-threatening dysrhythmias in the elderly is the same as in younger people, but older persons are more susceptible to cardiogenic shock.

13. The total number of pacemaker cells in the sinoatrial node decreases with aging, which decreases the inherent rhythmicity of the heart. Atrial dysrhythmias may occur from focal thickening and infiltration of fat in and around the region of the sinoatrial node.

14. The resting heart rate changes minimally with age, whereas the maximum attainable heart rate declines. Once the maximum heart rate is achieved, the heart requires a longer time to return to baseline or resting rate.

15. Third-degree heart block (complete heart block) occurs when there is no relationship between the P wave and the QRS complex. The ventricular rate is usually slow and cardiac output is decreased. This potentiates the occurrence of lethal ventricular dysrhythmias, cardiac standstill, and Stokes-Adams attack.

16. Dysrhythmias are serious in the elderly because they further compromise the blood supply to organs that already may be impaired by age-related changes and/or disease.

17. Temporary cardiac pacemaker insertion is indicated when a client has symptomatic bradydysrhythmias and there is a potential for severe bradycardia or ventricular standstill.

18. Temporary pacing restores a more normal heart rate by providing artificial electrical stimulation to the heart muscle when its intrinsic conduction system fails to stimulate a contraction within a specific time period. An external temporary pacemaker may be used in an emergency situation while the client is awaiting insertion of the temporary pacing wire (catheter). Age is usually not a factor in selecting pacemaker intervention.

CASE STUDY

Mr. Holmes, 79 years old, is admitted to a coronary care unit in no acute distress. He has no history of previous cardiovascular problems. The evening before admission, Mr. Holmes developed chest discomfort after supper, which he attributed to indigestion. He describes the discomfort as dull and midsternal, lasting approximately 2 hours. Mr. Holmes took Mylanta and went to bed but did not sleep well. When he awakened about 6:00 AM, he felt weak and dizzy. His chest felt sore, but the previous pain or discomfort was gone. Mr. Holmes called his physician, who met him in the emergency room. Findings: blood pressure, 98/62; pulse, regular at 42 beats/min; rhythm showing third-degree heart block; 12-lead electrocardiogram (ECG) showing acute inferior infarction; initial CK-MB isoenzyme, 600 mU/ml (normal in this hospital for males: 57-374 mU/ml). Mr. Holmes is alert and oriented to time and place. He states: "My wife tried to get me to call the doctor last night, but I thought it was just a good old case of indigestion." Admitting orders include bed rest with bedside commode, continuous electrocardiographic monitoring, IV heparin lock, and having the client sign a permit for temporary pacemaker insertion.

ASSESSMENT CRITERIA
Physical

History and nature of onset, precipitating factors, course of problem, patterns of the symptom
   Where were you/what were you doing when the pain started?
   Was the pain abrupt or gradual?
   Have you had this type of pain/discomfort previously?
Description of chest pain
   Location
   Duration
   Quality
Accompanying symptoms
   Lightheadedness
   Dizziness
   Syncope
   Orthopnea
   Diaphoresis
   Dyspnea
   Nausea and/or vomiting
   Abdominal bloating
   Palpitations

Alleviating factors
  Pain relief by rest
  Medications used with or without relief
  Position change
Personal health history
  Previous heart problems/heart attack
  Hypertension
  Stroke
  Diabetes
  Vascular disease
  Fatigue
  Presence of cardiac risk factors: dietary habits, smoking history, obesity, hyperlipidemia, stressors
  Medications, including over-the-counter preparations, and problems with adherence
Family health history
  General health of client's siblings and parents
  Age and cause of death of deceased family members
Vital signs
Heart sounds: auscultation with stethoscope for extra (abnormal) heart sounds, murmurs, irregular rhythm
Lung sounds: auscultation with stethoscope for crackles, rhonchi, etc.
Jugular vein distension
Skin: cool, clammy, diaphoretic, color
Edema: pedal/sacral
Pulses: presence or absence, quality of carotid, radial, femoral, and pedal pulses (and compare side to side)
Neurovascular: alert and oriented to time, place, and person
Gastrointestinal: nausea and/or vomiting, bowel sounds present in all four quadrants
Cardiac rhythm: dysrhythmia interpretation by rhythm strips; if dysrhythmias present, note patient tolerance (e.g., blood pressure, skin color and moisture, mentation)

Psychosocial

Life-style
  Description of typical day
  Recreation/leisure profile
  Occupational profile
  Living environment profile
Knowledge of heart condition and treatment course
Client's perception of and reaction to the problem
Perception of stressors and interpersonal conflicts/problems

Resources/support systems used
Concerns regarding sexuality and sexual function

Spiritual

Client's religious practices/beliefs
Effect of illness/hospitalization on belief system
Need for spiritual assistance

Initial denial of chest pain, as in Mr. Holmes's case, is often seen. Indigestion, hiatal hernia, gallbladder disease, and musculoskeletal pain frequently mimic chest pain.

Feelings of weakness and dizziness may accompany acute myocardial infarction. These symptoms indicate decreased perfusion because of myocardial damage and the heart's inability to pump blood as effectively. Other classic symptoms, which Mr. Holmes did not have, include nausea and/or vomiting, diaphoresis, and palpitations.

Mr. Holmes's blood pressure is low. Sympathetic stimulation secondary to pain may cause an increase in blood pressure and heart rate. Decreased cardiac output secondary to ischemia may cause lowered blood pressure.

Mr. Holmes's heart rate of 42 beats/min is congruent with the diagnosis of third-degree heart block. During the course of the night, his rhythm most likely progressed from first-degree to second-degree to third-degree heart block, with a gradual decrease in heart rate. Had Mr. Holmes sought treatment earlier, and had progression into second-degree heart block been noted, a temporary pacemaker would have been indicated.

The diagnosis of acute inferior infarction involves decreased right coronary blood flow, which predisposes the heart to conduction disturbances. The right coronary artery normally supplies oxygen and nutrients to the conduction system of the heart.

Mr. Holmes's CK-MB is 600 mU/ml, which is indicative of acute myocardial infarction (see Knowledge Base, no. 8).

NURSING CARE PLAN: ACUTE MYOCARDIAL INFARCTION, DYSRHYTHMIAS, AND TEMPORARY PACEMAKER INSERTION

Nursing diagnoses	Expected client outcomes	Nursing strategies

Potential for altered comfort: chest pain; related to myocardial ischemia/infarction	Client will experience no chest pain or will experience relief from symptoms	Instruct client to report pain immediately
		Obtain and record detailed description of pain, including:
		  Onset/duration
		  Location
		  Quality/intensity
		  Radiation
		  Associated symptoms
		Assess blood pressure and heart rate with each pain episode
		Administer oxygen at 2-4 liters/min by nasal cannula or mask, as prescribed
		Obtain 12-lead ECG during episode of chest pain
		Remain with client during pain episode, monitoring blood pressure and pulse every 5 minutes
		Monitor for side effects of analgesics (narcotics: excess sedation, constipation, nausea and vomiting, acute confusional state, dry mouth, respiratory depression, hypotension)

Potential decreased cardiac output, related to mechanical disorder of acute myocardial infarction and structural disorder of age-related changes	Client will demonstrate improved/normal cardiac output	Monitor ECG to detect dysrhythmias and blocks, and report any significant changes to physician Auscultate lung sounds and heart sounds when assessing routine and as indicated vital signs Assess skin for color, temperature, and dryness Inspect for signs of peripheral or dependent edema and jugular vein distention Monitor urine output and weight Assess mental status and behavior
Potential fear, related to change in health status, threat of death	Client will experience an increase in psychological comfort, as evidenced by verbal and nonverbal communications	Establish rapport with client and maintain confident, consistent manner Assess and acknowledge presence of fear; ask open-ended questions to facilitate communication Explain the illness, routine procedures, and expected activities as the client is ready; use simple terminology, clarify, repeat as necessary, and use positive approach Support and encourage information sharing between client and family; answer family's questions factually Support use of usual coping skills
Potential activity intolerance, related to insufficient oxygenation secondary to decreased cardiac output	Client will identify factors that increase workload of the heart Client will perform activities of daily living within established cardiac tolerance guidelines	Organize care to allow for adequate rest and take advantage of peak energy levels Promote bed rest, with chair/bedside commode; activities as tolerated Allow client to participate in and complete self-care activities as tolerated; instruct client to stop the activity if chest pain recurs Assist with progression of activity, and document responses before, during, and after activity, including blood pressure, heart rate and rhythm, respiration, and tolerance of activity Instruct client to avoid straining during bowel movements

NURSING CARE PLAN: ACUTE MYOCARDIAL INFARCTION, DYSRHYTHMIAS, AND TEMPORARY PACEMAKER INSERTION—cont'd

Nursing diagnoses	Expected client outcomes	Nursing strategies
Decreased cardiac output, related to electrical conduction disorders	Client will maintain regular heart rate and rhythm and normal cardiac output	Monitor heart rate and rhythm with cardiac monitor Document and report rate or rhythm disturbances, ectopy, and changes in the S & T segment Determine the type of dysrhythmia, and document with rhythm strip Check vital signs during dysrhythmias and note associating signs and symptoms. Report any significant changes or dysrhythmias to physician

Before temporary pacemaker insertion

Nursing diagnoses	Expected client outcomes	Nursing strategies
Knowledge deficit regarding insertion of temporary pacemaker, related to lack of previous experience	Client will understand the need for temporary pacemaker and procedure of insertion	Explain procedure to client and family, and assist with signing appropriate permission form(s) 　Purpose for insertion of temporary pacemaker in relation to dysrhythmias and infarction 　Function and use of pacemaker 　Insertion procedure under local anesthesia

After temporary pacemaker insertion

Nursing diagnoses	Expected client outcomes	Nursing strategies
Potential decreased cardiac output, related to pacemaker failure, improper stimulation, or improper sensing	Client will maintain regular heart rhythm within prescribed rate	Monitor vital signs and heart rhythm by cardiac monitor, noting whether rhythm is paced or unpaced Identify pacemaker parameters and maintain as prescribed 　Rate (between 60 and 80 beats/min) 　Milliamperes (mA) (the energy output) 　Mode (demand or asynchronous) 　Sensitivity (the amplitude of R or P wave) 　Battery check (sufficient battery life) Monitor appropriateness of pacemaker functioning; assess for pacemaker malfunction if problems noted with rate, capture, or sensing
Potential for injury related to temporary pacemaker insertion	Client will not experience complications as a result of microshock	Assess for electrically safe environment 　Electric bed is grounded or unplugged 　Environment is dry 　All electrical equipment in the room is grounded
Potential for infection related to invasive procedure and catheter	Client will not develop infection at site of pacemaker catheter (wire) insertion	Adhere to hospital policies and procedures regarding aseptic technique and infection control Maintain aseptic wound care, and change dressing as indicated 　Observe wound for redness, swelling, drainage 　Be careful not to dislodge catheter during wound care
Impaired physical mobility, related to limitations imposed by temporary pacemaker	Client will demonstrate adaptation to limited mobility while temporary pacemaker is used	Explain the rationale for limited mobility as a precaution to prevent dislodgment of the catheter Assist with active range-of-motion exercises Assist with increased mobility, as permitted; secure external pulse generator and extension cable to client's gown to prevent tension on the pacemaker catheter Assess skin for pressure every 2 hours Apply pressure relief device/surface per institution protocol

Continued.

NURSING CARE PLAN: ACUTE MYOCARDIAL INFARCTION, DYSRHYTHMIAS, AND TEMPORARY PACEMAKER INSERTION—cont'd

Nursing diagnoses	Expected client outcomes	Nursing strategies
Knowledge deficit regarding follow-up care, related to lack of previous experience	Client will display willingness to learn about health disorder and follow-up care	Assess client's desire to learn and knowledge level regarding client's health disorder and follow-up care Use teaching methods and materials at a level consistent with client's ability (e.g., videos, heart model, pamphlets); intersperse teaching with nursing care activities, rather than giving information just prior to discharge Teach in small increments, in a quiet environment, at a pace the client can tolerate

	Client will verbalize understanding of risk factors, medications, signs and symptoms to report, diet, activity level and restrictions	Explain the following, with appropriate rationale as needed:
		  Risk factors (e.g., obesity, hypertension, smoking)
		  Medications prescribed—name, dose, frequency, therapeutic effects, side effects
		  Signs and symptoms to report (e.g., chest pain unrelieved by nitroglycerin, syncope, palpitations)
		  Diet (e.g., low sodium, cholesterol, and fat)
		  Activity level and restrictions (e.g, progression, work, sexual activity)
		  Follow-up care
		  Community resources available (e.g., cardiac rehabilitation, support groups)

EVALUATION

1. The client verbalizes no complaints or expresses relief from chest pain.
2. The client does not experience extension of myocardial infarction, as evidenced by:
   a. Stable vital signs
   b. No further episodes of prolonged chest pain
   c. Cardiac enzyme levels returning to normal range
   d. 12-lead ECG showing resolution of acute myocardial infarction.
3. The client maintains clear lungs and has no abnormal heart sounds.
4. The client verbalizes understanding of the rationale for temporary pacemaker insertion.
5. The client's heart rate is regular and within the prescribed range. The temporary pacemaker functions adequately, with no malfunctioning.
6. The client experiences no complications as a result of temporary pacemaker insertion and its intervention.
7. The client limits activities as necessary and tolerates a steady progression of activity without complications.
8. The client displays and verbalizes a reduction in or resolution of fear relating to myocardial infarction.
9. The client comprehends and verbalizes understanding of the following: heart disease, risk factors, prescribed medications, signs and symptoms to report, dietary and activity-level regimen, physician or clinic follow-up, and available community resources.

NURSING ALERTS

1. Anticoagulation therapy is a commonly used intervention for acute myocardial infarction. Close observation for signs of bleeding is essential in the elderly because of an increased risk of cerebral, pericardial, renal, or gastrointestinal bleeding resulting from the anticoagulants.
2. Digitalis therapy should be used with caution in the elderly. Digitalis toxicity with resultant dangerous dysrhythmias can occur more readily because of the following age-related changes: loss of lean muscle mass, decrease in glomerular filtration rate, and reduced blood flow to the kidneys. These changes result in an increased half-life for the drug.
3. Respiratory depression or hypotension may occur in the elderly when excessive sedation or analgesia is used for chest pain.
4. Cardioversion for rapid dysrhythmias must be used with caution in the elderly. Cardioversion may cause a fatal sinus arrest.

5. Confusion and disorientation may occur when an elderly person is admitted to a coronary care unit, is isolated, and experiences disruption of normal sleeping and eating habits. The following suggestions can assist in decreasing confusion and disorientation:
   a. Be sure the client wears hearing aid and/or glasses
   b. encourage and allow more frequent visits by relatives
   c. allow the client to keep a few personal items in the room
   d. use clock, television, calendar, and verbal communication to assist in orientation to time and place
   e. Provide opportunities to participate in decisions regarding care
6. Denial and depression are common reactions to myocardial infarction. These reactions should not be ignored, but openly explored as normal responses.
7. Severe chest pain occurring after the initial infarction may indicate extension of the infarction and/or other complications, such as pericarditis or pulmonary embolus. Delayed reporting of such pain by the client may interfere with pain relief and require greater doses of medications to achieve relief.
8. Chest soreness is a common phenomenon during the acute infarction phase and does not necessarily require pain medication.
9. For severe chest pain, intravenous morphine sulfate is the analgesic of choice. For less severe attacks, sublingual nitroglycerin is used. The principal effects of nitroglycerin are to dilate the coronary arteries and/or collateral vessels, which increases circulation to the heart muscle (unless the coronary arteries are severely atherosclerotic), and to dilate the peripheral blood vessels, which reduces afterload. For bedside use of nitroglycerin by the client, please refer to the care plan on ischemic heart disease, p. 118.
10. Oxygen therapy (e.g., by nasal cannula) should be discontinued after chest pain subsides. Prolonged use will cause dryness of nasal passages, thereby increasing client discomfort. Also, assessment of whether the client is primarily a mouth breather or a nose breather will assist in deciding if a nasal cannula versus a mask should be used for the treatment.
11. During assessment of heart sounds, abnormal heart sounds of S_3, S_4, and murmurs may be noted. An S_4 is commonly seen in the elderly because of age-related decreased compliance of the heart musculature. An S_4 may also occur as a result of myocardial damage; it may be transient or intermittent during the acute phase and/or may become a permanent extra sound. The onset of a new S_3, diastolic murmur, or holosystolic murmur is serious and should be reported immediately.

12. Heart sounds may be "distant" and difficult to hear upon admission, and then become more audible as healing occurs (usually within 24 to 72 hours).
13. Avoid giving intramuscular injections, since these will alter serum enzyme levels.
14. The client should avoid straining during bowel movements. Any Valsalva maneuver may result in bradycardia caused by vagal stimulation, thereby temporarily decreasing cardiac output.
15. Changes in sensorium may accompany dysrhythmias as inadequate cerebral perfusion secondary to decreased cardiac output occurs.
16. When a temporary pacemaker is being used, the client's heart rate should remain within the prescribed and set limits of the pacemaker generator. A ventricular response should be noted with each pacemaker stimulus, and the pacemaker should not release a stimulus when the client's own heart rhythm is noted.

Bibliography

Chung EK: Arrhythmias associated with acute myocardial infarction, Physician Assistant 12(4):53, 1988.

Doenges ME, Moorhouse F, and Geissler AC: Nursing care plans: guidelines for planning patient care, ed 2, Philadelphia, 1989, FA Davis Co.

Eliopoulos C: Gerontological nursing, ed 2, Philadelphia, 1987, JB Lippincott Co.

Eliopoulos C: A guide to the nursing of the aging, Baltimore, 1987, Williams & Wilkins.

Gulanick M, Klopp A, and Galanes S: Nursing care plans: nursing diagnosis and intervention, St Louis, 1986, The CV Mosby Co.

Guzzetta CE and Dossey BM: Cardiovascular nursing: body-mind tapestry, St Louis, 1984, The CV Mosby Co.

Jacobs DS et al: Laboratory test handbook with key word index, Cleveland, 1988, Lexi-Comp/Mosby.

Lewis SM and Collier IC: Medical-surgical nursing: assessment and management of clinical problems, ed 2, New York, 1987, McGraw-Hill Book Co.

Matteson MA and McConnell ES: Gerontological nursing: concepts and practice, Philadelphia, 1988, WB Saunders Co.

Misinski M: Role of conventional management and alternative therapies in limiting infarct size in acute myocardial infarction, Heart and Lung, 16(6):746, 1987.

Ramsden CS: Management of the acute myocardial infarction patient receiving fibrinolytic therapy with activase, Califon, NJ, 1988, Gardiner-Caldwell SynerMed.

Swearingen PL, Sommers MS, and Miller K: Manual of critical care: applying nursing diagnoses to adult critical illness, St Louis, 1988, The CV Mosby Co.

Atherosclerotic Heart Disease

Shirley A. Saunders

KNOWLEDGE BASE

1. Atherosclerosis is a very common systemic arterial disorder. The lesion consists of yellowish plaques of cholesterol, lipids, and cellular debris involving the inner layer of the large and medium-sized arteries. These atheromatous plaques are major causes of angina and myocardial infarction.
2. The pathogenesis of atherosclerosis is unclear, but hyperlipidemia (as a result of dietary intake) and faulty carbohydrate metabolism are two factors associated with its development.
3. There is a moderate increase in the systolic blood pressure with advancing age, causing the development of atherosclerosis to be accelerated.
4. Aging leads to a greater increase in systolic blood pressure during exercise.
5. Calcification of the tunica media layer and loss of elasticity of the muscular and coronary arteries occur with age.
6. These age-related changes can combine with other variables, making the older population more susceptible to myocardial ischemia.
7. The ability of the left ventricle to pump blood may be reduced, which can result in decreased cardiac output and coronary artery filling.
8. The heart rate does not respond as readily to stress or sudden effort; therefore it takes longer for the heart rate to return to baseline after exercise or exertion.
9. The valves in the veins become less efficient, leading to an abnormal accumulation of blood in the lower extremities.
10. The metabolic rate decreases, leading to lowered calorie requirements, weight gain, higher percentage of body fat, and a decrease in the amount of oxygen used by the tissues.
11. Immunity is impaired, thereby making elderly clients more susceptible to infections and multiple diseases.
12. The ability to recuperate from illness is reduced.
13. Because physical activity and conditioning decrease as a result of less exercise and activity, there is a decrease in endurance, muscle tone, and muscle strength.
14. Perception of some types of pain diminishes, resulting in an inability to discriminate pain sensations, and a higher prevalence of referred pain from one part of the body to another.
15. The gastric mucosa atrophies and hydrochloric acid secretion is reduced, causing anorexia, poor nutritional intake, and malabsorption of vitamins and minerals.
16. Peripheral vascular resistance increases and cardiac output decreases, leading to decreased blood flow to the kidneys, altered fluid and electrolyte balance, decreased secretion, and early toxicity to drugs.
17. The respiratory muscles weaken and the rib cage becomes less flexible, leading to decreased vital capacity, decreased oxygen in the blood, and inefficient ventilation.
18. The bones lose calcium and become more brittle, ligaments calcify, and cartilaginous joint surfaces erode, leading to stiff joints, increased fatigue, and inactivity.
19. Psychological stress often increases because of the multiplicity and frequency of losses.

CASE STUDY

Mrs. Morgan, 70 years old, has been hospitalized for evaluation of recurrent chest discomfort at rest and following minimal exertion. During the past 8 months, these episodes have occurred with increasing frequency and duration.

The preliminary assessment data revealed an alert and oriented female who was pain free and in no acute distress. Vital signs on admission were as follows: blood pressure, 180/100; heart rate, 108 beats/min; heart rhythm slightly irregular because of ventricular ectopic beats; temperature, 37° C; respiratory rate, 24 breaths/min; breathing shallow and slightly labored.

Assessment of her risk factors and life-style revealed the following findings: a history of glucose intolerance; hypertension of 10 years' duration; two packs per day of cigarette usage for 40 years; obesity, gout, elevated cholesterol level, and a sedentary life-style. She admits to being under a lot of stress imposed by monetary problems and poor health. She has a history of noncompliance with medical treatment, nonadherance to prescribed diet, and lack of regular exercise. Her family history was significant in that her father died of a myocardial infarction (MI) at age 56 and her maternal grandmother died of complications resulting from uncontrolled diabetes mellitus at age 68.

Mrs. Morgan undergoes coronary arteriography 2 days after admission, which confirms the presence of atherosclerotic heart disease. Her left anterior descending artery was 50% occluded, and her circumflex artery was 75% occluded. Further evaluation showed that an angioplasty might be beneficial for this client.

Mrs. Morgan's home medications include nifedipine (Procardia), 20 mg every 6 hours, for angina and blood pressure control and 15 units of NPH insulin plus 10 units of regular insulin (mixed) given subcutaneously every morning and evening. Bowel sounds are present in all four quadrants, with pronounced protuberance. She has a productive cough, and diffuse coarse crackles bilaterally. Her skin is warm and dry with poor turgor and slight tenting. Peripheral pulses are diminished at 1+, and a right carotid bruit is present. There is a 2+ pitting edema of her feet.

Laboratory blood test results on admission were as follows: glucose, 260 mg/dl; sodium, 126 mEq/L; chloride, 116 mEq/L; potassium, 3.4 mEq/L; coenzyme 2, 26; serum creatinine, 1.9 mg/dl; creatine kinase (CK), 198; CK-MB, <4; cholesterol, 290 mg/dl; triglycerides, 200 mg/dl; high-density lipoprotein (HDL), 18 mg/dl; low-density lipoprotein (LDL), 188 mg/dl; blood urea nitrogen (BUN), 28 mg/dl; LDH-1 < LDH-2; serum glutamic-oxaloacetic transaminase (SGOT), 60; serum glutamic-pyruvic transaminase (SGPT), 50; hematocrit, 30; Hemoglobin, 10 g/dl; white blood cells (WBCs), 14,000/cu mm; and uric acid, 17 mg/dl. Arterial blood gas results were as follows: pH, 7.30; P_{CO_2}, 30 mm Hg; P_{O_2}, 75 mm Hg.

Urinalysis results were as follows: negative ketones, 2+ glucose, 1+ protein, 1+ blood.

Admission orders included the following: vital signs every 4 hours; nifedipine, 30 mg every 6 hours; Nitropaste, 1 inch applied topically three times a day; 20 units of NPH insulin and 10 units of regular insulin every morning and evening; furosemide (Lasix), 40 mg twice a day; enteric-coated aspirin, 325 mg every day; dipyridamole (Persantine), 25 mg every 6 hours; Accuchecks four times a day; daily weights; 1800-calorie American Dietetic Association (ADA) diabetic diet, with low cholesterol and 2-g/day sodium restriction; CK-MB every 12 hours; daily SMA 6, SMA 12, and chest x-ray; bedside commode; and 2 liters of oxygen per day by nasal cannula.

Mrs. Morgan lives with her 75-year-old husband, who has failing health. She has three adult children, who live in another state. Except for a few elderly friends, she has very little support. She was formerly a regular churchgoer, but has had to remain at home because of transportation problems, limited funds, her husband's illness, and her poor health state. Despite her problems she has been able to care for herself and her husband.

ASSESSMENT CRITERIA
Physical
Cardiovascular
  Presence of dysrhythmias on electrocardiogram (ECG)
  Presence of bruits over major arteries
  Quality of peripheral and central pulses (compare side to side)
  Abnormal blood pressure
  Presence of orthostatic blood pressure changes
  Abnormal heart sounds (S_3, S_4, murmurs)
  History of angina
  History of myocardial infarction
Respiratory
  Abnormal breath sounds
  Mild to moderate dyspnea on exertion
  Orthopnea
  Paroxysmal nocturnal dyspnea
  Reduced vital capacity
Gastrointestinal
  Increased weight
  Dietary patterns and tolerance
  Nausea/vomiting
  Presence of bowel sounds
  Stools (color, amount, consistency, occult blood)
Genitourinary
  Nocturia
  Frequency of voiding, quantity and quality of urine

Integument
   Capillary refilling
   Presence of vascular or diabetic skin lesions
   Presence of peripheral edema
   Presence of nicotine stains on nails and fingers
   Skin vital signs: color, temperature, and moisture
   Xanthomata
Musculoskeletal
   Ability to perform activities of daily living (ADLs)
   Muscle tone and strength
   Joint range of motion
   Fatigue
   Level of activity
   Presence of intermittent claudication
Neurological
   Communication skills (ability to express feelings)
   Hearing, speech, thought processes
   Recent and remote memory
   Vision changes
Diagnostic tests
   Arterial blood gases
   Serum creatine
   Lipid levels: HDL, LDL, cholesterol, and triglyceride
   Electrolytes
   BUN
   Urinalysis
   CK and CK-MB isoenzymes
   Liver function studies: SGOT, SGPT, lactate dehydrogenase (LDH) isoenzymes
   Uric acid
   Blood glucose
   Hemoglobin and hematocrit
   Thyroid function tests: thyroid-stimulating hormone (TSH), triiodothyronine (T_3), and thyroxine (T_4)
   Chest x-ray
   Exercise stress test
   12-lead ECG
   Technetium pyrophosphate scan
   Cardiac catheterization

Psychosocial

Habits: smoking; alcohol intake greater than 2 ounces per day
Support systems
Degree of drive and hostility
Response to stress and anxiety level
Mood disturbances
Recent life stresses/interpersonal problems
Risk factors: gout, diabetes, obesity, hyperlipidemia
Sleep disturbances
Cultural beliefs

Spiritual

Presence of ambivalent feelings about religious beliefs
Concern with the meaning of life or death
Participation in usual religious practices
Desire for spiritual assistance

General

Age
Educational level
Vital signs, including height and weight
Allergies
Medications, including over-the-counter preparations and problems with adherence
Past medical illnesses
Family health history
Knowledge of disease and treatment
Tolerance to exercise stress test

Mrs. Morgan is having increased angina because her coronary arteries are affected by the atherosclerotic lesions. The fact that the episodes are increasing in frequency and duration indicates a possible acceleration of the atherosclerotic process in the coronary arteries. Her peripheral pulses are diminished, and she has a carotid bruit, which also suggests significant arterial vascular disease.

Mrs. Morgan's elevated blood pressure indicates that her hypertension is not presently controlled, resulting in an increased work load on the heart and further reduction in coronary blood flow. The rapid heart rate of 108 beats/min is further reducing the coronary artery filling that occurs during diastole and thus increasing the likelihood that angina will occur.

Mrs. Morgan's irregular heart beat and premature ventricular contractions (PVCs) are probably secondary to the low potassium level and/or ongoing ischemia of the myocardium.

The bibasilar crackles and labored respiration that Mrs. Morgan is experiencing could be due to any one or combination of the following: (1) a decrease in circulating oxygen secondary to lung damage from cigarette abuse, (2) fluid imbalance, (3) obesity, (4) lowered activity tolerance, and (5) inability of the coronary arteries to meet the demands of the myocardium. The blood gas results indicate partially compensated metabolic acidosis with an acceptable Po_2.

The elevated glucose level, excess weight, and elevated blood pressure could be indicators of noncompliance with medical therapies. Because of the stress this client is experiencing relative to finances and the health problems of herself and her husband, there is a need to examine the factors that may cause noncompliance and to involve support services in her care.

The fact that Mrs. Morgan has a positive family history and long-standing hypertension indicates a need to reduce modifiable risk factors.

The low CK-MB levels and normal LDH-1 to LDH-2 ratios may indicate that Mrs. Morgan has not yet suffered a myocardial infarction. Serial blood tests are indicated, since these enzymes take hours to leak into the bloodstream after myocardial damage has occurred. A technetium pyrophosphate scan could help to identify the presence of a previous MI in the presence of normal enzyme studies.

Mrs. Morgan's abnormally low hemoglobin level and hematocrit could cause angina secondary to decreased oxygen-carrying capacity of the blood. Since Mrs. Morgan has a positive fluid imbalance, hemodilution should be considered a possible cause of the low values. The fact that her stools are guaiac negative is also important to note.

Mrs. Morgan's elevated lipid levels put her at greater risk for acceleration of the atherosclerosis, and may be a consequence of nonadherence to recommended dietary restrictions, inadequate glucose control, and/or genetic predisposition.

The elevated white blood cell count could be the result of an infectious process, stress, or the invasive cardiac procedures she has undergone during hospitalization.

Mrs. Morgan has not complained of anginal pain while in the hospital. However, it is important to note that diabetic clients may have silent MIs or other anginal equivalents that are silent because of loss of sensory function secondary to diabetic vascular neuropathy.

NURSING CARE PLAN: ATHEROSCLEROTIC HEART DISEASE

Nursing diagnoses	Expected client outcomes	Nursing strategies
Activity intolerance related to chest pain (angina) secondary to decreased coronary reserve	Client will be able to participate in graduated forms of exercise without experiencing angina	Determine limitations for exercise on the basis of diagnostic tests and physician orders
	Client will verbalize less difficulty when carrying on routine ADLs	Question client about the amount of activity that precipitates chest discomfort; then progressively increase activities to tolerance as per orders
	Client will recognize the precipitating events that may cause anginal attacks	
	Client will have fewer anginal attacks	Teach client ways to minimize precipitating events (e.g., exercise, stress, overeating, exposure to cold, or hot humid conditions)
	Client will be able to describe activity and modify activity plans so as to prevent anginal symptoms	Develop activity plans that will balance myocardial oxygenation demands with supply and help the client to adjust activity level below that which causes anginal symptoms
	Client's angina or anginal equivalent will be promptly identified and treated effectively	Assess client frequently for signs of discomfort and the need for analgesics by noting facial and verbal expressions and restlessness
		Monitor blood pressure, heart rate, respiratory rate, and ECG during exercise/activity, and stop if symptoms or ECG changes appear or at the achievement of an age-predicted maximum heart rate
	Client will incorporate rest periods into her daily routine to prevent overexertion and fatigue	Assist client in developing daily activity routine that takes advantage of peak energy levels and allows for adequate rest
		While client is hospitalized, space rest periods with exercise or performance of ADLs to take advantage of peak energy levels

Continued.

NURSING CARE PLAN: ATHEROSCLEROTIC HEART DISEASE—cont'd

Nursing diagnoses	Expected client outcomes	Nursing strategies
Altered nutrition: more than body requirement for fats, cholesterol, calories; related to decreased caloric requirements with aging and to a lack of knowledge regarding nutritional needs	Client or significant other will verbalize knowledge of the relationship between food intake, metabolism, exercise, and body weight	Assess for potential obstacles to adherence to recommended dietary changes, basic nutritional knowledge, ethnic or cultural values affecting food intake, and current eating patterns
	Client will eat 1800-calorie ADA diet, with low cholesterol and 2-g/day sodium restriction	Provide teaching materials appropriate to client's educational level and sensory capabilities Initiate teaching based on identified obstacles and concerns expressed by client: Explain basic nutritional concepts Explain hazards of obesity as related to client's medical problem Explain benefits of exercise
	Client will have lower serum lipid levels and a blood glucose level within an acceptable range	Instruct client about a diet that is low in saturated fats, cholesterol, and salt and high in complex carbohydrates and fiber; emphasize the positive aspects of dietary intervention (e.g., what the client can eat rather than what she cannot eat) Refer client to diabetic support group
Knowledge deficit: modifiable risk factors of atherosclerotic heart disease (cigarette smoking, diabetes mellitus, obesity, hypertension, lack of exercise, stress) and diagnostic tests, medications, and other treatment modalities; related to lack of previous experience	Client and significant other will identify the risk factors associated with the disease Client will take steps to modify risk factors: cease or reduce smoking, increase activity level, and recognize relationship between coping strategies and the resulting outcomes	Assess client and significant other for readiness to learn, level of knowledge about the reduction of risk factors, diagnostic tests, and medical treatment and medications prior to instruction Teach client and significant other about risk factors associated with the development of atherosclerotic heart disease Teach the effects of smoking on oxygen transport, coronary risk factors, and the HDL/LDL ratios; the relationship between energy expenditure and weight; and physiological manifestations of stress
	Client and significant other will demonstrate understanding of prescribed diagnostic tests and procedures	Explain in simple terms the purpose, rationale, and preparation for diagnostic testing and treatment plans
	Client and significant other will verbalize knowledge of prescribed medications	Teach client the name, dose, frequency, action, and side effects of prescribed medications Use efficient and effective teaching strategies appropriate to the situation (e.g., pamphlets, audiovisual aids, repetition, discussion, demonstration, return demonstration) Allow time for review and reinforcement of materials presented
Anxiety related to change in health status	Client and significant other will exhibit less anxiety and be able to discuss fears and concerns openly	Assess the client and significant other's level of anxiety Teach stress-reduction or relaxation techniques or constructive problem solving Use support services and persons when providing reassurance and support Give simple explanations, in terms the client can understand, at appropriate times and as often as necessary Allow client and significant other to discuss their fears and concerns regarding heart disease, hospitalization, and treatment

NURSING CARE PLAN: ATHEROSCLEROTIC HEART DISEASE—cont'd

Nursing diagnoses	Expected client outcomes	Nursing strategies
Potential for decreased cardiac output related to decreased myocardial contractility secondary to atherosclerotic heart disease	Client will not develop signs of decreased cardiac output: decreased blood pressure, increased heart rate, decreased urine output, cool clammy skin, or heart failure	Assess the client's blood pressure, pulses, ECG, and respiratory status to determine baseline Assess heart sounds, lung sounds, and vital signs every 2-4 hours or as indicated by client's status; weigh daily; monitor intake and output and electrolytes Assess skin for color, temperature, dryness; inspect for signs of peripheral or dependent edema Assess for jugular vein distention (JVD); assess mental status

EVALUATION

1. The client describes plans for pacing activity, rest, and exercise after discharge.
2. The client participates in a prescribed progressive activity plan within established guidelines.
3. The client reports an increase in physical endurance and stamina.
4. The client and/or significant other discuss measures that will decrease the likelihood of chest pain occurring during activity.
5. Coronary circulation has improved as a result of regular exercise, as evidenced by the client's ability to participate in moderate forms of activity without chest discomfort.
6. The client verbalizes acceptance of the dietary revisions as part of her every day life-style and demonstrates compliance with the diet.
7. The client maintains desired changes in her diet as evidenced by normal lipid levels and acceptable blood glucose levels for her age.
8. The client and significant other demonstrate adequate knowledge regarding low-cholesterol, complex-carbohydrate diets; calorie consumption in relation to body requirements; an exercise program; stress and ways to reduce it; and the role of life-style changes in the reduction of risk factors for atherosclerotic heart disease.
9. The client has ceased smoking, and is no longer dyspneic on exertion.
10. The client has modified her life-style and eliminated risk factors to reduce the chances of sustaining another myocardial infarction.
11. The client verbalizes understanding of prescribed tests and procedures.
12. The client can state the name, dose, frequency, purpose, action, and side effects of each prescribed medication.
13. The client experiences less anxiety, and her sense of well-being has improved.
14. The client is optimistic about her prognosis.
15. The client has optimal cardiac output.

NURSING ALERTS

1. The physician should be consulted in the development of an exercise program for the client.
2. Sexual activity is frequently neglected in teaching; it is an area that should be discussed with the client.
3. Persons with a history of chest pain at rest or during minimal activity are at risk for an infarction or death during exercise testing.

Bibliography

Brunner LS and Suddarth DS, editors: Textbook of medical-surgical nursing, ed 5, Philadelphia, 1984, JB Lippincott Co.

Diethrich EB: Condemned: is there an alternative for the patient with severe coronary disease? Critical Care Nurse Quarterly 9(4):8, 1987.

Gelfant B: Stress assessment of the M.I. patient, The Journal of Practical Nursing 10:44, 1984.

Gettrust Kathy, Ryan SC, and Engelman D, editors: Applied nursing diagnosis: guides for comprehensive care planning, New York, 1985, John Wiley & Sons, Inc.

Hudak C et al: Critical care nursing, ed 2, Philadelphia, 1981, JB Lippincott Co.

Long BC and Phipps WJ, editors: Medical-surgical nursing: a nursing process approach, ed 2, St Louis, 1985, The CV Mosby Co.

Luckmann J, and Sorensen KC: Medical-surgical nursing: a psychophysiologic approach, ed 3, Philadelphia, 1987, WB Saunders Co.

Michaelson CR: Bedside assessment and diagnosis of acute left ventricular failure, Critical Care Quarterly 4(3):1, 1981.

Nesbitt B: Nursing diagnosis in age-related changes, Gerontological Nursing 14(7):7, 1988.

Schroeder SA et al, editors: Current medical diagnosis and treatment, Norwalk, Conn, 1989, Appleton & Lange.

Solack SD: Assessment of psychogenic stresses in the coronary patient, Cardiovascular Nursing 15(4):16, 1979.

Thompson JM et al: Mosby's manual of clinical nursing, ed 2, St Louis, 1989, The CV Mosby Co.

Vitello-Cicciu J: Risk-factor modification in the prevention of coronary heart disease, Journal of Cardiovascular Nursing 1(4):67, 1987.

Wyngaarden JB and Smith LH Jr: Cecil textbook of medicine, vol 1, ed 18, Philadelphia, 1988, JB Lippincott Co.

Ischemic Heart Disease and Cardiac Catheterization

Sharon Bowles

KNOWLEDGE BASE

1. Angina can be differentiated from the pain that results from myocardial infarction (see Table 3). However, older persons do not always exhibit the expected signs and symptoms. Look for a blunted or atypical presentation.
2. The occurrence of coronary artery disease increases with advanced age, as a result of calcification of the tunica media layer and loss of elasticity of the arteries. Most persons age 70 and over have the disease in some form.
3. The aged heart has relatively less blood in the coronary arteries because the venous vessels and sinusoids dominate. In childhood, the capillary network and coronary arteries dominate.
4. At age 60, the maximum coronary blood flow is estimated to be 35% less than that of a younger adult.
5. Angina pectoris, or angina, is chest pain or discomfort resulting from an imbalance between oxygen supply and oxygen demand of the heart muscle.
6. As increased oxygen is needed with an increase in exercise, consumption of a heavy meal, exposure to cold, or excessive emotional stress or excitement, the supply may decrease, thereby causing symptoms of anginal pain. The decreased supply may be due to the formation of atherosclerotic plaques in the arteries as well as to conditions of generalized vasoconstriction, orthostatic hypotension, hypertension, hypovolemia, or valvular disorders.
7. Names associated with angina include stable or unstable angina, crescendo angina, preinfarction angina, progressive angina, the intermediate syndrome, anginal decubitus, nocturnal angina, and Printzmetal's angina. The nurse should consult a cardiac textbook for differentiation and further information.
8. Angina is not commonly seen in the 80-and-over age group, possibly because of reduction in physical activity in this population.
9. Diagnostic tests for angina include laboratory work, electrocardiographic and/or Holter monitoring, exercise electrocardiography (stress test), nuclear imaging, and cardiac catheterization.
10. Cardiac catheterization, also called coronary angiography and angiocardiography, is used to determine the presence and extent of coronary artery disease as the etiology of chest pain. Cardiac catheterization is an invasive procedure involving insertion, under fluoroscopy, of a radiopaque catheter through an artery and/or vein into the heart. Determinations of intracardiac pressures, oxygen levels, and cardiac output can be made. Radiopaque dye is injected to discern structure and motion of the chambers and valves as well as patency of the coronary arteries.
11. Complications of cardiac catheterization include myocardial infarction, cardiac tamponade, pulmonary embolism, and cerebral embolism. These complications rarely occur. Less severe complications include dysrhythmias, dye reactions, infection, hematoma and/or internal bleeding at the catheter insertion site, and impaired distal perfusion of the catheterized extremity.
12. The nurse's role with a client having cardiac catheterization primarily involves care before and after the procedure, since the procedure takes place in a specialized laboratory. It would be helpful for a nurse who cares for such clients to observe a cardiac catheterization procedure.
13. Cardiac catheterization may be performed on an elective or emergency basis and as an outpatient or inpatient procedure. Mortality following elective catheterization is less than 1%.
14. Cardiac catheterization can be performed safely in the aged but carries a higher risk than in younger clients.
15. When nitroglycerin is prescribed, its principal effects are to dilate the coronary arteries and/or collateral vessels, which increases circulation to the heart muscle (unless the coronary arteries are severely atherosclerotic), and to dilate the peripheral blood vessels, which reduces afterload.
16. Activity restrictions and life-style modifications are aimed at reducing oxygen demands on the heart.
17. If hypothyroidism is a concurrent condition, caution should be used in administering replacement thyroid hormone, since it may aggravate angina.

Table 3 **Differentiation of pain: angina versus myocardial infarction**

	Angina	Myocardial infarction
Description/location	Mild to moderate, usually similar with each attack; substernal, retrosternal	Severe, crushing, squeezing, burning, sharp
	More diffuse and not as easily located	Radiation to neck, jaw, arms, back
	May radiate	May be associated with dyspnea, diaphoresis, nausea/vomiting, apprehension
Precipitating factors	Usually brought on by exertion, heavy meal, emotional distress, etc.	Not necessarily brought on by precipitating factors
Onset/duration	Onset either gradual or sudden	Onset is sudden
	Usually brief pain; lasts 15 minutes or less	May last 20-30 minutes up to 2-3 hours
	Relieved by rest, nitroglycerin	Not relieved by rest or nitroglycerin

CASE STUDY

Mr. Pantel is a 68-year-old retired banker. Two weeks before admission, Mr. Pantel was vacationing with his wife and experienced a sudden onset of chest pain while sight-seeing. The pain was substernal, with some radiation to the left arm, and was accompanied by diaphoresis and pallor. He was examined at a local hospital, diagnosed with angina, and released with sublingual nitroglycerin tablets. The physician recommended that Mr. Pantel see his regular physician upon returning home. Mr. Pantel has continued to have attacks of chest pain on exertion (e.g., walking long distances and yard work), each lasting approximately 10 minutes and accompanied by diaphoresis. The pain is relieved with 1 to 2 nitroglycerin tablets and rest. Mr. Pantel has seen his regular physician and now enters the hospital with a diagnosis of ischemic heart disease. He is to have a cardiac catheterization. Admission blood pressure is 124/86, pulse is regular at 76 beats/min, and respiration is unlabored at 18 breaths/min. Mr. Pantel denies chest pain at this time. He states: "I hope this problem with my heart gets straightened out. I'm finally retired and the wife and I want to travel to all the places we didn't get to in our younger years."

ASSESSMENT CRITERIA
Physical

History of problem onset
  Date, time, and setting
  Slow or abrupt; noticeable to others?

Description of pain
  Location and radiation
  Quality
  Severity
  Timing
  Duration
  Associated symptoms (diaphoresis, dizziness, syncope, nausea and/or vomiting)
  Precipitating factors (exercise induced, during rest or sleep, after meals, stress induced, or on exposure to cold)
  Alleviating factors (rest, position change, nitroglycerin—note amount taken, frequency, side effects)
Personal health history
  Previous heart problems
  Hypertension/stroke
  Diabetes
  Vascular disease
  Fatigue
  Presence of cardiac risk factors: dietary habits, smoking history, obesity, hyperlipidemia, stressors
  Medications, including over-the-counter preparations, and problems with adherence
  Other health problems
Family health history
  General health of client's children, siblings, and parents
  Age and cause of death of deceased family members
Physical assessment
  Vital signs: if irregular pulse noted, obtain rhythm strip by ECG machine or ECG monitor to assess dysrhythmias
  Heart sounds: auscultation with stethoscope for extra (unusual) heart sounds, murmurs, irregular rhythm
  Lung sounds: auscultation with stethoscope for crackles, rhonchi, etc.
Jugular vein distension (JVD)

Skin: color, temperature, turgor

Edema: pedal/sacral

Pulses: presence/absence and quality of carotid, radial, femoral, popliteal, and dorsalis pedis, and compare side to side

Neurovascular: alert and oriented to time, place, and person

Gastrointestinal: nausea/vomiting; bowel sounds present in all four quadrants

Psychosocial

Life-style: description of typical day, recreation/leisure profile, occupational profile, living environment profile

Perception of and reaction to heart condition, assessment and treatment modalities

Knowledge of heart condition and treatment course

Perception of stressors and interpersonal conflicts/problems

Resources/support systems used

Concerns regarding sexuality and sexual function

Spiritual

Religious practices/beliefs

Effect of illness/hospitalization on belief system

Need for spiritual assistance

Angina pectoris pain is transient. It is usually linked to emotional or physical stress and often subsides with cessation of the stress. Nitroglycerin tablets dilate the coronary arteries and have been effective in pain relief for Mr. Pantel.

There is a familial tendency toward heart disease. Mr. Pantel has one brother who had an uncomplicated heart attack at age 60.

Mr. Pantel's essentially unremarkable initial assessment is a common phenomenon. However, further and more extensive assessment procedures may result in identification of problems that contribute to his ischemic heart disease.

Angina pectoris causes ischemia of the heart muscle but not necrosis. Pain is usually substernal, often radiating up the neck to the jaw and/or the left arm and hand. The presence of diaphoresis and pallor with anginal pain is common.

Mr. Pantel's "will to live" and desire for health are evident by his comments on admission.

NURSING CARE PLAN: ISCHEMIC HEART DISEASE AND CARDIAC CATHETERIZATION

Nursing diagnoses	Expected client outcomes	Nursing strategies
Potential decreased cardiac output, related to mechanical disorder of ischemic heart disease and structural disorder of age-related changes	Client will demonstrate improved or normal cardiac output	Monitor blood pressure, pulse, respiration, and temperature Auscultate lung sounds for crackles, rhonchi, etc. Auscultate heart sounds for abnormal (extra) heart sounds, murmurs; note: the onset of a new S_3 should be reported immediately Assess skin for color, warmth, and dryness Inspect for signs of peripheral or dependent edema Assess for presence of jugular vein distension Assess mentation

Potential for altered comfort: chest pain, related to anginal attacks	Client will experience no chest pain or discomfort or will have relief from symptoms	Instruct client to report pain immediately
		Obtain and document detailed description of pain, including:
		  Onset
		  Location and radiation
		  Quality
		  Timing
		  Duration
		  Severity
		  Associated symptoms
		Assess blood pressure, heart rate, and respiration with each pain episode; assess blood pressure and pulse every 5 minutes or as ordered until pain has subsided
		Administer nitroglycerin and analgesics as ordered
		Administer oxygen at 2-4 liters/min by nasal cannula, as prescribed
		Remain with client during pain episode

NURSING CARE PLAN: ISCHEMIC HEART DISEASE AND CARDIAC CATHETERIZATION—cont'd

Nursing diagnoses	Expected client outcomes	Nursing strategies

Knowledge deficit: self-administration of sublingual nitroglycerin; related to lack of previous experience	Client will verbalize knowledge and demonstrate proper use of sublingual nitroglycerin	Instruct client on purpose and use of sublingual nitroglycerin tablets
		  Place tablet under the tongue at the onset of pain
		  Stop activity with the onset of pain, and sit or lie down
		  Monitor time: take a second nitroglycerin tablet after 5 minutes and a third tablet in another 5 minutes if the pain is unrelieved
		  A tingling or burning sensation under the tongue indicates that the tablet is activated
		  Head throbbing, headache, and/or flushing may be felt, and is a normal side effect
		  Caution the client not to sit or stand suddenly after nitroglycerin administration
		  Report the pain immediately

Potential activity intolerance, related to ischemic heart disease and/or anginal attacks	Client will identify factors that increase myocardial demands for oxygen Client will perform activities of daily living within established cardiac guidelines	Explain to client: Relationship between increased work of the heart and increased oxygen demand; causes of increased heart oxygen demand Teach energy conservation methods for activities Allow client to participate in and complete self-care activities as tolerated Organize care to allow for adequate rest, and take advantage of peak energy levels Assist with progression of activity and document responses before, during, and after activity, including blood pressure, heart rate, respiration, and tolerance Instruct client to stop an activity if anginal pain occurs
Potential anxiety, related to change in health status	Client will experience an increase in psychological comfort as evidenced by both verbal and nonverbal communications	Establish rapport with client and maintain confident, consistent manner Assess and acknowledge anxiety/ ask open-ended questions to facilitate communication Explain the illness/disease, routine procedures, and expected activities as the client is ready; use simple terminology, clarify and repeat as necessary, and use positive approach Support and encourage information sharing between client and family; answer family's questions factually Support use of usual coping skills

Before cardiac catheterization
Potential anxiety, related to unknown experience of heart catheterization
	Client will experience a decrease in anxiety after gaining knowledge of cardiac catheterization procedure	Assess level of knowledge of procedure; explain the following, as needed:
		Purpose of the cardiac catheterization
		Pre-catheterization preparation:
		  Pre-testing such as chest x-ray, 12-lead ECG, blood tests
		  Necessity for taking nothing by mouth or for limited fluid intake
		  Attire (e.g., hospital gown, dentures in, eye glasses on if preferred, hearing aid in; note: check with catheterization laboratory personnel regarding specific protocol)
		  Use of bathroom prior to premedication

Continued.

NURSING CARE PLAN: ISCHEMIC HEART DISEASE AND CARDIAC CATHETERIZATION—cont'd

Nursing diagnoses	Expected client outcomes	Nursing strategies

Potential anxiety, related to unknown experience of heart catheterization—cont'd	Client will experience a decrease in anxiety after gaining knowledge of cardiac catheterization procedure—cont'd	Premedication and possible side effects (e.g., dry mouth, blurred vision)
		 Mode of transportation to catheterization laboratory
		 Expected length of procedure (1½-3 hours)
		   Expected experience in the catheterization laboratory:
		     Hard bed with large equipment surrounding client
		     Attire of personnel in laboratory (e.g., masks, gowns)
		     IV inserted; client attached to constant ECG monitoring
		     General overview of procedure, including compliance requests:
		       Will be instructed to cough (after dye injected) and breathe deeply at intervals
		       Should immediately report if chest pain occurs
		     Any pain or discomfort to be expected:
		       Local skin anesthetic at catheter insertion site feels like a "bee sting"
		       Sensation of hot flash or flushing when dye injected
		       May feel urgency to urinate when dye injected
		       Tenderness/soreness at catheter insertion site after catheter removed
		   Post-catheterization interventions:
		     Frequent vital signs
		     Sandbag or pressure dressing on catheter insertion site
		     Bed rest for 6-12 hours
		     Allow time for clarification and questions

After cardiac catheterization

Nursing diagnoses	Expected client outcomes	Nursing strategies
Potential decreased cardiac output, related to heart catheterization procedure	Client will demonstrate normal or improved cardiac output	Monitor vital signs at frequent intervals (e.g., every 15 minutes for 4 times, then every 30 minutes for 4 times, then every 1-4 hours as needed and/or prescribed); for other assessment parameters, see first nursing diagnosis in this table Obtain ECG rhythm strip or 12-lead ECG if persistent abnormal rhythm noted with pulse Instruct client to report chest pain immediately; see second nursing diagnosis in this table Encourage fluid intake, unless contraindicated (e.g., potential congestive heart failure)

Potential for injury related to invasive catheter insertion	Client will comply with limited activity; perfusion to affected extremity will remain normal	Instruct the client to remain on bed rest 6-12 hours, as prescribed
		   Encourage turning side-to-side
		   Leg or arm of affected extremity should remain straight
		   Encourage frequent flexing of ankle and toes or fingers and wrist of affected extremity
		 Use precautionary measures (side rails; bed in low position), since client will be sleepy from premedication and fatigued from procedure

NURSING CARE PLAN: ISCHEMIC HEART DISEASE AND CARDIAC CATHETERIZATION—cont'd

Nursing diagnoses	Expected client outcomes	Nursing strategies
Potential for injury related to invasive catheter insertion—cont'd	Client will comply with limited activity; perfusion to affected extremity will remain normal—cont'd	Observe catheter insertion site for bleeding or hematoma 　Use pressure as indicated (e.g., sandbag, pressure bandage) 　Change dressing as per physician's order Assess distal peripheral pulses of affected extremity at frequent intervals (same regimen as vital signs) 　Popliteal and dorsalis pedis pulses for leg 　Radial pulse for arm 　Compare with pulses in opposite extremity Note strength of pulses and immediately report if pulses are absent or strength is diminishing
Potential for infection related to invasive catheter insertion	Client will experience normal healing process at site of catheter insertion	Adhere to hospital policies and procedures relating to aseptic techniques and infection control Maintain aseptic wound care and change dressings as indicated; observe wound for redness, swelling, drainage, and heat Note and report temperature elevation
Potential anxiety, related to unknown outcome of heart catheterization	Client will verbalize feelings of anxiousness concerning heart catheterization outcome Client will use effective coping skills in managing anxiety	Demonstrate you are available to help; listen attentively; offer support and reassurance as client talks Be supportive of healthy coping skills exhibited; provide options for managing anxiety Be with client when physician explains results of heart catheterization to client and family Reinforce and clarify explanation as needed
Knowledge deficit: post-catheterization and discharge regimen; relates to lack of previous experience	Client will communicate knowledge and understanding of self-care adjustments and resources after discharge	Explain to client: 　Care of wound and signs and symptoms to report (e.g., redness, swelling, drainage, heat) 　Signs and symptoms related to ischemic heart disease to report (e.g., shortness of breath, chest pain unrelieved by nitroglycerin tablets, dizziness, syncope, palpitations, excessive fatigue) 　Physician follow-up appointments 　Prescribed medications, including name, dosage, frequency, therapeutic effects, side effects 　Instructions related to use of sublingual nitroglycerin tablets; see nursing strategies for nitroglycerin instruction, plus the following: 　　Always carry nitroglycerin 　　A tablet may be taken before strenuous exercise or in emotionally stressful situations that usually precipitate anginal attacks 　　If pain is not relieved after client has taken 3 tablets, medical attention should be sought 　　Store tablets in a dark, airtight container and replenish supply every 6 months or before expiration date 　Instructions related to nitroglycerin skin patches: 　　How to apply 　　Skin care

Continued.

NURSING CARE PLAN: ISCHEMIC HEART DISEASE AND CARDIAC CATHETERIZATION—cont'd

Nursing diagnoses	Expected client outcomes	Nursing strategies

Knowledge deficit: post-catheterization and discharge regimen; relatres to lack of previous experience—cont'd	Client will communicate knowledge and understanding of self-care adjustments and resources after discharge—cont'd	Need for site rotation and preferred sites of application
		Frequency of changes
		Caution not to sit or stand suddenly
		Sublingual nitroglycerin may be used in addition to skin patches if needed
		  Dietary modifications (e.g., sodium restriction, low fat/low cholesterol diet)
		  Activity restrictions, if any (including client's own precipitating factors and ways to decrease):
		    Ingestion of heavy meals
		    Extremes of temperature
		    Sexual activity
		    Emotional stress
		    Prophylactic nitroglycerin
		  Life-style modifications to reduce cardiac risk factors (e.g., stress, hypertension, smoking, obesity)
		  Community resources available (e.g., cardiac rehabilitation, support groups)
		Provide the family members an opportunity to share their concerns and comprehend the client's self-care adjustments

EVALUATION

1. The client maintains adequate cardiac output as evidenced by normal vital signs; clear lungs; normal heart sounds; skin that is warm, dry, and pink; no edema or JVD; and usual mentation.
2. The client verbalizes knowledge and complies with appropriate use of prescribed nitroglycerin for anginal attacks.
3. The client limits activities as necessary.
4. The client displays and verbalizes a reduction in or resolution of anxiety.
5. The client verbalizes comprehension of heart catheterization, including care before and after the procedure.
6. The client's cardiac output remains unchanged after cardiac catheterization.
7. The client experiences no complications as a result of cardiac catheterization, including hemorrhage or excessive bleeding at the catheter insertion site, infection, or decreases in peripheral pulses of the affected extremity.
8. The client verbalizes understanding of the results of the cardiac catheterization and the physician's recommendations.
9. The client verbalizes comprehension of the postdischarge regimen
   a. Wound care and signs and symptoms of complications to report
   b. Heart disease and accompanying signs and symptoms to report
   c. Follow-up appointments(s) with the physician
   d. Prescribed medications, including use, dose, frequency, therapeutic effects, side effects
   e. Dietary modifications
   f. Activity restrictions
   g. Risk factors and life-style modifications
   h. Available community resources
10. The client's family is knowledgeable concerning the client's heart disease, follow-up care, and self-care regimen.

NURSING ALERTS

1. An elderly client may give less expression to pain than a younger client would. Shortness of breath, extreme fatigue, or syncope may be the presenting symptoms. This may be due partly to a decreased sensory ability in the elderly. Indigestion, hiatal hernia, ulcer, gallbladder disease, and muscular pain are often mistakenly diagnosed when the correct diagnosis is angina.
2. In the assessment of heart sounds, abnormal heart sounds of S_3, S_4, and murmurs may be noted. An S_4 is commonly seen in the elderly as a result of age-related decreased compliance of the heart musculature. The onset of a new S_3, a diastolic murmur, or a holosystolic murmur is serious.
3. When administering oxygen therapy (e.g., by nasal cannula), the nurse should discontinue its use when symptoms subside. Prolonged use will

cause dryness of nasal passages, thereby increasing client discomfort. Also, assessment of whether the client is primarily a mouth breather or a nose breather will assist the nurse in deciding whether a nasal cannula versus a mask should be used for the treatment.

4. Nitrate therapy should be used with caution in the elderly. Loss of vasomotor and baroreceptor activity increases the possibility of orthostatic hypotension, so a lower dose may be necessary.

Bibliography

Amsterdam E: Unstable angina: ischemic chest pain that mimics MI, Consultant 28(4):127, 1988.

Doenges ME, Moorhouse F, and Geissler AC: Nursing care plans: guidelines for planning patient care, ed 2, Philadelphia, 1989, FA Davis Co.

Eliopoulos C: Gerontological nursing, ed 2, Philadelphia, 1987, JB Lippincott Co.

Eliopoulos C: A guide to the nursing of the aging, Baltimore, 1987, Williams & Wilkins.

Gulanick M et al: Nursing care plans: nursing diagnosis and intervention, ed 2, St Louis, 1990, The CV Mosby Co.

Johanson BC et al: Standards for critical care, ed 3, St Louis, 1988, The CV Mosby Co.

Kee JL: Laboratory and diagnostic tests with nursing implications, ed 2, Norwalk, Conn, 1987, Appleton & Lange.

Lewis SM and Collier IC: Medical-surgical nursing: assessment and management of clinical problems, ed 2, New York, 1987, McGraw-Hill Book Co.

Long BC and Phipps WJ, editors: Medical-surgical nursing: a nursing process approach, ed 2, St Louis, 1989, The CV Mosby Co.

Matteson MA and McConnell ES: Gerontological nursing: concepts and practice, Philadelphia, 1988, WB Saunders Co.

Miller CL: Medications in Angina, Focus on Critical Care 15(4):22, 1988.

Pagana KD and Pagana TJ: Diagnostic testing and nursing implications: a case study approach, ed 3, St Louis, 1989, The CV Mosby Co.

Swearingen PL, Sommers MS, and Miller K: Manual of critical care: applying nursing diagnoses to adult critical illness, St Louis, 1988, The CV Mosby Co.

Ulrich SP, Canale SW, and Wendell SA: Nursing care planning guides: a nursing diagnosis approach, Philadelphia, 1986, WB Saunders Co.

Ventrua B: What you need to know about cardiac catheterization, RN 9:24, 1984.

Heart Failure

Shirley A. Saunders

KNOWLEDGE BASE

1. Structural and functional age-related changes of the heart increase impedance to left-ventricular ejection during exercise and stress, resulting in decreased cardiac output.
2. Sympathetic responsiveness decreases with advancing age, reducing the ability to augment heart rate and cardiac function under the stress of depressed left-ventricular function. Thus it takes longer for the heart rate to normalize after exertion.
3. Myocardial muscle contraction is prolonged and relaxation is delayed in the aged heart, leading to a possible reduction in subendocardial myocardial blood flow because of shortened diastole in certain cardiac diseases.
4. The mortality rate for heart failure increases with age.
5. The myocardium becomes more rigid, so it is slower in recovering its contractility and irritability. Consequently stress and tachycardia are poorly tolerated.
6. Blood more readily accumulates in the lower extremities because the valves in the veins become less efficient.
7. The aldosterone and renin responses to upright posture and sodium restriction are altered.
8. The respiratory muscles weaken and the rib cage becomes less flexible, causing a reduction in vital capacity and possibly a decrease in oxygen supply in the blood.
9. Reduced serum albumin levels lead to a decrease in the binding of some drugs, causing an increased serum availability of the free (active) form of some drugs.
10. The ability to fight off infection is reduced with age because of fewer lymphocytes and an impaired antibody response.
11. Heart failure may be caused by decreased myocardial contractility and/or by extreme demands placed on the myocardium.
12. The backward effects of left-ventricular pump failure are manifested by increased left-atrial pressure, increased pressure and volume in the left ventricle, increased pressure in the pulmonary capillary bed, and subsequent pulmonary edema.
13. The forward effects of left-ventricular pump failure are manifested by a decrease in cardiac output and a resultant reduction in perfusion of the vital organs and tissues.

14. The backward effects of right-ventricular pump failure are manifested by increased right-ventricular end-diastolic volume, increased right-atrial pressure, and increased congestion in the systemic venous circulation and organs.

15. The forward effects of right-ventricular pump failure are manifested by a decrease in blood flow to the lungs and right heart and a resultant decrease in cardiac output.

16. When the blood pressure is low, the renin-angiotension-aldosterone mechanism is activated, causing an increase in the resorption of sodium, chloride, and water.

17. Sympathetic stimulation during heart failure causes vasoconstriction in an attempt to increase the blood pressure and the perfusion to vital organs.

18. The heart rate increases during heart failure to increase cardiac output.

19. Decreased perfusion of the kidneys causes activation of the renin-angiotensin-aldosterone system, which results in an increase in the renal absorption of sodium, water, and chloride.

20. The reflex vasoconstriction that occurs during heart failure increases the resistance to ejection, lowers cardiac output, and increases the work load on the heart.

21. During heart failure hepatic blood flow is reduced, leading to reduced degradation of aldosterone and an increase in its concentration in the body.

22. Arteriolar vasodilators may be used during heart failure to decrease resistance to ventricular emptying, thereby increasing cardiac output.

23. Diuretics and venous dilators may be used to reduce preload, reduce ventricular filling pressures, and ultimately decrease pulmonary congestion.

24. Inotropic drugs may be given to a client in heart failure to improve ventricular contraction and increase cardiac output.

25. The intraaortic balloon pump may be used in severe cases of heart failure because of its ability to increase perfusion pressure through the coronary arteries, decrease left-ventricular work load, decrease myocardial oxygen consumption, and decrease resistance to left-ventricular emptying.

26. Progressive heart failure leads to severe hypoperfusion and cardiogenic shock and/or death.

27. Myocardial pump failure may result from a myocardial infarction, excess blood or fluid administration, valvular dysfunction, hypovolemia, renal dysfunction, constrictive myocardial muscle disorders, severe anemia, or endocrine disorders.

28. Hemodynamic monitoring allows for the measurement of cardiac pressures and assists in the evaluation of therapy in cardiac failure.

29. When the heart is failing, the myocardial fibers begin to stretch in an attempt to increase cardiac contractility. The result is dilatation of the ventricular chambers and an increase in the oxygen demand of the hypertrophic heart.

30. Anticoagulants are frequently administered because of the increased susceptibility to thromboembolism resulting from venous stasis, hemoconcentration after diuresis, and atrial dysrhythmias.

31. With advancing age blood flow to the kidneys decreases because of a decrease in cardiac output and an increase in peripheral vascular resistance. The resultant decrease in renal function predisposes the older adult to drug toxicities.

32. Supraventricular and ventricular dysrhythmias increase in frequency as a result of increased catecholamine release, myocardial ischemia, and distension of the heart chambers.

33. When cardiac output decreases, oxygen supply decreases. The tissues try to compensate for this by extracting more oxygen from the hemoglobin, causing venous oxygen saturation (SvO_2) to decrease.

34. The arteriovenous oxygen content difference may be widened when cardiac output is decreased.

35. The venous oxygen content represents the sum of oxygen attached to hemoglobin and that dissolved in plasma.

36. When oxygen consumption is constant (stable temperature, no change in musculature work), extraction per unit volume of blood decreases as cardiac output increases.

37. In pulmonary edema there is an imbalance between ventilation and perfusion, causing hypoxemia.

38. Renal failure can cause the excretion of calcium and the retention of phosphorus.

39. When the extracellular fluid becomes acidic, the kidneys reabsorb bicarbonate, shifting the pH toward normal; chloride ions are exchanged for bicarbonate ions and are excreted in the urine.

40. By the time peripheral edema is noticeable, a client will have accumulated approximately 10 pounds of extra fluid.

41. Gross pulmonary edema usually presents as acute alveolar hyperventilation with hypoxemia.

42. Peripheral edema may be caused by hypoproteinemia or chronic venous insufficiency.

43. Atrophic changes in the skin may make the skin turgor assessment less reliable.

44. Normal arterial blood gas (ABG) values: pH, 7.40; PCO_2, 35-45 mm Hg; bicarbonate, 22-26 mEq/L; PO_2, 80-100 mm Hg; oxygen saturation (SO_2), >95%

45. Normal mixed venous blood gas values: pH, 7.36; PCO_2, 45; PO_2, 35-45; SvO_2, 70-75%

46. Normal hemodynamic values:
    Cardiac output: 4-8 L/min; cardiac index: 2.5-4.5 L/min/m²
    Systemic vascular resistance represents the total resistance to blood flow in the systemic circulation. Normal: 900-1200 dynes/sec/cm^{-5}
    Pulmonary vascular resistance represents the total resistance to blood flow in the pulmonary circulation. (Normal: 150-250 dynes/sec/cm^{-5}

CASE STUDY

Mr. Nolan, a 70-year-old widower, had three myocardial infarctions 2 years ago. Despite compliance with medical therapy, his cardiac status has become increasingly more debilitating; he now gets severely dyspneic during minimal activity. His son states that Mr. Nolan has not eaten for over 4 days and is unable to care for himself. He is being admitted to the hospital for a cardiac workup and subsequent treatment. He presents in moderate respiratory distress. The initial assessment reveals the following findings:

Blood pressure, 180/110 mm Hg

Heart rate, 110 beats/min

Respiratory rate, 32 breaths/min

Sinus tachycardia with greater than 5 premature ventricular beats/min

Peripheral and central cyanosis

Productive cough of frothy, pink sputum

Moist crackles two thirds of the way up the lung fields

Generalized pitting peripheral edema up to the knees

Jugular vein distension of 6 cm

Positive hepatojugular reflex

Pronounced S_3 and S_4 gallop rhythm

Cool, diaphoretic extremities

Inappropriate verbal responses

Disorientation to time and place

Restlessness

Mr. Nolan's chest roentgenogram shows cardiomegaly and pulmonary congestion. His electrocardiogram (ECG) shows a pattern of left-ventricular hypertension. The client is diagnosed as having biventricular heart failure.

Mr. Nolan is started on supplemental oxygen at 40%, given by mask, and admitting laboratory specimens are drawn. Initial medical therapy consists of intravenous furosemide (Lasix) and morphine sulfate. Because of his critical status, this client is transferred to the coronary intensive care unit for hemodynamic monitoring and further medical management.

Initial laboratory data are as follows (normals are in parentheses):

Sodium, 128 mEq/L (135-145)

Potassium, 4.9 mEq/L (3.5-5.5)

Chloride, 85 mEq/L (96-106)

HCO_3^-, 26 mEq/L (22-25)

Total CO_2, 29 mEq/L (25-27)

BUN, 50 mg/dl (8-25)

Serum creatine, 3.7 mg/dl (.6-1.5)

Glucose, 148 mg/dl

Calcium, 8.6 mg/dl (8.9-10.3)

Phosphate, 8.0 mg/dl (2.3-4.3)

Magnesium, 2.5 mEq/L (1.5-2.5)

Plasma total protein, 6.0 g/dl (6.5-8.5)

Albumin, 2.9 g/dl (3.6-5)

Cholesterol, 280 mg/dl (0-239)

Alkaline phosphatase, 290 IU/L (38-126)

SGPT, 63 IU/L (7-53)

SGOT, 58 IU/L (11-47)

LDH, 280 IU/L (99-237)

CK-MB, <4 IU/L (0-12)

Creatine kinase, <27 IU/L (3-220)

Digoxin, 2.3 ng/ml (0.5-2)

RBC, 3,000,000/cu mm (4,500,000-5,700,000)

Hemoglobin, 12 g/dl (13-18)

Hematocrit, 31.5% (40.7-50.3)

MCH, 30 cu/mic (26.7-33.7)

MCHC, 33.3 g/dl (of whole blood) (32.7-35.5)

WBC, 15,200/cu mm (3800-9800)

Lymphocytes, 3% (20-54.3)

Granulocytes, 85% (38.7-74.5)

Monocytes, 2.5%, (2.7-9.8)

PT, 21.9 sec (12-15)

Pt ratio, 1.75 sec

PTT 60 sec (39-53)

Platelets, 490,000/cu mm

Urine specific gravity, 1.040 (1.000-1.035)

Urine pH, 5 (4.5-8)

Urobilinogen, 0.1 mg/dl (.1-1)

Urine albumin, negative

Ketones, negative

Occult blood, 3+

ABGs on a 40% mask: pH, 7.53; PCO_2, 28 mm Hg; PCO_2 23 mm Hg; PO_2, 64 mm Hg; Saturation, 92%

Mixed venous ABGs: pH, 7.37; PCO_2, 45 mm Hg; PO_2, 33 mg Hg; Cal HCO_3, 27 mm Hg; SvO_2, 60%

Arterial oxygen content (CaO_2: $(1.36 \times 10.3 \times 0.92) + (0.40 \times 0.003) = 12.889$

Mixed venous oxygen content (CvO_2: $(1.36 \times 10.3 \times 0.60) + (0.40 \times 0.003) = 8.406$; $CaO_2 - CvO_2 = 12.889 - 4.406 = 8.483$

$PAO_2 = (FiO_2 \times (BP - 47) - (1.25) \times PaCO_2$; $PAO_2 = 0.40 \times (760 - 47) - (1.25 \times 28) = 250.20$

a/A ratio = $PaO_2/PAO_2 = 64/250.29 = 0.26$ (Normal, >0.75; an a/A ratio less than 0.75 may indicate a low ventilation/perfusion (V/Q) ratio or a shunt.

A Swan-Ganz catheter was inserted. Opening pressures were as follows: PAS, 70; PAD, 35; RV, 65/9; RA, 11; PAOP, 26. Body surface area, 2.0 m²; cardiac output, 3.0 L/min; cardiac index, 1.6 L/min/m² (normal, 2.5-4.5); systemic vascular resistance, 3262 dynes/sec/cm^{-5} (normal, 900-1200); pulmonary vascular resistance, 551 dynes/sec/cm^{-5} (normal, 150-250); stroke volume, 27 ml/beat; stroke index, 14 ml/min/m^2.

A Foley catheter was inserted to monitor renal response. The initial drainage was 60 ml of dark, amber, concentrated urine.

After the above data were obtained, the following medications were started: dobutamine (Dobutrex) at 5 µg/kg/min, nitroprusside (Nipride) at 2 µg/kg/min, and heparin at 1000 units/hr.

ASSESSMENT CRITERIA
Physical
Brief history of problem onset and course
Respiratory
    Dyspnea on exertion or at rest
    Orthopnea
    Paroxysmal nocturnal dyspynea
    Cough (frothy white or pink-tinged sputum)
    Respiration: rate and rhythm, depth, equality, symmetry, labored, use of accessory muscles, retractions
    Breath sounds: bilateral corresponding areas for rales and wheezes
    Pleural effusions
    Respiratory alkalosis
Neurological
    Level of consciousness
    Mental status: orientation, attention and concentration, judgment, memory, thought content and processes, mood and affect
Cardiovascular
    Electrocardiogram for dysrhythmias
    Jugular venous pressure at 45-degree angle
    Inspect anterior chest wall for contour, pulsations, retractions, heaves
    Palpate precordium at apex, left sternal border, and base for thrill, point of maximal impulse (PMI)
    Auscultate all heart areas for systolic or diastolic murmurs, S_3, S_4, or pericardial friction rub
    Angina
    Blood pressure and pulse
Hemodynamic pressures
    Right-atrial pressures
    Pulmonary artery pressures
    Cardiac output (CO) and cardiac index (CI)
    Systemic vascular resistance (SVR)
    Pulmonary vascular resistance (PVR)
    Stroke volume (SV) and stroke index
Integument: color, moisture, temperature, turgor, edema
Musculoskeletal
    Activity intolerance
    Weakness and fatigue

Gastrointestinal
    Nausea, vomiting
    Abdominal distension
    Anorexia
    Constipation
    Hepatojugular reflex
    Splenomegaly
Genitourinary
    History of weight changes
    Oliguria
    Nocturia
    Elevated blood urea nitrogen (BUN), serum creatinine, and serum electrolytes

Psychosocial
Client's perception of and reaction to diagnosis, and regimen for treatment
Resources/support systems currently available to client and family
Life-style
    Description of typical day
    Recreation/leisure profile
    Occupational profile
    Living environment profile (obtain from collateral sources if client condition warrants)
    Family profile

Spiritual
Usual religious practices/beliefs
Effect of illness and hospitalization on belief system
Need for spiritual assistance

General
Serum sodium level
Hemoglobin and hematocrit values
Blood coagulation studies

Mr. Nolan has become increasingly more dyspneic during minimal activity because his heart is no longer able to keep up with the oxygen demands of the body. In addition, lowering his head below 90 degrees further compromises his respiratory status, causing extreme anxiety and dyspnea.

This client's rapid and labored respiration is caused by a decrease in ventilatory capacity secondary to lung congestion.

The audible lung crackles two thirds of the way up his lung fields and the S_4 gallop represent failure of the left ventricle to adequately pump its contents into the systemic circulation.

The production of pink frothy sputum indicates the accumulation of mucus in the lungs, thereby causing a ventilation/perfusion mismatch.

The ABG values indicate that Mr. Nolan has acute alveolar hyperventilation and mild hypoxemia. The chest x-ray film confirms the presence of pulmonary congestion and dilatation of the heart chambers.

The widened arteriovenous oxygen difference coincides with the low cardiac output and cardiac index.

This client has a low a/A ratio, indicating a low ventilation/perfusion (V/Q) ratio or a shunt.

The restlessness and inappropriate verbal responses indicate inadequate perfusion of the brain and arterial hypoxemia.

The client's blood pressure and heart rate are abnormally elevated because of sympathetic stimulation secondary to hypoperfusion and vasoconstriction. These findings indicate that his body is attempting to compensate for the decrease in cardiac output.

The ventricular ectopy is probably due to myocardial ischemia resulting from decreased coronary artery perfusion.

Mr. Nolan is in atrial fibrillation, probably because of distension of the atrial muscle fibers.

Mr. Nolan is prone to emboli and mural thrombi because of venous stasis and atrial dysrhythmias, and therefore needs to be treated prophylactically with intravenous heparin.

The atrial and ventricular gallop sounds confirm the presence of heart muscle dysfunction.

Despite the fact that Mr. Nolan is at risk for angina during this bout of heart failure, he has not yet complained of angina or one of its equivalents.

Hemodynamic monitoring is indicated in this client because of the failure of both sides of the heart and the need for aggressive intravenous therapy to optimize his cardiac output.

The increased pulmonary capillary wedge pressure is due to the excessive pressures in the left side of the heart and lungs secondary to fluid retention and decreased pumping ability of the heart.

The right-atrial pressures are elevated as a result of depressed right heart functioning.

The high systemic vascular resistance, low cardiac output, and low cardiac index are further indicators of hypoperfusion, despite the elevated blood pressure of 180/110 mm Hg.

The presence of the Swan-Ganz catheter will enable the medical team to more effectively assess this client's venous and arterial oxygenation status.

The peripheral edema and jugular vein distension represent failure of the right side of the heart in pumping its contents to the pulmonary system for oxygenation.

The pitting edema indicates an increase in preload, which is commonly seen in clients with severe fluid imbalance and overload.

The cool, diaphoretic extremities indicate that blood is being diverted to the visceral organs as a result of vasoconstriction of the peripheral vessels, which increases peripheral vascular resistance.

The peripheral and central cyanosis represent pronounced tissue hypoxia secondary to the shunting of blood in the pulmonary circulation.

This client becomes more dyspneic with minimal activity. In addition, he is weak and appears to be exhausted as a result of the increased work of breathing.

Although bowel sounds are audible, Mr. Nolan has some abdominal distension, thought to be secondary to liver congestion and fluid accumulation. The hepatojugular reflex is present, indicating that the right side of the heart cannot tolerate an increase in blood flow without a corresponding increase in venous pressure, and it suggests right heart failure.

The low albumin and calcium levels suggest a nutritional deficit.

Mr. Nolan's urinary output has decreased because the renal system is attempting to compensate for decreased renal perfusion by preventing the excretion of water, chloride, and sodium.

His electrolytes are abnormal because of an acid-base imbalance resulting from to respiratory difficulties and altered renal perfusion.

The elevated BUN, serum creatinine, and digoxin levels indicate decreased renal perfusion. Hypoperfusion states lead to concentrated urine with a specific gravity greater than 1.025 and a low urine sodium level.

Although this client has not weighed himself lately, his wife states that he has become progressively more "swollen" over the past several weeks. Mr. Nolan's urinary output is being measured via a Foley catheter. Despite intravenous furosemide, he has excreted only 20 ml of urine during the first hour after the injection. More aggressive diuresis is indicated.

Because of his altered mental status resulting from hypoperfusion of the brain, Mr. Nolan will probably not be able to respond appropriately to assessment questions. However, he still needs to be made aware of what is happening to him, with frequent repetition of information.

This client's respiratory and cardiovascular difficulties are limiting his ability to participate in his usual religious practices.

The abnormally low sodium, hemoglobin, and hematocrit values could be a manifestation of hemodilution resulting from fluid overload. The prolonged partial thromboplastin time (PTT) is secondary to treatment with intravenous heparin.

 ## NURSING CARE PLAN: HEART FAILURE

Nursing diagnoses	Expected client outcomes	Nursing strategies

Decreased cardiac output related to electrical conduction disorders	Client will have optimal cardiac output as evidenced by:
	  Vital signs within normal range
	  Optimal hemodynamic pressures and cardiac output and adequate tissue perfusion
	  Normal fluid balance
	Client will have optimal respiratory function
	Client will demonstrate a reduction in cardiac work load
		Establish baseline vital signs
		Monitor vital signs as indicated by client's status and treatment
		Auscultate heart sounds for gallops and murmurs as indicated by client status changes and treatment
		Monitor hemodynamic parameters (pulmonary artery and pulmonary capillary wedge pressures, central venous pressure, cardiac output, cardiac index, stroke volume, intraarterial pressure, systemic vascular resistance, pulmonary vascular resistance) in response to treatment and as per orders
		Monitor positive and negative fluid status
		Weigh client daily with the same scale, at the same time, and with the same clothing, and report significant gains or losses
		Maintain sodium and fluid restrictions as per orders
		Administer diuretics (thiazides, loop diuretics, potassium-sparing diuretics) as ordered, and assess effectiveness
		Monitor electrolytes, edema, and vital signs in response to prescribed diuretic therapy
		Assess lung sounds; determine need to clear the airway (via suctioning) of retained secretions
		Monitor for orthopnea, paroxysmal nocturnal dyspnea, and dyspnea
		Assess effectiveness of treatment by monitoring arterial blood gases, arterial saturation, a/A ratio, arteriovenous oxygen content difference, mixed venous oxygen content, and hemoglobin
		Provide supplemental oxygen as ordered
		Inform client of need for bed rest and provide for same
		Administer preload and afterload reducers as ordered, and assess effectiveness
		Administer cardiac glycosides (digoxin), sympathomimetics (dopamine, dobutamine), and other positive inotropic drugs (amrinone) as per orders, and monitor effectiveness
		Administer stool softeners, and instruct client to avoid the Valsalva maneuver by exhaling when he moves about in bed, exercises, or moves his bowels

NURSING CARE PLAN: HEART FAILURE—cont'd

Nursing diagnoses	Expected client outcomes	Nursing strategies
Decreased cardiac output related to electrical conduction disorders—cont'd		Monitor actions of all prescribed drugs in terms of therapeutic effects, adverse effects, and toxic effects Maintain client in semi-Fowler's or high Fowler's position Plan care to provide frequent and adequate rest periods
Impaired gas exchange: decreased; related to altered capacity of blood to carry oxygen	Client will experience improved gas exchange as evidenced by comfortable breathing and less orthopnea and paroxysmal nocturnal dyspnea	Perform ongoing assessment of breathing Place client in semi-Fowler's position Place a pillow lengthwise behind the shoulders and back as indicated for dyspnea Support the arms on a pillow or over a bedside table Restrict participation in self-care activities as necessary Auscultate lung sounds, and determine the need to clear the airway via suctioning of retained secretions or facilitating cough Check peripheral pulses, skin temperature and color, and capillary filling time at regular intervals Monitor arterial and venous blood gases: arterial and venous saturations, a/A ratio, arteriovenous oxygen content difference Provide supplemental oxygen as per orders Detect and treat acid-base imbalances early as per orders Monitor for signs of hypoxia: changes in mental status, irritability, restlessness
Anxiety related to breathlessness and unknown outcome	Client will experience increased psychological comfort as evidenced by self-report of relaxed state Client will be able to identify anxiety and associated feelings Client and significant others will demonstrate ability to openly discuss concerns and feelings Client will use relaxation techniques	Provide supplemental oxygen as per orders Remain with client and provide reassurance during episodes of respiratory distress; be calm, consistent Decrease external stimulation, but allow presence of supportive family member or significant other Assist client with assessing situation and gaining insight into feelings, identifying coping skills Give frequent, realistic reassurance and let the client know that his feelings are normal Monitor the environment for hospital- and treatment-related stressors (e.g., noise, visitors, interruption in sleep patterns) Provide consistent caregivers, decrease stimulation, encourage family/significant other interaction, and provide distraction Discuss plans for improving cardiac functioning through cardiac rehabilitation program with client and significant other Develop trust and rapport by being nonjudgmental and genuine Promote verbal expressions of feelings and assist client in recognizing anxiety Encourage family members or significant others to verbalize concerns Demonstrate useful relaxation techniques such as rhythmic breathing, imagery Assess need for additional support services and counseling: clergy, social services, etc.

Continued.

NURSING CARE PLAN: HEART FAILURE—cont'd

Nursing diagnoses	Expected client outcomes	Nursing strategies

Potential altered thought processes, related to hypoxia and multiple stresses associated with hospitalization	Client will maintain cognitive functioning	Frequently assess mental status for:
		  Appropriate verbal responses
		  Orientation to person, place, and time
		  Ability to concentrate
		  Adequate recall of recent and past events
		  Ability to sleep soundly
		  Ability to participate in self-care
		Detect hypoxemia and acid-base imbalances so that treatment can be initiated promptly
		Provide supplemental oxygen as indicated (per orders) to keep arterial PO_2 greater than 60 mm Hg and oxygen saturation greater than 95%
		Monitor vital signs and respiratory status for changes that may precede mental status changes
		Provide meaningful sensory input; reduce nonessential stimuli
		Promote optimal hearing and vision
		Schedule care to provide for adequate rest and sleep periods
		Explain all procedures and activities
		Provide constant reassurance through a calm and caring presence

Potential for impaired skin integrity related to decreased tissue perfusion and prescribed immobility	Client will maintain skin integrity	Assess for risk factors associated with skin breakdown Assess all skin surfaces for lesions, and document Gently wash, dry, and apply lotion to skin surfaces daily and as needed Change position at least every 2 hours, and inspect areas of pressure for erythema, blanching, warmth, and tissue bogginess Assess need for preventive pressure-relief surface, and obtain order from physician Monitor laboratory values (albumin, sodium, BUN, uric acid, ABGs) as indicated Elevate edematous extremities If client is incontinent, cleanse perineum with a product that will not alter skin pH, and apply a protective-barrier product Avoid friction and shear with position changes and transfers
Activity intolerance related to insufficient oxygenation	Client will regain optimal activity tolerance Client will verbalize the rationale for activity restrictions	Optimize rest and restrict activities during the acute phase of the illness Explain reasons for prescribed therapeutic regimen and its effect on activity Assess usual activity pattern prior to acute event Assist client with passive exercise regimen As condition improves, progress activity slowly from dangling, to sitting, to walking under supervision; initiate physical therapy consultation as needed Assist client in adapting and progressing self-care activities during recovery; provide opportunities for participation in and decision making regarding activity Allow for independent functioning within client tolerance and prescribed limitations to prevent exacerbation of illness Note tolerance of activity by monitoring the client's heart rate and rhythm, blood pressure, and respiratory status during activity

NURSING CARE PLAN: HEART FAILURE—cont'd

Nursing diagnoses	Expected client outcomes	Nursing strategies
Knowledge deficit: prevention and treatment of heart failure; related to lack of previous experience	Client will verbalize understanding of: Causes of heart failure Its prevention Signs and symptoms Dietary and activity modifications Medical treatment Diagnostic tests	Implement teaching when client's condition permits (i.e., absence of dyspnea, discomfort, pain, etc.) Assess client's level of understanding about content to be taught Present information in small increments, in a quiet environment, at a pace the client can tolerate, on the following topics relative to heart failure: Causes of heart failure Risk factors Reportable signs and symptoms Dietary and activity modifications Medications Diagnostic tests Medical follow-up Use teaching methods and materials at a level consistent with client's ability

EVALUATION

1. Vital signs are within normal levels for this client.
2. Pulmonary artery pressures, cardiac output, cardiac index, and systemic and pulmonary vascular resistance are normal for this client.
3. The client's body weight is within his normal range.
4. Serum electrolytes are within normal levels.
5. Urine output is normal for this client and greater than 30 ml/hr.
6. The client reports less dyspnea and the ability to rest comfortably.
7. The client experiences normal arterial and venous blood gas values and an absence of hypoxia.
8. The lungs are clear to auscultation.
9. The skin is warm and dry, without cyanosis.
10. The client reports less anxiety.
11. The client expresses a positive attitude about his health state and eventual recovery.
12. The client discusses concerns openly and with less anxiety.
13. The client successfully uses relaxation techniques.
14. The client is able to openly discuss issues and concerns.
15. The client demonstrates appropriate contact with reality.
16. The client experiences no pressure sores or evidence of skin breakdown.
17. The client does not show signs of cardiac decompensation during activity.
18. The client performs all of his self-care activities without complaining of fatigue and dyspnea.
19. The client verbalizes accurate and appropriate information on the following topics: the causes of heart failure, ways to prevent its occurrence, signs and symptoms, necessary dietary modifications, activity restrictions, prescribed medications, medical treatment, and diagnostic tests.

NURSING ALERTS

1. Although an oximeter can be useful in continuously assessing the oxygenation status of a client, periodic arterial blood gas determinations need to be made for correlation.
2. Sudden changes in oxygen saturation shown by oximetry signal the need to follow up with arterial blood gas measurements.
3. The client's physician should be involved in any exercise program planned for the client.
4. Cardiac function during activity should be monitored by experienced personnel.
5. An anemic client can have a normal arterial oxygen pressure (PaO_2), but a reduced arterial oxygen content (CaO_2), causing hypoxia.
6. CvO_2, PvO_2, and SvO_2 values cannot be used to ensure adequacy of tissue oxygenation in all individuals.
7. Aggressive diuresis can cause complications such as volume depletion, hyponatremia, hypokalemia, hypomagnesemia, contraction metabolic alkalosis (resulting from sodium and chloride depletion), orthostatic hypotension, and prerenal azotemia.
8. Rapid aspiration of mixed venous blood from the pulmonary artery catheter can result in pulmonary capillary blood being mixed with the pulmonary artery blood, causing a false increase in the oxygen content.
9. Placing in the flat position a client who may be going into pulmonary edema subsequent to heart failure may precipitate a crisis.
10. Clients with gastrointestinal disease or digitalis toxicity may have the same gastrointestinal signs and symptoms as a client with severe right-sided heart failure.
11. Clients who have an acute hypotensive event are at high risk for skin breakdown secondary to tissue hypoperfusion, necessitating immediate attention to pressure-relief needs.

12. Acute confusional states are a frequent occurrence in the older adult population as a result of physiological, environmental, and psychosocial etiologies. Treatment must be aimed at the cause.

Bibliography

Brunner LS and Suddarth DS, editors: Textbook of medical-surgical nursing, ed 5, Philadelphia, 1984, JB Lippincott Co.

Darovic GO: Hemodynamic monitoring: invasive and non-invasive clinical applications, Philadelphia, 1987, WB Saunders Co.

Diethrich EB: Condemned: is there an alternative for the patient with severe coronary disease? Critical Nurse Quarterly 9(4):8, 1987.

Gelfant B: Stress assessment of the M.I. patient, The Journal of Practical Nursing 10:44, 1984.

Gettrust K, Ryan SC, and Engelman D, editors: Applied nursing diagnosis: guides for comprehensive care planning, New York, 1985, John Wiley & Sons.

Goldschlage NF: Congestive heart failure. In Luce JM and Pierson DJ: Critical care medicine, Philadelphia, 1988, WB Saunders Co, pp 81-87.

Hess D: Bedside monitoring of the patient on a ventilator, Critical Care Nurse Quarterly 6(2):23, 1983.

Hudak C et al: Critical care nursing, ed 2, Philadelphia, 1981, JB Lippincott Co.

Huang SH et al: Coronary care nursing, ed 2, Philadelphia, 1989, WB Saunders Co.

Long BC and Phipps WJ, editors: Medical-surgical nursing: a nursing process approach, ed 2, St Louis, 1989, The CV Mosby Co.

Luce JM and Pierson DJ: Critical care medicine, Philadelphia, 1988, WB Saunders Co.

Luckmann J and Sorensen KC: Medical-surgical nursing: a psychophysiologic approach, ed 3, Philadelphia, 1987, WB Saunders Co.

Michaelson CR: Bedside assessment and diagnosis of acute left ventricular failure, Critical Care Quarterly 4(3):1, 1981.

Nesbitt B: Nursing diagnosis in age-related changes, Gerontological Nursing 14(7):7, 1988.

Schroeder SA et al, editors: Current medical diagnosis and treatment, Norwalk, Conn, 1989, Appleton & Lange.

Shapiro BA, Harrison RA, and Walton JR: Clinical application of blood gases, ed 2, Chicago, 1978, Year Book Medical Publishers.

Solack SD: Assessment of psychogenic stresses in the coronary patient, Cardiovascular Nursing 15(4):16, 1979.

Thompson JM et al: Mosby's manual of clinical nursing, ed 2, St Louis, 1989, The CV Mosby Co.

Vitello-Cicciu J: Risk-factor modification in the prevention of coronary heart disease, Journal of Cardiovascular Nursing 1(4):67, 1987.

Wyngaarden JB and Smith LH Jr: Cecil textbook of medicine, vol 1, ed 18, Philadelphia, 1988, JB Lippincott Co.

Intraaortic Balloon Pump

Shirley A. Saunders

KNOWLEDGE BASE

1. The intraaortic balloon pump (IABP) counterpulsation device assists a failing heart by (a) increasing coronary artery perfusion during diastole by means of inflation of a balloon in the thoracic aorta and (b) decreasing afterload by deflation of the balloon at the onset of systole. Use of an IABP is a temporary measure done as an adjunct to medical therapy.

2. Balloon insertion can be performed as an emergency procedure at the bedside or under fluoroscopy. The most common method of placement of the intraaortic balloon catheter is percutaneous insertion via the femoral or iliac artery. Once passed through the introducer sheath into the thoracic aorta, the catheter is attached to the pump console, which has three basic components: a monitoring system, an electronic trigger mechanism, and a drive system that pumps gas in and out of the balloon by alternating pressure and vacuum.

3. The balloon is inflated during diastole, concurrent with aortic valve closure. The blood in the aortic arch above the level of the balloon is displaced back toward the aortic root, thus increasing diastolic coronary arterial blood flow and myocardial oxygen supply. In an alternating fashion, the balloon is deflated immediately before opening of the aortic valve, causing a space or vacuum toward which blood can flow during systole. This decreased afterload facilitates ventricular emptying and decreases myocardial oxygen demand. The R wave of the patient's electrocardiogram (ECG) is the trigger that signals the balloon to inflate with each cardiac cycle.

4. Cardiovascular system monitoring is critical in determining the effectiveness of IABP therapy. Variations in heart rate of 10 or more beats/min require possible timing readjustments. The pulmonary capillary wedge pressure (PCWP) provides an early indication of volume depletion or overload. Systolic, peak-diastolic, and end-diastolic blood pressure readings all require careful monitoring during IABP therapy to ensure acceptable therapeutic values.

5. Weaning from the balloon catheter can begin as soon as the client is hemodynamically stable: cardiac index (CI) greater than 2 L/min/m², PCWP less than 20 mm Hg, and systolic blood pressure greater than 100 mm Hg. Also, vasopressor support should be minimal. There should be evidence of good coronary artery perfusion and adequate cardiac function.

6. The elderly are less able to ward off infection, because of reduced numbers of lymphocytes and impaired antibody response. This predisposes the older client to the complication of infection at the catheter insertion site.

7. Structural and functional age-related changes of the heart increase impedance to left-ventricular ejection during exercise and stress, resulting in decreased cardiac output.

8. Sympathetic responsiveness decreases with advancing age, reducing the ability to augment heart rate and cardiac function under the stress of depressed left-ventricular function. Consequently, it takes longer for the heart rate to return to normal after exertion.

9. Myocardial muscle contraction is prolonged and relaxation is delayed in the aged heart, leading to a reduction in subendocardial myocardial blood flow because of shortened diastole in certain cardiac diseases.

10. Blood flow to the kidneys decreases secondary to a decrease in cardiac output and an increase in peripheral vascular resistance. The resultant decrease in renal function predisposes the older adult to drug toxicities.

11. Supraventricular and ventricular arrhythmias increase in frequency with advancing age.

12. Arteries become less elastic and compliant with age; insertion of the balloon catheter in a client with severe atherosclerotic vascular disease can result in arterial perforation or occlusion. Valves in the veins become less efficient, resulting in blood more readily accumulating in the lower extremities.

13. The myocardium becomes more rigid, so it is slower in recovering its contractility and irritability. Consequently, stress and tachycardia are poorly tolerated.

14. Because respiratory muscles weaken and the rib cage becomes less flexible, ventilation is less efficient.

15. Reduced serum albumin levels lead to a decrease in the binding of some drugs, causing an increased serum availability of the free (active) forms of these drugs.

16. Psychological stress often increases because of personal losses, loss of physical endurance, deaths of family members and friends, retirement, reduced income, and perceived loss of self-worth. When these factors are coupled with the stressors associated with acute illness, the older adult is at high risk for coping problems.

CASE STUDY

Mr. Simmons, a 65-year-old retired electrician, is admitted to a coronary care unit after an acute anterolateral myocardial infarction, complicated by hypotension and moderately severe chest pain that persists despite treatment with morphine sulfate and intravenous nitroglycerin. Initial assessment findings are as follows: blood pressure, 70 mm Hg (Doppler); heart rate, 125 beats/min, with more than 5 multiformed premature ventricular contractions (PVCs) per minute; respiratory rate, 30 breaths/min (labored); skin, cool and diaphoretic; urinary output, less than 5 ml (Foley catheter) over the past 2 hours. Despite inotropic support with dopamine and diuretic therapy, the client's condition continues to deteriorate. A Swan-Ganz catheter is inserted, as an emergency procedure, for hemodynamic monitoring. The client's opening PCWP is 30 mm Hg, and his CI is 1.2 L/min/m². To stabilize the patient, the physician obtains permission to insert an IABP. Medical diagnoses: intractable angina and cardiogenic shock.

Within an hour after insertion of the assist device, Mr. Simmons' cardiovascular status has improved: chest pain has subsided, urinary output has been 75 ml, the CI has increased to 2.5 L/min/m², and the respiratory rate has decreased to 20 breaths/min. The dopamine drip rate is decreased to 3 µg/kg/min, and the nitroglycerin rate is maintained at 20 µg/min.

ASSESSMENT CRITERIA
Physical
Brief history of problem onset and course related to angina pectoris
Respiratory
    Dyspnea on exertion or at rest
    Orthopnea
    Cough (frothy white or pink-tinged sputum)
    Paroxysmal nocturnal dyspnea
    Respiration
        Rate and rhythm
        Depth

Equality
Symmetry
Labored or unlabored
Use of accessory muscles
Retraction
Breath sounds (assess bilateral corresponding areas for rales and wheezes)
Central cyanosis (lips, earlobes, and buccal mucosa)

Neurological
  Level of consciousness
  Mental status
    Orientation
    Attention and concentration
    Judgment
    Memory
    Thought content and processes
    Mood and affect

Cardiovascular
  Peripheral pulses (for rate, rhythm, amplitude, and equality); color and temperature of extremities
  Heart rate, blood pressure, and mixed venous oxygen saturation (SvO_2) on a continuous basis
  Jugular venous pressure (JVP)
  Inspect anterior chest wall for contour, pulsations, retractions, heaves
  Palpate precordium at apex, left sternal border, and base for thrill, point of maximal impulse
  Auscultate all heart areas for systolic murmur, S_3, S_4, or pericardial friction rub
  Monitor electrocardiogram for changes indicative of ischemia, ST and T wave changes, premature ventricular beats
  Monitor:
    Pulmonary artery pressure (PAP)
    Pulmonary artery mean pressure
    Pulmonary capillary wedge pressure (PCWP)
    Systemic vascular resistance (SVR)
    Pulmonary vascular resistance (PVR)
    Cardiac output (CO) and cardiac index (CI)
    Urine output

Integument
  Color
  Moisture
  Temperature
  Turgor
  Edema

Gastrointestinal
  Symptoms resulting from splanchnic congestion
    Nausea
    Anorexia
    Vomiting
    Abdominal distention
  Constipation, fecal impaction
  Hiccups

Psychosocial

Client's perception of and reaction to diagnosis, purpose for IABP, and procedure for insertion
Resources/support systems currently available to client and family
Life-style
  Description of typical day
  Recreation/leisure profile
  Occupational profile
  Living environment profile (obtain from collateral sources of information on client condition)
Use of alcohol, tobacco, and caffeine

Spiritual

Usual religious practices/beliefs
Effect of illness and hospitalization on belief system
Need for spiritual assistance

Diagnostic tests

Urinalysis: pH, specific gravity, protein, cells, casts, blood, ketones, glucose
Blood chemistry: sodium, potassium, chloride, carbon dioxide, glucose, calcium, phosphorus, uric acid, blood urea nitrogen (BUN), serum creatinine
Serum enzymes: creatine phosphokinase (CK), serum glutamic-oxaloacetic transaminase (SGOT), lactate dehydrogenase (LDH)
Chest x-ray
Electrocardiogram
Arterial blood gas (ABG) determinations

The unstable angina and cardiogenic shock that Mr. Simmons experienced subsequent to his acute myocardial infarction are common indications for the use of an IABP. His drop in blood pressure, increased heart rate, and minimal urinary output, PCWP, and CI were all manifestations of cardiogenic shock. By increasing left-ventricular pressure and workload, and improving cardiac output, the IABP therapy quickly interrupted the shock cycle.

NURSING CARE PLAN: INTRAAORTIC BALLOON PUMP

Nursing diagnoses	Expected client outcomes	Nursing strategies
Anxiety/fear related to IABP procedure, stress of acute, life-threatening illness, and uncertain outcome	Client will experience increased psychological comfort	Observe for restlessness and increasing anxiety resulting from subsequent to treatment plans and activity restrictions
	Client will understand the purpose of the balloon pump	Simply and calmly explain the following to the client if he or she is able to comprehend (include family member): purpose of the balloon pump, usual routines before insertion of IABP and after the procedure, sensations during the procedure, and discomfort after the procedure
	Client will be able to openly discuss his or her fears	Encourage and provide time for the client, family member, and/or significant other to discuss their fears regarding the disease process and treatment plans
		Offer frequent reassurance and emotional support; use touch as tolerated; provide additional emotional support to client and family members, if indicated, by calling in other support persons: clergy, social worker
		Reassure client that the staff is prepared to act quickly in an emergency
		Prepare family members for activities of the day and control visitors
		Monitor the environment for stressors: excessive light or noise, multiple caregivers, unusual equipment, and interruption in sleep patterns/usual routine
	Client will utilize relaxation techniques to reduce anxiety	If appropriate, demonstrate useful relaxation techniques
Potential for systemic or local infection related to invasive procedure	Client will not develop wound infection or sepsis secondary to procedure	Use meticulous hand-washing technique before and after contact with the client; change dressings, tubes, and IV lines (per hospital protocol), using aseptic technique
		Assess for signs of infection: redness, local tenderness, edema, purulent drainage, pain, elevated white blood cell (WBC) count, fever
		Tape Foley catheter to the leg opposite the dressing, and thoroughly clean stool from the perineal area
Potential for decreased cardiac output related to improper or ineffective balloon pump timing	Client will maintain an adequate cardiac output while the balloon is in place, as evidenced by hemodynamic pressures within normal limits, normal renal functioning, and optimal respiratory functioning	Monitor hemodynamic pressure parameters, vital signs, mental status, and ECG rhythm according to client status changes, medication therapy, protocol, or physician orders
		Assess respiratory status per protocol or physician orders or as indicated by patient status changes: respiratory rate, lung sounds, cough, peripheral or central cyanosis, arterial blood gases, mixed venous blood gases, arteriovenous oxygen content difference, arterial/alveolar ratio, and chest x-ray results
		Provide supplemental humidified oxygen per orders
		Instruct and encourage client to cough and deep breathe at least every 2 hours, and assess the need for incentive spirometry; monitor hemoglobin and hematocrit values daily
		Monitor intake and output hourly; serum electrolytes, BUN, and creatinine daily
		Examine the 12-lead ECG to identify the lead that maximizes the R wave and minimizes other waveforms

Continued.

NURSING CARE PLAN: INTRAAORTIC BALLOON PUMP—cont'd

Nursing diagnoses	Expected client outcomes	Nursing strategies
Potential for decreased cardiac output related to improper or ineffective balloon pump timing—cont'd	Client will maintain an adequate cardiac output while the balloon is in place, as evidenced by hemodynamic pressures within normal limits, normal renal functioning, and optimal respiratory functioning—cont'd	Assess for conditions that may prevent the use of ECG triggering: atrioventricular sequential pacing, tachyarrhythmias, inability to locate a suitable ECG lead, or various intraventricular conduction defects Time inflation and deflation according to the arterial waveform and the site of the arterial catheter: Radial artery: set inflation just before the dicrotic notch, or 40-50 milliseconds prior to the dicrotic notch Central aortic: inflate immediately after the aortic valve closes, or at the dicrotic notch Femoral arterial: 120 milliseconds prior to the dicrotic notch Check timing on 1:2 assist at least every 1-2 hours or in the following situations: if cardiac index decreases, when triggering mode is changed, during arrhythmias, if there is a 20% increase or decrease in the heart rate When adjusting timing, adjust balloon inflation before adjusting deflation Assess for and prevent late inflation and early deflation of the balloon Assess for and prevent late deflation and early inflation of the balloon Restrict patient participation in self-care activities if dyspnea, fatigue, hypotension, or arrythmias are present
Potential decrease in peripheral tissue perfusion, related to obstruction of artery by catheter or thrombus	Client will demonstrate adequate peripheral tissue perfusion as evidenced by normal extremity pulses, color, sensations, capillary filling time, and motor function	Assess vital signs, including peripheral pulses, at least every 1-2 hours per protocol or physician orders or as indicated by status changes Assess affected extremities for adequate pulses, color, temperature, sensation, and mobility no less often than every 15 minutes for 1 hour, every 30 minutes for 1 hour, and hourly thereafter; notify physician immediately if there are changes Prevent flexion at the hip of the involved extremity; restrain as needed; keep the head of the bed at 30 degrees or less; perform passive foot exercises with hip bending hourly; apply antiembolism hose Instruct client on performing passive range-of-motion exercises of arms, ankles, and unaffected leg at least every 2 hours if condition has stabilized Note results of chest x-ray Maintain patency of the arterial pressure line Observe for increased frequency of balloon filling and volume changes, and presence of blood in tubing Maintain anticoagulation therapy as per orders (heparin, dextran, or aspirin) Monitor prothrombin time and partial thromboplastin time (1½ to 2 times normal) During console failure or cardiac arrest, manually inflate and deflate the balloon rapidly with a syringe, using half the balloon volume, several times every 10 minutes

NURSING CARE PLAN: INTRAAORTIC BALLOON PUMP—cont'd

Nursing diagnoses	Expected client outcomes	Nursing strategies
Potential for injury related to risk of bleeding as a result of anticoagulation therapy and balloon catheter in the aorta	Client will demonstrate no evidence of bleeding problems	Monitor vital signs at least every 1-2 hours or as indicated by status change, protocol, physician orders, or medication therapy Assess hematocrit, hemoglobin, prothrombin time, partial thromboplastin time, and platelet count daily Frequently assess for presence of internal or retroperitoneal bleeding: hypotension, tachycardia, cool clammy skin, decreased level of consciousness, dyspnea, decreased hematocrit and hemoglobin, low pack pain, absence of pulse in involved extremity, ecchymosis or swelling at the balloon insertion site, tarry stools, hematuria Test all excretions for blood After removal of the balloon catheter, place a pressure dressing and/or sandbag over the insertion site, assess frequently for evidence of bleeding, and instruct client to notify staff if pain develops or if dressing becomes wet
Potential for sleep pattern disturbance related to stimulation of environment, anxiety and fear, and prescribed immobility	Client will have periods of uninterrupted sleep	Provide comfort measures and try to simulate some of client's usual bedtime routines when preparing him for nighttime Limit disruptions and create an environment that has minimal noise Minimize physical and emotional stress, and allow for sufficient rest periods between activities Plan activities around client's rest periods; organize care to provide periods of uninterrupted sleep during the night When possible, offer client choices regarding self-care activities
Potential impairment of skin integrity related to enforced bed rest, limited mobility, impaired circulation	Client maintains normal skin integrity	Assess surfaces every 2 hours for redness or ulcerations over bony prominences and areas of pressure Change client's position at least every 2 hours, using logrolling techniques and keeping balloon leg extended Keep skin clean and dry Obtain order for air fluidized therapy bed Ensure adequate nutritional intake; consult with physician about most appropriate means (i.e., enteral or parenteral) Monitor laboratory values (albumin, sodium, BUN, uric acid, calcium, phosphate, and ABGs) as indicated

EVALUATION

1. The client experiences less anxiety and fear after explanation of IABP therapy and related care.
2. The client openly discusses concerns and fears.
3. The client expresses confidence in the staff and exhibits less anxiety about the staff's ability to handle emergencies.
4. The client is aware of his stress response, reduces that response, and maintains control over it through the use of relaxation techniques.
5. The client remains afebrile, with normal WBC counts and negative cultures.
6. The client's hemodynamic status is stabilized by the IABP, as evidenced by normal systemic vascular resistance and pulmonary vascular resistance, adequate cardiac output, normal preload, normal heart rate, a decrease in or absence of arrhythmias, normal blood gas values, decreased respiratory rate, normal urine output, warm, dry skin, and alert and oriented mental status.

7. The client reports no chest pain during IABP therapy.
8. The client has adequate perfusion of the affected leg.
9. The client reports that periods of sufficient sleep are being obtained.
10. The client's skin is free of pressure sores.

NURSING ALERTS

1. A consent form must be obtained before insertion of the IABP.
2. It may be necessary to turn off the pump so that lung sounds, heart sounds, and bowel sounds can be auscultated. Consult the physician.
3. During cardiopulmonary resuscitation, balloon pumping must be synchronized with cardiac compression.
4. Proper balloon timing must be done by means of an arterial waveform, since systole and diastole are mechanical events.
5. Notify the phsyician immediately if peripheral pulses diminish or become absent.
6. Obtain chest x-ray film with the client in the position he frequently assumes to confirm proper placement of the IABP.
7. During the weaning process, the client's clinical status should be monitored very closely to detect acute cardiac deterioration.
8. For 4 to 6 hours after removal of the IABP, coughing may stimulate bleeding from the insertion site.
9. If bleeding occurs, remove the dressing, apply manual pressure, and notify the physician.
10. The majority of clients undergoing IABP therapy will also require intubation and mechanical ventilation.
11. Nutrition must be an early consideration to maintain and promote strength and healing.
12. Small amounts of gas will normally diffuse out of the balloon, necessitating evacuation and refilling about every 3 to 4 hours. An increase in refilling frequency may indicate a serious leak. In such a situation, notify the physician immediately.

Bibliography

Brunner LS and Suddarth DS, editors: Textbook of medical-surgical nursing, ed 5, Philadelphia, 1984, JB Lippincott Co.

Diethrich EB: Condemned: is there an alternative for the patient with severe coronary disease? Critical Care Nurse Quarterly 9(4):8, 1987.

Gelfant B: Stress assessment of the M.I. patient, The Journal of Practical Nursing 10:44, 1984.

Gettrust K, Ryan SC, and Engleman D, editors: Applied nursing diagnosis: guides for comprehensive care planning, New York, 1985, John Wiley & Sons, Inc.

Hudak C et al: Critical care nursing, ed 2, Philadelphia, 1981, JB Lippincott Co.

Kleehammer P, Fundaro J, and Hancock, L: Pumps that bolster a failing heart, RN 48(5):44, 1985.

Long BC and Phipps WJ, editors: Medical-surgical nursing: a nursing process approach, ed 2, St Louis, 1989, The CV Mosby Co.

Luckmann J and Sorensen KC: Medical-surgical nursing: a psychophysiologic approach, ed 3, Philadelphia, 1987, WB Saunders Co.

Michaelson CR: Bedside assessment and diagnosis of acute left ventricular failure, Critical Care Quarterly 4(3):1, 1981.

Nesbitt B: Nursing diagnosis in age-related changes, Gerontological Nursing 14(7):7, 1988.

Purcell J: Intra-aortic balloon pump therapy, American Journal of Nursing 5:775, 1983.

Schroeder S et al, editors: Current medical diagnosis and treatment, Norwalk, Conn, 1989, Appleton & Lange.

Shively M: The physiologic principles of intra-aortic balloon counterpulsation, Critical Care Quarterly 4(2):83, 1981.

Solack SD: Assessment of psychogenic stresses in the coronary patient, Cardiovascular Nursing 15(4):16, 1979.

Thompson JM et al: Mosby's manual of clinical nursing, St Louis, 1989, The CV Mosby Co.

Vitello-Cicciu J: Risk-factor modification in the prevention of coronary heart disease, Journal of Cardiovascular Nursing 1(4):67, 1987.

Weinberg LA: Buying time with an intra-aortic balloon pump, Nursing '88 9:6, 1988.

Wyngaarden JB and Smith LH Jr: Cecil textbook of medicine, vol 1, ed 18, Philadelphia, 1988, JB Lippincott Co.

Primary Hypertension

Elaine E. Steinke

KNOWLEDGE BASE

1. Hypertension is the most prevalent cardiovascular disease in the elderly. Incidence of the disease is correlated with race, with blacks being more likely to experience hypertension than whites.
2. Impaired distensibility of the walls of large vessels influences the development of hypertertension in the older adult. There is increased stiffness and loss of arterial elasticity, increased peripheral resistance, and possibly decreased renal blood flow. Decreased renal blood flow activates the renin-angiotensin system, which compounds the problem.
3. Hypertension places the elderly person at risk for stroke, renal failure, transient ischemic attacks, and myocardial infarction. Hypertensive effects on the microcirculation result in retinal, kidney, and brain changes.
4. Pharmacokinetic changes in the absorption, distribution, metabolism, and excretion of drugs in the older adult are important considerations for drug therapy.
5. Side effects of medications should be closely monitored, since drug toxicity can occur quickly. These side effects may also inhibit compliance with drug therapy.
6. The client and a family member should be taught to take the blood pressure and keep a record. The blood pressure should be taken regularly and at the same time of day in order to make more accurate comparisons between readings.
7. The cost to an elderly person who must take multiple medications is significant. Most elderly people pay out-of-pocket for medications and may not be able to afford medications as well as other costs of living.
8. Life-style changes for an elderly client may include weight reduction, a salt-restricted diet, adherence to a medication regimen, development of a weight-control program when appropriate, and promotion of adequate rest and activity.

CASE STUDY

Mr. Conover is a 68-year-old black male with whom you regularly interact during blood pressure screening at a local senior clinic. Two months ago his blood pressure reading was 202/100, and you referred him to his local physician for treatment. Currently his hypertension is controlled with methyldopa, chlorothiazide, and potassium chloride. Today his blood pressure is 158/94. On questioning, Mr. Conover tells you that on days that he feels well he does not take his methyldopa. He states, "I don't like taking so many pills, and they are just too expensive. I can barely make ends meet." He also complains that food is "tasteless" without salt. Further discussion reveals that Mr. Conover is experiencing erectile dysfunction.

ASSESSMENT CRITERIA
Physical

Vital signs, including bilateral lying, sitting, and standing blood pressure readings
Signs of headache, flushing, vertigo, blurred vision, orthostatic hypotension
Cardiac risk factors
    Diet
    Obesity
    Smoking history
    Alcohol intake
    Stressors
Knowledge about hypertension
Medications
    Name, purpose, frequency, side effects
    Reasons for variable use of medications
Dietary patterns
Cardiovascular and respiratory systems assessment
    Gallops and/or murmurs, S_3, S_4, irregular rhythm
    Breath sounds for rales
    Bruits, particularly in carotid arteries
    Weight, and pattern of changes or stability
    Presence of peripheral edema
    Fundoscopic examination for papilledema, exudates, hemorrhages, or arteriovenous nicking

Psychosocial

Life-style
    Description of typical day
    Recreational/leisure profile
    Living environment profile
Family profile

Resources/support systems used
Client's perception of and reaction to the health
   problem
Client's approaches to control hypertension
Perceptions of stress and stressful events
Concerns regarding sexuality and sexual function

Mr. Conover is exhibiting signs of noncompliance with medication and diet, with resulting poor control of his hypertension. Erectile dysfunction can result both from uncontrolled

hypertension and as a side effect of methyldopa. Mr. Conover may have a limited understanding of his disease process and treatment.

Mr. Conover's compliance with his treatment is hindered by financial resources that are insufficient to meet his need for medications. He also has some health beliefs about medication-taking that need to be explored. He is probably experiencing changes in relationship patterns related to his sexual dysfunction. This can be viewed as a stressor that could increase his hypertension.

NURSING CARE PLAN: PRIMARY HYPERTENSION

Nursing diagnoses	Expected client outcomes	Nursing strategies
Potential knowledge deficit regarding disease and treatment plan, related to lack of previous exposure and negative side effects of medication	Client will verbalize understanding of hypertension, including causes, potential complications, and control measures	Identify current level of knowledge about hypertension and its management and treatment; proceed with teaching based on assessment findings Use a variety of teaching methods and materials at level consistent with client's ability Teach in small increments, in a quiet environment, and at a pace client can tolerate

	Client will demonstrate understanding of risk factors, diet, medications, and reportable signs and symptoms	Explain the following, with appropriate rationale as needed:
		   Risk factors (i.e., diet, smoking, obesity, stressors)
		   Signs/symptoms to report (i.e., shortness of breath (SOB), discomfort on exertion (DOE), paroxysmal nocturnal dyspnea (PND), edema)
		   Ways to minimize hypotensive reactions to antihypertensive medication (e.g., moving slowly from lying to sitting position, lying down with feet elevated)
		Review with client a list of foods appropriate for sodium restriction
		Help client/family to develop meal plans:
		   Suggest use of spices and salt substitutes
		   Avoid foods high in sodium and prepackaged foods
		   Avoid processed meats such as lunchmeat, weiners, and bacon
		   Include more fresh fruits and vegetables
		   Limit alcohol consumption
		   Incorporate ethnic preferences
		Encourage weight reduction and exercise as needed
		Emphasize the benefits of following the diet as prescribed
		Explore with client specific reasons for nonadherence to medication regimen
		Review name, purpose, dose, frequency, and side effects of prescribed medications
		Provide written instructions for each medication, and develop a schedule for taking medications for the next week

NURSING CARE PLAN: PRIMARY HYPERTENSION—cont'd

Nursing diagnoses	Expected client outcomes	Nursing strategies
Potential knowledge deficit regarding disease and treatment plan, related to lack of previous exposure and negative side effects of medication—cont'd	Client will demonstrate understanding of risk factors, diet, medications, and reportable signs and symptoms—cont'd	Emphasize the benefits of following the medication regimen closely, and provide positive reinforcement Assess client's willingness to comply with medication and diet, including motivating factors (e.g., increased longevity, quality of life) Identify community resources that might help provide economic help Suggest relaxation techniques and biofeedback as supportive strategies Contract with the client to review his success with following the diet and medication plan in 1 week

Sexual dysfunction (impotence) related to side effects of antihypertensive medications	Client will have improved sexual function and/or adapt to changes in function	Explore Mr. Conover's perception of the problem
		Encourage Mr. Conover to discuss the problem with his physician to determine if other drugs might be used
		Discuss alternative means of achieving sexual satisfaction
		  Partner can assist with "stuffing" a somewhat soft penis into the vagina; the penis may harden even with partial entry
		  Oral-genital contact if it is acceptable to the couple
		  Couples can explore each other's bodies to discover other areas that are arousing
		  Sharing sexual fantasies and feelings
		  Sexual behaviors such as touching, kissing, holding, lying close together
		Refer to sexual counselor if needed

EVALUATION

1. The client is able to explain the disease process of hypertension, including causes, potential complications, risk factors, treatment regimen, and reportable signs and symptoms at a follow-up visit after 1 week.
2. The client maintains a low-sodium meal plan as evidenced by a 7-day diet log.
3. The client is able to correctly state the name, purpose, dose, frequency, and side effects of medications prescribed for treatment of hypertension.
4. The client reports a sexually satisfying relationship.

NURSING ALERTS

1. A reliable determination of the presence of hypertension requires repeated blood pressure readings in both arms over a period of time, with the client lying, sitting, and standing.
2. Emphasize in client teaching that hypertension is a chronic disease that is controlled but not cured by medication, diet, control of stress, and a balance between activity and rest.
3. Unless it is severe, hypertension may be asymptomatic, so careful subjective and objective assesssment is essential.
4. Do not assume that sexual performance and function are unimportant to an older client. The nurse must be adept at eliciting the effects of drug therapy as related to libido.

Bibliography

Carnevali DL and Patrick M: Nursing management for the elderly, ed 2, Philadelphia, 1986, JB Lippincott Co.

Carpenito LJ: Nursing diagnosis: application to clinical practice, ed 2, Philadelphia, 1987, JB Lippincott Co.

Kirkendall WM, Weber MA, and Weinberger MH: Which drug for the aging hypertensive? Patient Care 22(1):133, 1988.

Matteson MA and McConnell ES: Gerontological nursing concepts and practice, Philadelphia, 1988, WB Saunders Co.

Steinke EE: Older adults' knowledge and attitudes about sexuality and aging, Image: Journal of Nursing Scholarship 20(2):93, 1988.

Steinke EE and Bergen MB: Sexuality and aging: a review of the literature from a nursing perspective, Journal of Gerontological Nursing 12(6):6, 1986.

Taylor CM and Cress SS: Nursing diagnosis cards, Springhouse, Pa, 1987, Springhouse Corp.

Walz WH and Blum NS: Sexual health in later life, Lexington, Mass, 1987, Lexington Books.

Yurick AG et al: The aged person and the nursing process, ed 3, Norwalk, Conn, 1989, Appleton & Lange.

Orthostatic Hypotension

Roberta Purvis Bartee

KNOWLEDGE BASE

1. Orthostatic hypotension is a significant problem among older people. One in ten hospitalized elders has orthostatic (postural) hypotension.
2. Orthostatic hypotension is defined as a fall in arterial blood pressure on standing of such magnitude that symptoms result from inadequate end-organ perfusion.
3. Effective compensation during positional change depends on the competence of pressure-regulating mechanisms.
4. Normally upon standing, the arterial pressure in the head and upper body falls; however, the falling pressure at the baroreceptors elicits an immediate reflex, resulting in strong sympathetic discharge throughout the body, which causes vasoconstriction of the arteries in the lower extremities, maintaining pressure in the head and upper body.
5. Aging affects the efficiency of blood pressure regulators.
   a. The efficiency of the autonomic nervous system may be decreased.
   b. Baroreceptor sensitivity diminishes or even fails.
   c. Myelin degeneration and neuronal loss slow conduction.
   d. Rigid vasculature compromises compliance.
   e. Inactive renin is not as readily converted to active renin.
6. Symptoms of orthostatic hypotension are those of decreased cerebral perfusion, such as sudden dizziness, vertigo, tinnitus, disturbances of vision and balance, limpness, and syncope.
7. Persistent orthostatic hypotension suggests autonomic dysfunction if the following are present:
   a. Decreased blood pressure without increased heart rate
   b. Manifest aberrancies of bowel, bladder, thermoregulation, and gait; physiological sexual impotence; and nasal stuffiness
8. Drugs that depress the central and sympathetic nervous systems and those affecting fluid volume are likely culprits in the clinical picture of orthostatic hypotension. Examples include the following:
   a. Antihypertensives, diuretics, sedatives
   b. Tricyclic antidepressants, phenothiazines, levodopa, vasodilators, hypnotics, antihistamines
   c. Over-the-counter drugs such as diet pills, cold preparations, decongestants
9. Orthostatic hypotension may occur in the absence of drug use. Serum sodium levels at or below the normal limit are seen in a significant percentage of clients with orthostatic hypotension.
10. Health problems contributing to events of orthostatic hypotension are as follows:
    a. Neurogenic disorders of afferent pathways (diabetes, peripheral neuropathy), efferent pathways (alcoholism, bronchial, pancreatic, and breast cancer), or the central nervous system (brain: Parkinson's disease, cerebrovascular accident (CVA); spinal cord: syringomyelia)
    b. Elimination or respiratory problems creating circumstances for the Valsalva maneuver or vasovagal response
    c. Varicosities and incompetent valves that threaten peripheral vascular integrity
    d. Cardiovascular system's inability to compensate for decreased venous flow
    e. Anemia, which decreases the oxygen-carrying capacity of the blood and potentiates the hypotensive effect
11. Changes in internal environments influencing the amount and location of fluid volume may induce orthostatic hypotensive events. Examples include the following:
    a. Vasodilation that reduces circulatory volume, which may be caused by warm weather, hot baths or showers, fever, hypokalemia, or postprandial release of vasoactive substances
    b. Postprandial events, including the blood shift to hepatic and splanchnic beds and reduced baroreceptor sensitivity from insulin. Most postprandial orthostatic hypotensive events represent subclinical autonomic dysfunction.
12. A suggested protocol to determine the presence of orthostatic hypotension is to take three sequential sets of blood pressure measurements along with pulse rates. The first set is taken after the client has been supine for an hour. The second and third sets follow 2 minutes of sitting and 2 minutes of standing, respectively.
13. Use of the same protocol among team members increases reliability of the results.

14. The suggested criterion for establishing the presence of orthostatic hypotension is a drop in systolic pressure greater than 10 mm Hg after positional changes, with an accompanying 10-beat pulse increase and subjective reports of dizziness.
15. The literature shows various protocols for measurement and various criteria for identification of orthostatic hypotension.
16. Responses to decreased blood pressure are variable. In some elders, small pressure drops may cause symptoms; others may be asymptomatic with significant drops in blood pressure.
17. Blood pressure findings vary daily.
18. During morning hours, baroreceptors are sluggish and thus less sensitive.
19. The following are some of the effects of orthostatic hypotension.
    a. Injuries caused by falls compromise mobility.
    b. Experiences of falls may erode confidence levels and increase fear.
    c. Decreased cerebral perfusion resulting from the hypotension may cause confusion.
    d. Decreased venous return compromises perfusion of the heart, brain, and cochlea, thus increasing vulnerability to myocardial infarction, CVA, seizure, and hearing loss.
20. Client teaching is the major focus in the management of orthostatic hypotension. The following instructions should be included in client teaching:
    a. Getting out of bed should be done in stages: (1) Do bed exercises before sitting up in bed; movement of all extremities increases vascular tone. (2) Come to a sitting position very slowly; if dizziness occurs, lie down and start the bed exercises again. (3) After sitting on the side of the bed without dizziness, slowly come to a standing position.
    b. Avoid prolonged sitting and leg crossing. Intermittent periods of leg elevation and chair exercises increase venous return and cardiac output, decreasing hypotensive episodes.
    c. Avoid bending and stooping followed by a sudden righting. Pausing between positional changes and slowing postural changes decrease the symptoms.
    d. Be alert to the symptoms and quickly lower your head if they occur. If a fall is imminent, learn how to fall without injury.

CASE STUDY

Sadie Daniels, a 74-year-old retired harpist, normally wakes up earlier in the summer than during the rest of the year. She spends the extra time doing needlework. One morning while she was completing a needlepoint piece, the telephone rang. She fainted while dashing to answer the call. She regained consciousness immediately and seemed to be unhurt, but the experience was frightening.

Mr. Daniels brought her to a hospital clinic. She had a history of anemia and diabetes, and 4 months ago she began taking a diuretic for hypertension. Sadie recalled previous weak spells, which she had disregarded until now. Last week, when leaving a restaurant after lunch with friends, she felt faint. After she sat down for a moment, the episode passed. She also remembered being dizzy sometimes when she got out of bed in the morning. Sadie had attributed feeling faint to the warm weather and the dizziness to waking up too early.

Consecutive blood pressure measurements and pulse rates were obtained as Sadie assumed supine, sitting, and standing positions. During the maneuver, her heart rate significantly increased while systolic and diastolic pressures fell. Sadie reported feeling slightly dizzy while standing. She felt better after being assisted onto the examination table. Specimens for laboratory work were obtained, and Sadie was admitted for further observation of orthostatic hypotension.

ASSESSMENT CRITERIA
Physical

Medical, surgical history
Coexisting health problems
Current over-the-counter and prescribed medications
Nutritional status
Height
Usual, ideal, current weight
Nutrient intake; 1-day recall
Laboratory data: creatinine, hemoglobin, hematocrit, complete blood count, electrolytes, protein
Hydration
Cardiopulmonary
  Vital signs
  Lung sounds
  Heart sounds
  Shortness of breath
  Cough
  Sputum
  Edema
  Pain
Neurological
  Tremor
  Paresis/paralysis
  Seizures
  Speech

Peripheral vascular
    Color
    Warmth
    Pulses
    Capillary refilling
    Edema
    Claudication
    Pain
    Varicosities
Mobility
    Gait
    Balance
    Coordination
    Muscle strength
    Endurance
History of falls
    Pattern
    Frequency
    Surrounding events
Usual rest-activity patterns; recent changes
Symptoms indicative of cerebral anoxia: patterns/
    duration
Integrity of the autonomic nervous system
Vision
Level of auditory acuity
Effect of position (supine, sitting, standing) on con-
    secutive blood pressure measurements and pulse
    rates

Psychosocial

Role in family and community
Impact of health problem on well-being and sense of
    self
Methods of coping with current health problem
Life-style and health practices
    Alcohol intake
    Smoking
    Substance abuse
    Caffeine intake
    Socializing
    Exercise
Support system and relationships
Environment
    Recent changes
    Safety hazards
    Maintenance
Economic status and resources

Spiritual

Religious practices
Philosophical beliefs about the process of aging

The correlation of Sadie's activities with incidents of orthostatic hypotension indicates her vulnerability and a need for health teaching. Needlework is a sedentary activity that promotes venous pooling in lower extremities and contributes to orthostatic hypotension.

Sadie's admitting event occurred in the morning. She reported dizziness when getting out of bed. She fainted while dashing to answer the telephone. Both symptoms indicate diminished cerebral perfusion. Sadie's faintness after lunch may have been a combination of the mealtime sedentary circumstances and postprandial phenomena, including a blood shift to the mesentery and release of vasoactive substances.

Other conditions that may contribute to Sadie's problem are being investigated. Sadie could be hypovolemic from recent diuretic therapy and summertime diaphoresis, so her hydration status is being evaluated. A decrease in the oxygen-carrying capacity of blood contributes to orthostatic hypotension; thus anemia would need to be ruled out, since she had been anemic in the past. She may be having episodes of hypoglycemia.

In the incident in her home, Sadie regained consciousness while in the supine position as cerebral perfusion was restored. At the clinic, positional changes raised her heart rate and lowered her blood pressure. The increased heart rate was compensatory. Return to the supine position relieved the dizziness she had during maneuvers for sequential vital sign measurements. Transient ischemic attacks (TIAs) also cause dizziness, so further examination is needed.

The incident of fainting was frightening; she could have been injured during the episode. Sadie's psychological well-being may be threatened by loss of confidence because of orthostatic incidents. Without health teaching, she may tend to become more sedentary to avoid injury or embarrassment.

NURSING CARE PLAN: ORTHOSTATIC HYPOTENSION

Nursing diagnoses	Expected client outcomes	Nursing strategies
Altered tissue perfusion (cerebral, cardiac) related to rapid fall in blood pressure secondary to diminished baroreceptor and autonomic responses	Client will enhance cerebral and cardiac tissue perfusion	Concurrently measure blood pressure and pulse in supine, sitting, and standing positions Assess for signs of cerebral anoxia; teach the client how to recognize the symptoms and to take quick action
	Client will be free of elimination problems that may cause vasovagal or Valsalva responses	Assess bowel and bladder function for situations that may cause a vasovagal response or Valsalva maneuver Assess heart sounds and report abnormalities Evaluate medication and health problem that may be contributing to baroreceptor and autonomic dysfunction Assess frequency pattern of and contributing factors to hypotensive episodes Monitor laboratory values for evidence of low sodium, potassium, and serum osmolality, and report abnormalities to the physician Assess for neurological or cardiovascular deficits Instruct client to sleep with head elevated and feet lowered to encourage autoregulation of cerebral flow and maintain regulatory reflex activity Increase salt and fluid intake to expand fluid volume if not contraindicated
	Client will state ways that tissue perfusion can be compromised	Instruct client to avoid crossing legs, wearing tight clothing on lower extremities, standing or sitting for long periods of time Teach client how to monitor episode occurrence progression and to report changes to health care provider Include significant others in teaching Document outcome of client teaching
Potential for activity intolerance related to hypotensive episodes	Client will increase tolerance to activity	Assess current activity level; document for baseline Request physical therapy consultation to plan exercise program with the client
	Client, with assistance, will design a plan for safely increasing levels of activity	Evaluate client management of orthostatic hypotensive events; teach importance of lowering head to increase cerebral blood flow Assess frequency, circumstances of episodes Assess client's medications for implications in regard to orthostatic hypotension
	Client will relate hypovolemia to orthostatic events	Teach impact of diarrhea or emesis on blood volume status and the effect on orthostatic hypotension

	Client will explain strategies to prevent pooling of blood	Teach how to avoid pooling of blood:
		  Perform calf flexion, leg and arm exercises prior to getting out of bed
		  Wear waist-high support hose (properly fitted, applied) during the day to increase venous return; remove during the night to prevent central volume pooling
		  Avoid prolonged sitting, standing, or bed rest
		Teach how to avoid sudden position changes:
		  Get out of bed gradually, pausing between each stage and being prepared to lower head should symptoms occur
		  Avoid popliteal pressure while dangling
		Teach that standing is the most vulnerable time for an orthostatic hypotensive event; avoid hyperextending knees, and do frequent knee flexions when standing

Continued.

NURSING CARE PLAN: ORTHOSTATIC HYPOTENSION—cont'd

Nursing diagnoses	Expected client outcomes	Nursing strategies
Potential for activity intolerance related to hypotensive episodes—cont'd		Encourage client to drink coffee for its caffeine effect
		Encourage exercise as tolerated; avoid isometrics, which could induce a blood pressure drop
		Teach client to avoid holding breath when straining, coughing, or lifting
		Teach that climbing stairs may induce orthostatic hypotensive events
	Client and significant other will demonstrate taking blood pressure and radial pulse	Teach client and significant other how to take the blood pressure and a radial pulse
		Request them to assess blood pressure and pulse three times a week and submit results for evaluation of progress
		Document outcome of client teaching
Potential for injury related to decreased cerebral blood flow	Client will remain free from preventable injury	Assess times, circumstances of episodes
		Assess management of episodes
	Client will identify mornings as a vulnerable time for orthostatic event	Teach that mornings are a vulnerable time
		Evaluate need for grab bars in the home bathroom
	Client will explain methods of safely attending to activities of daily living, including morning events	Instruct client to get out of bed gradually after performing bed exercises
		Instruct client to avoid hot showers/baths during the morning
		Instruct client not to shave immediately in the morning
	Client will report injuries to significant other and health care provider	Teach importance of reporting injuries to significant others and health care provider
	Client will state reasons for consuming caffeine and limiting postprandial activity	Teach impact of meals on circulating volume (avoid large meals)
		Encourage client to consume caffeine after meals if not contraindicated
		Teach client to avoid rigorous activity for 2 hours after meals, especially after breakfast
		Instruct client to avoid the Valsalva maneuver during bowel and bladder evacuation
		Instruct client to avoid vasodilation (prevent overheating during warm weather; report fever to health care provider)
		Document outcome of client teaching
Sensory/perceptual alterations (disrupted neurological and auditory integrity) related to decreased blood flow to the brain and cochlea	Client will demonstrate methods of restoring cerebral blood flow	Assess neurological and auditory status
		Assess client management of orthostatic hypotensive events
		After episodes, assess neurological function for residual deficits suggesting TIA or CVA
		Use seizure precautions; decreased blood supply may trigger seizure activity
	Client will report no change in auditory status	Assess hearing status and client's perception of auditory function
		Instruct client to report persistent deficits or changes in hearing to health care provider
		Document outcome of client teaching
Altered body image, related to the loss of confidence and the relationship of activity to syncope	Client will verbalize feelings related to body image	Assess impact of orthostatic hypotension on daily life
		Assess client's perception of self and body competence
		Identify client's concerns regarding activities
		Reinforce client's role in resolving problems
	Client will verbalize concerns regarding activities	Teach safety practices and reassure client that she will be safe if they are followed
		Encourage client to monitor effects of medication and discuss with physician options for changing amount, frequency, or administration time

EVALUATION

1. The client's vital signs reflect increased stability with postural change.
2. The client sleeps with the head of the bed elevated.
3. The client explains how tissue perfusion is compromised by orthostatic hypotension.
4. The client explains the importance of monitoring episodes and reporting changes in the number of episodes to the health care provider.
5. The client describes safe management of orthostatic hypotensive episodes (i.e., putting her head down to increase cerebral flow).
6. The client performs exercises within the range of tolerance.
7. The client demonstrates safety precautions while getting out of bed.
8. The client names activities that could induce orthostatic hypotension.
9. The client explains the relationship of venous pooling to orthostatic hypotension.
10. The client demonstrates pulse and blood pressure measurement and recording.
11. The client and significant other identify times of increased vulnerability, explaining methods for reducing the threat of orthostatic hypotension.
12. The client reports the occurrence of diminished auditory function.
13. The client manifests confidence by increased participation in the treatment plan, activities, and control over hypotensive episodes.

NURSING ALERTS

1. Before sequential measurements of blood pressure and pulse, evaluate the client's risk of experiencing cerebrovascular or cardiovascular compromise during the maneuvers. If necessary, halt the maneuvers to preserve the physical safety of the client.
2. Use the same measurement techniques for each evaluation of orthostatic hypotension.
3. Assess elderly clients with auditory deficits for a history of orthostatic hypotension.
4. Significant drops in blood pressure may be caused by raising the arms above the shoulders.
5. Diagnostic testing that requires a client to take nothing by mouth increases the risk for hypotensive episodes.

Bibliography

Agate J: Common symptoms and complaints. In Rossman I, editor: Clinical geriatrics, ed 3, Philadelphia, 1986, JB Lippincott Co, pp 138-149.

Anderson WF: Teaching geriatrics in the United Kingdom. In Somers AR and Fabian DR, editors: The geriatric imperative: an introduction to gerontology and clinical geriatrics, New York, 1981, Appleton-Century-Crofts, pp 283-293.

Aronow WS et al: Prevalence of postural hypotension in elderly patients in a long term health care facility, American Journal of Cardiology 62:336, 1988.

Barrows JJ: Nursing role in management: blood pressure disturbances. In Lewis SM and Collier IC: Medical-surgical nursing: assessment and management of clinical problems, ed 2, New York, 1987, McGraw-Hill Book Co, pp 729-766.

Birdsall C, Pizzo C, and Muller B: What are orthostatic BP changes? American Journal of Nursing 85:1062, 1985.

Bowen J: Orthostatic hypotension, Comprehensive Therapy 14(10):6, 1988.

Caird FI, Dall JLC, and Williams BO: The cardiovascular system. In Brocklehurst, editor: Textbook of geriatric medicine and gerontology, ed 3, Edinburgh, 1985, Churchill Livingstone, pp 230-267.

Campese VM: Orthostatic hypotension: idiopathic and uremic, Kidney International 34 (suppl 25): S-152, 1988.

Cerebrovascular Disease: Thrombus, Embolus, Hemorrhage

Dixie M. Flynn

KNOWLEDGE BASE

1. "Stroke," the lay term for cerebrovascular accident (CVA) is one of the leading causes of death, exceeded only by heart disease and cancer. There are well over 400,000 new cases of stroke each year in the United States, with most of them occurring in individuals over the age of 50.
2. A diagnosis of stroke can be determined by CT scan (magnetic resonance imaging [MRI] if necessary), carotid Doppler studies, and neurological changes (e.g., weakness on one side).
3. There are a number of events that typically cause strokes in the elderly. Atherosclerotic changes represent an underlying condition in all types of CVAs.
4. There are three types of strokes: thrombotic, embolic, and hemorrhagic. The most common type is thrombotic.
5. In the thrombotic stroke, atherosclerotic plaques form in the arteries, most commonly at the branchings of blood vessels. When a blood vessel becomes so narrowed that flow is slowed or interrupted, a stroke results.
   a. High blood pressure and diabetes appear to be the most common risk factors.
   b. Such strokes are often preceded by the appearance of one or more transient ischemic attacks (TIAs).
   c. The stroke itself may have a stuttering course, with neurological impairment developing over hours or days.
6. Embolic stroke occurs when a thrombus forms in a large vessel such as the carotid artery or in the heart. The thrombus breaks off and travels with the circulating blood to the brain, where it lodges in a smaller vessel, or it may break up and disperse, causing little or no damage.
   a. Older individuals may develop an embolic stroke following or simultaneously with a myocardial infarction, atrial fibrillation, or other arrhythmia.
   b. The underlying cause must be treated, as well as the stroke.

7. Hemorrhagic stroke results from the rupture of a blood vessel, usually a deep one in the brain. Blood extravasates into the tissue, and blood flow to the area is interrupted.
   a. Neurological impairment is usually sudden and severe, often resulting in immediate coma and respiratory compromise.
   b. Massive hemorrhage into the ventricles or brainstem is usually fatal within 24 hours.
   c. In clients who survive, recovery of function is apt to be protracted.
8. The life-threatening phase of stroke is usually confined to the first week. Of the majority of clients who survive this initial period, over one third live for more than 5 years after the stroke, and over one fifth live 8 to 10 years longer.
9. Although some patients recover completely from a CVA, many suffer some degree of permanent disability. Even with long-term rehabilitation, in many cases only partial success is achieved in reversing the associated loss in neurological capabilities, especially in regard to mobility and communication.
10. The location of the injury in the brain determines the resultant effects on the body. Damage to the left side of the brain will result in injury to the right side of the body; damage to the right side of the brain will result in injury to the left side of the body.
11. A person with left cerebral damage will most generally manifest the following:
    a. Right hemiplegia
    b. Speech/language deficits (aphasia)
    c. Swallowing difficulties (dysphagia)
    d. Memory deficit (language)
    e. Behavioral style—slow, cautious
12. A person with right cerebral damage will most generally manifest the following:
    a. Left hemiplegia
    b. Spatial/perceptual deficits
    c. Memory deficits (performance)
    d. Unilateral neglect
    e. Behavioral style—quick, impulsive

13. Characteristics common to all persons who experience cerebral injury are as follows:
    a. Increased motor activity beyond necessary muscle use
    b. Perseveration—continuation of activities or sounds
    c. Apraxia—inability to perform certain tasks without cuing
    d. Hemianopsia—defect in which a portion of the visual field is missing
    e. Emotional lability—mood swings, with bouts of unexplained crying
    f. Agnosia—inability to recognize familiar objects
    g. Paresthesia on affected side
    h. Bowel and bladder incontinence
    i. High level of suggestibility
    j. Spasticity of the limbs
    k. Subluxation of limbs because of weak musculature
    l. Ataxia—loss of coordination of voluntary movement
    m. Anasognosia—denial of paralysis
14. Psychosocial problems experienced by a person after a stroke can be divided into two categories:
    a. Alterations in personality and emotional behavior—usually reflect how the person responds to the disabilities that result from the stroke
    b. Changes in intellectual abilities—usually result from actual brain damage
    Frequently the two kinds of changes interact.
15. The most common emotional state experienced by the client is depression, usually as a response to frustration, helplessness, change in body image, and/or change in role status. Family members of the stroke victim experience many of the same emotions, especially when they assume roles that the stroke victim can no longer assume.
16. The family will adapt to the changes in the family through five stages, similar to those of the Kübler-Ross model in regard to death and dying: denial, anger, bargaining, depression, and acceptance. Referral to social services or pastoral care may help the family identify these stages.
17. The goals of treatment are to minimize injury to the brain after the initial stroke (acute phase of care) and to return the client to his or her optimum level of self-care (rehabilitation).
18. The acute phase of care (in an intensive care unit and/or medical unit) generally lasts 5 to 7 days, depending on the severity of the stroke and the type of stroke. Recovery from a hemorrhagic stroke tends to take longer, because of the presence of cerebral edema prolonging acute symptoms.
19. In the presence of a cerebral thrombus, medical treatment generally includes bed rest and anticoagulation therapy to prevent further thrombus formation. Oxygen therapy ensures increased oxygen flow to brain cells. In the presence of cerebral emboli, the underlying medical problems are treated. In cerebral hemorrhage, the physician must ensure that the hemorrhage has stopped and then decrease the cerebral edema. In the event that large areas of hemorrhage in the brain occur and displace brain tissue, a craniotomy is done to reduce the cerebral pressure.
20. Nursing diagnoses must be considered in the physical, social, psychological, and spiritual realms, since a stroke causes multiple, complex, interacting problems.
21. In addition to nursing diagnoses related to a stroke, many clients will have problems caused by other chronic diseases or complications.
22. Stroke clients will have focal deficits, the nature of which depends on the area of the brain affected.
23. Families of stroke clients may demonstrate problems that must be addressed within the plan of care for the client, such as knowledge deficit, ineffective family coping, or spiritual distress.
24. The rehabilitation phase must begin as soon as the client is medically stable, so that morbidity and complications can be minimized or avoided. Treatment of the stroke client must be delivered on a continuum of care and through a multidisciplinary approach.

CASE STUDY

Mr. R., a 69-year-old white male, was admitted to a hospital after the sudden onset of right-sided hemiparesis, inability to talk, and inability to swallow. At the time his symptoms appeared, he was reading a newspaper while sitting in a living room recliner. Mr. R. has a history of adult-onset diabetes mellitus, which has been successfully controlled with oral hypoglycemic medication. He also has a history of essential hypertension, which has been controlled with one antihypertensive medication.

On admission to the emergency care area, his blood pressure was 168/100; temperature, 98.6° F; pulse rate, 68 beats/min; respiratory rate, 36 breaths/min. He was placed on bed rest with the head of his bed slightly elevated. Arterial blood gas values were obtained, and although they were within normal limits, oxygen was started at 2 liters/min by nasal cannula. Baseline complete blood count, urinalysis, and chemistry profile specimens were drawn. Also, specimens for determination of prothrombin and partial thromboplastin times were drawn. A CT scan of the head was completed immediately, as well as carotid Doppler studies. The laboratory results were essentially within normal limits for his age, except for a slightly elevated white blood cell count of 11,500 and a blood glucose level of 150. The CT scan showed a density in the left side of the brain consistent with a cerebral thrombus in the left hemisphere. The carotid Doppler studies showed 25% to 50% occlusion of the right and left internal carotid arteries.

Mr. R. was admitted to a medical unit. He was started on a heparin drip, piggy-backed into an IV of half-strength normal saline, 1000 ml over 12 hours. Within 48 hours of the initiation of the heparin, warfarin (Coumadin) was started, and the heparin was discontinued 24 hours later. Coumadin doses were altered daily according to prothrombin times.

Within 48 hours of the onset of symptoms, Mr. R.'s speech began to return. However, he continued to experience difficulty swallowing thin liquids and some foods. (Mr. R. was on an 1800-calorie American Dietetic Association [ADA] diet). He was alert and oriented to time, place, and person. He began to move his right arm in gross, uncontrolled actions (right hand dominant). He continued to be unable to move his right leg. His vital signs had remained stable for the last 48 hours. He began experiencing urinary incontinence, with which he had no prior problems.

Mr. R. is married and has no children. He lives in a two-story house in an affluent midwestern suburb. Mr. R. had recently retired; he had managed his own construction business. He and his wife have planned to travel extensively and have already gone to Europe and taken a Caribbean cruise. Mr. and Mrs. R. are active in the Baptist Church, where Mr. R. is a deacon.

Mr. R. has always managed the financial affairs of the household. Mrs. R. frequently visits Mr. R. in the hospital and is beginning to look fatigued. She refuses to leave Mr. R.'s bedside, even at the nurses' insistence. Mr. R. is demonstrating an increasing amount of frustration at not being able to move his right arm and leg. He also cries very easily, and Mrs. R. says this makes her feel helpless. She also says that Mr. R. has always been open with her, but now is withdrawn.

The social worker has spoken with Mr. and Mrs. R. about Mr. R.'s need for further reha-

bilitation and has suggested that he be transferred to the hospital's rehabilitation unit. Mr. and Mrs. R. have agreed. That transfer took place on the seventh day of Mr. R.'s acute-care stay.

ASSESSMENT CRITERIA
Physical
Neurological
  Mental status (level of consciousness, affect, insight, attention)
  Memory (recent, past)
  Cognitive status
  Orientation to time, place, person
  Ability to communicate
  Balance, gait, reflexes
  Sensory/motor function of the extremities
  Pupillary response
  Headache
  Nausea, vomiting, hiccups
Respiratory
  Airway maintenance
  Rate/rhythm
  Dyspnea
  Chest sounds
Cardiovascular
  Blood pressure
  Pulse
  Temperature
  Peripheral vascular status
  Carotid bruits
  Activity tolerance
  Fluid volume/electrolytes
Musculoskeletal
  Muscle tone/strength in neck and all extremities
  Joint strength, particularly on the affected side
  Presence of contractures, particularly on the affected side
  Transfer ability
Gastrointestinal
  Appetite
  Ability to swallow
  Percentage of food intake by food group
  Intake of fluids
  Status of oral cavity, including teeth, gums, tongue, buccal mucosa
  Bowel habits
  Nutritional status, height, present weight compared with ideal and usual
Genitourinary
  Ability to void
  History of voiding patterns
  Incontinence
  History of sexual function (impotence)
  Urinary output
  Urinary residual volume
  Functional ability to use toilet
  Cognitive ability to use toilet, urinal

Integument
   Integrity
   Lesions
   Turgor
Self-care ability
   Bathe
   Groom
   Dress
   Toilet
   Feed

Psychosocial

Life-style
Health perceptions
Health maintenance behaviors
Knowledge of disease/treatment
Usual coping mechanisms (self and spouse)
Adequacy of coping behaviors
Support systems
Risk factors (smoking, drinking, etc.)
Life goals/values
Self-concept
Ability to learn
Motivation
Roles

Spiritual

Ability to participate in religious practices
Trust
Religious affiliations

Mr. R. arrived at the emergency care area with the classic symptoms of a CVA. He also had two of the most commonly identified risk factors—diabetes mellitus and hypertension.

Mr. R.'s blood pressure was initially elevated. This condition is a compensatory mechanism of the body to increase cardiac output, which in turn increases cerebral circulation. Oxygen therapy was started to increase oxygen saturation of the blood, even though the arterial blood gas values were within normal limits, so that increased oxygen could be provided to the brain cells.

The initial diagnostic examinations revealed that the cause of the CVA was in fact a thrombus. Anticoagulation therapy was started accordingly to decrease the chances of further clot formation. Heparin, a rapidly acting anticoagulant, treats the immediate need. Coumadin, a slower-acting drug, is begun when initial anticoagulation is achieved. The efficacy of the anticoagulation therapy is tested by laboratory tests, partial thromboplastin times, and prothrombin times.

Carotid Doppler studies are performed to determine if occlusions exist in the external and internal carotid arteries. If occlusions are found, depending on the severity, carotid endarterectomies may be performed to remove them. This procedure can have major complications and usually is done only if medical treatment is not an option. In Mr. R.'s case the occlusions were minimal, and medical treatment was selected as the treatment of choice.

Mr. R. was stable enough to be treated on a medical floor, as opposed to the intensive care unit. Half-strength normal saline was given intravenously to ensure hydration of the client. This solution was selected over dextrose solution because dextrose solutions are hypotonic and can increase cerebral edema.

Mr. R.'s symptoms and sequelae—right arm and leg hemiplegia, dysphagia, and dysphasia—are characteristic of a left-hemisphere brain injury.

The effects of the stroke have left some obvious emotional and thought process disturbances in the client, such as the withdrawn behavior and the emotional lability.

Some apparent challenges to be considered in regard to Mr. R.'s return home involve his ability to successfully respond to rehabilitation, Mrs. R.'s ability to assist in his care, community services available, and the physical layout of the family home.

NURSING CARE PLAN: CEREBROVASCULAR DISEASE—THROMBUS, EMBOLUS, HEMORRHAGE

Nursing diagnoses	Expected client outcomes	Nursing strategies

Altered tissue perfusion related to disruption of blood flow to brain cells (thrombosis) and cerebral edema (first 48 hours)	Within 48 hours of admission to hospital, client will have optimum level of consciousness, and further cerebral injury will have been minimized, as demonstrated by return/maintenance of neurological status	Assess physical/neurological status to obtain baseline (see Assessment Criteria)
		Assess neurological status every hour for first 4-6 hours; then every 4 hours, if stable
		Maintain bed rest for first 48 hours
		Observe for acute or subtle changes in:
		  Level of consciousness
		  Progression of neurological deficits
		  Blood pressure/respiratory pattern
		Notify physician if neurological changes occur
		Facilitate venous return by:
		  Elevating head of bed 15 to 30 degrees
		  Preventing flexion rotation or hyperextension of head
		Prevent Valsalva maneuver:
		  Assist client to move in bed
		  Provide stool softener
		  Instruct client to avoid straining, coughing, sneezing, blowing nose
		  If suctioning necessary, limit to 15 seconds
		  Avoid rectal temperatures
		Maintain oxygen at 2 L/min by nasal cannula for 48 hours (per physician orders)
		Allow for adequate rest periods between activities
		Provide quiet environment
		Provide total care, including bathing, turning, toileting
		Monitor intake and output every 8 hours or per physician's orders; notify physician if output is less than intake
		Administer medications as ordered (document results/side effects as indicated):
		  Heparin
		  Coumadin
		  Oral hypoglycemic agents
		  Antihypertensive drug

Ineffective airway clearance (potential/actual) related to ineffective chewing/swallowing	Client will maintain patent airway at all times
	Client will experience prompt treatment for respiratory complications
		Request consultation for speech therapy to assist swallowing
		Assess for signs/symptoms of ineffective airway clearance (see Assessment Criteria and care plan for impaired swallowing, p. 87)
		Assess gag reflex
		Carefully administer oral food/fluids
		Keep head of bed elevated 30 to 45 degrees
		Keep throat suction machine at the bedside
		Monitor arterial blood gas values as ordered
		Observe for signs/symptoms of aspiration pneumonia:
		  Increased cough
		  Temperature (1° F over baseline)
		  Adventitious chest sounds
		Notify physician immediately if signs/symptoms occur

NURSING CARE PLAN: CEREBROVASCULAR DISEASE—THROMBUS, EMBOLUS, HEMORRHAGE—cont'd

Nursing diagnoses	Expected client outcomes	Nursing strategies
Altered nutrition: less than body requirements; related to ineffective chewing/swallowing and history of adult-onset diabetes (controlled with oral hypoglycemics)	Client will have adequate food/fluid intake as demonstrated by: Restoration/maintenance of ideal body weight Serum albumin within normal limits Blood glucose maintained between 100 and 140 mg/dl Urinary output of at least 30 ml/hr	Obtain baseline height/weight on admission Weigh twice a week thereafter Notify physician of weight loss of 2 pounds or more Observe for swallowing difficulty, and determine which food/fluid items client has most difficulty with Obtain order for speech pathologist evaluation Obtain dietary consultation, including calculation of: Ideal body weight Daily caloric requirements Daily protein/carbohydrate/fat requirements Daily fluid requirements Obtain consultation order for occupational therapist to develop a restorative feeding program and advice on assistive devices Provide dysphagia diet according to swallowing tolerance/capability of the client, as determined by speech therapist and dietician Add thickening to thin fluids as necessary Monitor fluid intake/urinary output every 8 hours Monitor food intake by food groups after each meal If food intake consistently falls below 50% in any major food group, perform nutrient count for 3 days If client is unable to take adequate nutrition, confer with the physician and health care team about prosthetic feeding devices (i.e., nasogastric tube, gastrostomy tube) Monitor blood glucose by "finger stick" 4 times a day for 2 days, then twice a day for 7 days, then daily in the morning thereafter
Impaired physical mobility related to neuromuscular deficit secondary to right hemiplegia	By time of dismissal from rehabilitation unit, client will: Sit up in bed without assistance Transfer from bed to chair and chair to bed with minimal assistance Ambulate with standby assistance of one person using an assistive device Perform right extremity exercises; progressing from passive to active assistance and from maximal assistance to minimal assistance Tolerate increased activity Turn self from side to side in bed with minimal assistance	As soon as client is medically stable, request evaluation from physical therapist regarding forumulation of plan of care Perform range-of-motion exercises, especially on affected side, every 2 hours Position extremities in neutral positions using protective/positioning devices (pillow, splint) Increase activity as client's endurance improves: Chair for meals Commode Chair in morning and afternoon Use walker/transfer belt to assist in transferring Alternate rest with activity Keep initial therapy sessions short and terminate them before client becomes fatigued or frustrated Follow physical therapist's plan of care to maintain consistency in care

Continued.

NURSING CARE PLAN: CEREBROVASCULAR DISEASE—THROMBUS, EMBOLUS, HEMORRHAGE—cont'd

Nursing diagnoses	Expected client outcomes	Nursing strategies
Self-care deficits (bathing, dressing, feeding, grooming, toileting) related to neuromuscular impairment secondary to right hemiplegia	Client will be able to bathe, dress, feed, groom, and toilet self with standby assistance by time of dismissal from rehabilitation unit Client will demonstrate safety practices	Assess client ability to perform self-care skills As soon as client is medically stable, obtain order for occupational therapist evaluation to determine degree of self-care deficits and formulate plan of care Follow occupational therapist's plan of care in helping client to use long-handle sponge, eating utensil, adaptive device Set realistic and achievable expectations regarding rehabilitation Maintain calm, stress-free environment as client performs self-care activities Apply protective devices to affected side to prevent contractures/injury during movement Require consistent approaches from all health team members

Altered urinary elimination patterns: incontinence; related to impaired central control micturation	Client will be able to identify "normal" voiding patterns
	Client will demonstrate knowledge of the rationale for his treatment plan
	Client will report symptoms of urinary tract infections
		Assess client's urinary status
		Accurately record intake and output every 8 hours
		Obtain urologic evaluation to determine exact reason for incontinence
		Establish bladder retraining program based on reason for incontinence:
		  Offer urinal every 2-3 hours
		  Check bladder for residual every 8 hours until bladder routine established
		  Administer anticholinergics, antispasmodics, calcium channel blockers as prescribed; observe for side effects (see Nursing Alerts)
		Manage any episodes of incontinence with matter-of-fact attitude, acknowledging feelings of client
		Observe for signs of urinary tract infection and treat as ordered:
		  Odor
		  Burning (may be absent)
		  Bleeding (NOTE: client taking anticoagulant)
		  Clarity

Altered thought processes: emotional lability; related to damage to brain structure	Client will demonstrate fewer "emotional" or inappropriate outbursts and ability to maintain or regain control	Assess frequency of emotional outbursts and length of time of catastrophic reactions Assess environment for precipitating events, and eliminate them or restructure the situation When events occur, "back off" and allow client to regain control Avoid scolding or shaming Explain to client and spouse about emotional lability, causes, solutions Offer comfort/support during and after episodes Always determine if episode is emotional lability as opposed to depression

NURSING CARE PLAN: CEREBROVASCULAR DISEASE—THROMBUS, EMBOLUS, HEMORRHAGE—cont'd

Nursing diagnoses	Expected client outcomes	Nursing strategies

Ineffective individual coping, frustration, withdrawal, related to sudden onset of devastating illness, loss of control, altered thought processes	Client's level of coping will increase as demonstrated by:
	    Less frustration with deficits
	    Willingness to share concerns with spouse, staff
	    Fewer episodes of emotional outbursts
	Client will verbalize chosen coping strategies
		Assess former coping style
		Be supportive of client
		Encourage client to share concerns, fears, frustration
		Promote positive coping strategies
		Set goals that are realistic and achievable
		Reinforce progress toward rehabilitation goals
		Obtain social services referral to:
		    Assist client and spouse in redefining family roles
		    Identify support systems or provide services to assist in life-style restructuring
		Encourage dialogue between client and spouse, particularly the honest expression of feelings
		See care plan for altered thought processes, p. 90
		Involve pastoral care/minister in supporting emotional recovery process

Ineffective coping by a spouse: lack of willingness to rest, verbalization of concerns about client's behavior, and feelings of helplessness; related to sudden need for drastically altered life-style and role changes	Spouse's level of coping will increase:
	    Exhibits fewer feelings of helplessness
	    Verabalizes understanding of client's withdrawn behavior/emotional lability
	    Shows willingness to rest and care for self away from hospital
	    Assumes increased role in family
	    Participates in client's plan of care
		Assess former style of coping and coping behaviors
		Listen attentively to spouse's concerns regarding client's behavior
		Explain disease process and effects of disease
		Encourage spouse to rest and care for self away from hospital
		Establish trust relationship between nursing staff and spouse (phone spouse; allow spouse to phone when she is gone to assure herself of client's condition)
		Obtain social services consultation to help spouse to redefine role functions in family and to identify support systems to assist in some of the role functions
		Gradually involve spouse in client's plan of care, especially rehabilitation
		Encourage dialogue between client and spouse, particularly the honest expression of feelings
		Encourage pastoral care/minister/friends to support emotional recovery process

Impaired verbal communication: aphasia; related to damage to left-hemisphere brain structure	Client will communicate needs, understanding, and feelings	Obtain consultation from speech pathologist to determine extent of speech impairment and develop plan of care Observe client's speech patterns for irregularities (see care plan for impaired verbal communication, p. 19) Allow client to speak at his own pace; do not hurry him Speak to client slowly and clearly in a normal tone of voice Observe client's facial expressions to determine understanding Observe client for follow-through after simple commands Use nonverbal communication/gestures Keep message concise; one idea to a sentence If frustration occurs, allow client to rest, and then restart communication Minimize changes in routines Suggest television programs for the client that are "action" shows (sports) as opposed to talk shows that require verbal cues

Continued.

NURSING CARE PLAN: CEREBROVASCULAR DISEASE—THROMBUS, EMBOLUS, HEMORRHAGE—cont'd

Nursing diagnoses	Expected client outcomes	Nursing strategies
Knowledge deficit (client and spouse) in regard to disabilities, treatment, and rehabilitation after stroke	Client and spouse will verbalize understanding of: Disease process, including causes, symptoms, short- and long-term effects, recovery expectations Diagnostic procedures and treatment, including medications and side effects, diet, activity Rehabilitation, including physical, occupational, and speech therapy, dietary needs, and social services Discharge planning, options, insurance benefits Client and spouse will demonstrate ability to: Transfer and ambulate safely Perform self-care activities Participate in bladder retraining program Take/administer medications appropriately	Assess knowledge level Explain to client and spouse: Disease process: causes, symptoms, short- and long-term effects, reasonable recovery Treatment modalities: medications (Coumadin, antihypertensive, hypoglycemics) and side effects; diet (dysphagia/ADA); activity (bed rest, gradual activity) Rehabilitation: physical, occupational, and speech therapy plans of care; diet preparation; social services plan of care Discharge planning: levels of care needed; Medicare/Medicaid coverage Involve client and spouse in plan of care with nursing staff and rehabilitation team to learn: Transfer techniques Performance of self-care activities Participation in bladder retraining program Medications, schedules, side effects
Impaired home maintenance management; related to role changes in management of household, and parts of home not being easily accessible by handicapped person (two-story house) secondary to cerebrovascular accident with right hemiplegia	Roles for client and spouse will be redefined, reflecting comprehensive management of household maintenance Home will be made accessible to client so that he can perform self-care activities independently and safely	Assess meanings of roles Obtain social services consultation to begin discharge planning, including: Social assessment (see Assessment Criteria) Financial and support systems available to client and spouse Care options available to client and spouse: Rehabilitation unit Skilled nursing unit or facility Home health care Nursing care facility Durable medical equipment Outpatient rehabilitation services Adult day services Present options to client and spouse; include them in planning Reevaluate client's progress during rehabilitation phase to determine if discharge plan is appropriate or needs to be changed Close to dismissal time, obtain occupational therapist's "home evaluation" to: Determine accessibility to house, bedroom, bathroom, kitchen Examine the need for grab bars, wider doors, assistive devices Determine safety measures, including removal of throw rugs, removal of furniture from pathways, etc.

EVALUATION

1. The client receives prompt treatment through the monitoring of vital signs, levels of consciousness, and neurological status.
2. The client maintains a patent airway and receives prompt treatment of respiratory infection.
3. The client maintains adequate food and fluid intake.
4. The client adequately performs the tasks of transferring and ambulating with the standby assistance of a quad-cane.
5. The client is able to perform activities of daily living with standby assistances.
6. The client maintains urinary continence and can report symptoms of a urinary infection.
7. The client exhibits progressively fewer inappropriate emotional outbursts and regains control within an optimum time.
8. The client exhibits increased levels of effective coping behavior.
9. The client's spouse exhibits increased levels of effective coping behavior.

NURSING ALERTS

1. This care plan is developed especially for the client with an injury of the left hemisphere of the brain. Give close attention to the special needs of the client with an injury of the right hemisphere or brainstem as determined diagnostically.
2. Concurrent disease conditions must be treated with special cautions:
   a. Hypertension: edema and ischemia may result in an increase in intracranial pressure, necessitating a somewhat elevated blood pressure to maintain cerebral blood flow. A too rapid reduction in blood pressure may result in an increase in the size of an infarct or a new stroke. Treatment will be conservative, including bed rest and a low-sodium diet. When the neurological condition has stabilized, use of antihypertensive drugs may be introduced.
   b. Diabetes: immobility, hospitalization, and change in life-style alter metabolic needs at the same time that dietary intake may be limited by swallowing and chewing difficulties and decreased appetite. Management requires frequent monitoring of blood glucose levels and frequent adjustments of diet and insulin dosage.
3. Anticoagulation therapy requires very frequent and meticulous monitoring. Clients who have a high likelihood of injuring themselves by falling or in other ways because of poor muscle control must be observed closely for bruising and must be protected from hitting limbs on bed rails or other objects.
4. Anticholinergics for treatment of urge incontinence must be used judiciously, with cardiac effects being monitored closely.
5. In the course of acute medical treatment, nutrition and diet are often overlooked. There is a high incidence of aspiration pneumonia resulting from inappropriate selection of diet. All stroke clients should be checked for swallowing capabilities by the speech pathologist and for nutritional status by the dietitian.
6. Urinary tract infection may not be detected because of the absence of sensation—that is, burning. Frequency and urgency may be viewed as incontinence.
7. All stroke clients should be evaluated for degree of cognitive deficits by each member of the health care team.
8. To secure the best results, rehabilitation services must be started as soon as the client is medically stable.

Bibliography

Adams GF: Cerebrovascular disability and the aging brain, Edinburgh, 1974, Churchill Livingstone.

Bray GP and Clark GS: A stroke family guide and resource, Springfield, Ill, 1984, Charles C Thomas, Publisher.

Groer MW and Shekleton ME: Basic pathophysiology: a holistic approach, ed 3, St Louis, 1989, The CV Mosby Co.

Kim MJ, McFarland GK, and McLane AM: Pocket guide to nursing diagnoses, ed 3, St Louis, 1989, The CV Mosby Co.

Rockstein M and Sussman M: Biology of aging, Belmont, Calif, 1979, Wadsworth Publishing Co.

Seidel et al: Mosby's guide to physical examination, St Louis, 1987, The CV Mosby Co.

Taylor JW: RN nursing management of stroke: acute care, part 1 and 2, Cardiovascular Nursing 21:1, 1985.

MUSCULOSKELETAL SYSTEM

Rheumatoid Arthritis

Janet T. Barrett

KNOWLEDGE BASE

1. Rheumatoid arthritis (RA) is a chronic systemic inflammatory disease of unknown cause for which there is no cure. Joint changes occur over time. The destructive process begins with inflammation of the synovial membrane. The thickened synovium, or pannus, develops and extends over the articular surface. This formation erodes and destroys articular cartilage and underlying bone. Fibrous ankylosis (subluxation and deformity of the joint) begins, and scar tissue is laid down, prohibiting normal joint movement. The last stage is bony ankylosis, in which solid bony union takes place in the joints, causing immobile of "fixed" joints. Indications of systemic involvement include anemia, pleurisy, pericarditis, peripheral neuropathy, and leg ulcers. The characteristic subcutaneous rheumatoid nodule is frequently seen around the elbows and fingers but is also observed in the bursas and tendon sheaths.

2. The onset of rheumatoid arthritis is usually insidious, with symptoms of malaise, weight loss, and vague periarticular pain and stiffness. Rheumatoid arthritis may be precipitated by anxiety, exposure to cold, overwork, or an acute infection.

3. Signs and symptoms are symmetrical joint stiffness, pain, warmth, and swelling. The pain and stiffness are prominent in the morning and subside with moderate use of the joint as the day progresses. Stiffness may increase after strenuous activity. Joint stiffness is an important indicator of inactive disease.

4. Any joint may be affected by RA, but the proximal interphalangeal and metacarpophalangeal joints of the fingers, wrists, knees, ankles, and toes are most typically involved.

5. With the advancement of rheumatoid arthritis, ocular manifestations such as uveitis and keratoconjunctivitis can occur as a result of dryness of the eyes.

6. Several laboratory tests may be used to help diagnose rheumatoid arthritis: rheumatoid factor (RF), erythrocyte sedimentation rate (ESR), latex fixation, agglutinin reactions, and immunoglobulins (IgM and IgG).

7. Synovial fluid aspiration may be used to diagnose rheumatoid arthritis. In persons with RA the fluid is opaque and sterile, with reduced viscosity and an elevated white blood cell count.

8. X-ray films of involved joints may show the progress of joint destruction.

9. Emotional disturbances, such as loneliness or grieving, may trigger exacerbation of RA. Keeping an older adult productive and active may lessen emotional disturbances.

10. Because RA is a systemic disease, fatigue, weakness, and anorexia may occur.

11. An elderly person with RA usually experiences morning stiffness, which increases his or her discomfort and thus the risk of accidents.

12. The major objectives of treatment are to reduce pain and inflammation, preserve function, and prevent deformity through rest, therapy, and drugs.

13. A balance between rest and activity is crucial in the older adult with RA. The use of strict bed rest is reserved for acute exacerbations, to prevent further damage to the inflamed joints.

14. Demineralization of the bone occurs with the aging process, as evidenced by decreased mass and density of bone. Lack of stress on all bones (resulting from pain with RA) can exacerbate osteoporosis. There is marked resorption of calcium in the fingers and hands. Calcium supplements may be needed if calcium intake in the diet is inadequate.

15. Intraarticular injections of steroids may be used for symptomatic relief if only one or two joints are affected.

16. Methotrexate, an immunosuppressive drug, has some effect on RA. It is used only when other therapies have been exhausted.

17. Aspirin is the drug of choice for treatment of RA, primarily because of its antiinflammatory effect. The proper dose is one that relieves symptoms without causing toxic effects. It should be taken during remission as well as exacerbations. Another group of medicines frequently prescribed is the nonsteroidal antiinflammatory drugs (NSAIDs), which include ibuprofen, fenoprofen, naproxen, tolmetin, sulindac, and piroxicam. The physician may also prescribe oral corticosteroids, gold, or one of the slow-onset agents such as sodium thromalate or D-penicillamine.

18. No special diet is needed, but adequate nutrition and fluids will help keep the joints and the body systems functioning. Adequate calcium is necessary to minimize the bone demineralization associated with the aging process.

CASE STUDY

When Mrs. Wilkerson was 35 years old, she noticed the first troubling changes in her body. At that time her feet, wrists, and fingers began to swell and become stiff. She also noticed generalized fatigue and a 10-pound weight loss. A diagnosis of rheumatoid arthritis was made. As the years went by, Mrs. Wilkerson was treated with a variety of medications, including gold salts, aspirin, penicillamine, and steroids.

Mrs. Wilkerson has experienced an average of one acute rheumatoid episode a year. During an episode she experiences an acute inflammatory reaction with symptoms of pain, swelling, redness, tenderness, and heat in the metacarpals, phalanges, and wrists. Sometimes she has the same inflammatory reaction in her elbows, hips, and cervical spine. Her physician usually prescribes rest, heat, and steroids during the acute exacerbations.

Over the years, joint thickening and destruction have occurred. Ulnar deviation, swan-neck deformities of the fingers, and several subcutaneous nodules on the elbows have gradually developed. Systemically, Mrs. Wilkerson has had two episodes of pleurisy, each requiring hospitalization. She has not developed any cardiovascular or neuropathic problems.

Now at age 75, Mrs. Wilkerson is living in a retirement home. The retirement community includes many friends who are important sources of support when an acute episode occurs. She maintains a small apartment with weekly cleaning services. She prepares her own meals using specialized assistive devices.

Physically Mrs. Wilkerson's hands look very deformed, with marked ulnar deviation. She has approximately 40% normal flexion and extension in her wrists. She has experienced a loss of strength in both hands and wrists. For about 60 minutes every morning on arising, her hands and wrists are very stiff. She takes medication daily to control the chronic pain on movement. Mrs. Wilkerson feels fortunate to have lived a long life and has been able to cope with her rheumatoid arthritis.

ASSESSMENT CRITERIA
Physical
Joints:
  Erythema, edema, or deformities
  Heat, pain, or crepitation
  Length of fingers, deviation, movement, and grip of both hands
  Morning stiffness and alleviating factors
  Muscle atrophy around affected joints
Skin
  Subcutaneous nodules
  Color
  Consistency
  Thickness
  Ulcers
  Dryness, including mucous membranes
Activity
  Degree of active and/or passive range of motion
  Exercise activities and ability to perform activities of daily living
  Activity tolerance
Height and weight
Vital signs, with emphasis on temperature
Head-to-toe assessment using inspection, palpation, percussion, and auscultation as appropriate on all body systems
Neurosensory assessment of hands and feet

Psychosocial
Description of typical day
Recreation/leisure profile
Occupational profile
Living environment profile
Family profile
Resources/support systems used
Knowledge of rheumatoid arthritis and specific treatment measures
Perceptions of stress and stressful events
Coping skills

Spiritual
Religious practices/beliefs
Incorporation of spiritual resources into personal support system

The initial joint changes Mrs. Wilkerson experienced are characteristic of rheumatoid arthritis. The fatigue and weight loss are frequently occurring systemic manifestations of the disease. There is characteristically peripheral, symmetrical joint swelling with associated stiffness, warmth, and tenderness. The course of the disease is unpredictable, with remissions and exacerbations. The aims of treat-

ment are a balance between rest and activity and control of pain through a variety of measures.

The pleurisy Mrs. Wilkerson developed is a typical systemic manifestation of RA. The connective tissues of the heart, lungs, pleura, and arteries are commonly affected. The hand deformities are due to the progression of the RA.

NURSING CARE PLAN: RHEUMATOID ARTHRITIS

Nursing diagnoses	Expected client outcomes	Nursing strategies
Chronic pain related to joint degeneration	Client will be able to effectively manage pain	Investigate all complaints of pain as to location, severity, precipitating factors, and emotional distress Recommend that client take a warm bath or shower upon arising to help decrease joint stiffness Apply heat and/or cold to affected joints Take medication as prescribed for pain Teach client never to massage an acutely inflamed joint Help client plan a daily exercise routine within the limits of pain tolerance and in association with a rest program
Impaired physical mobility related to joint edema and pain	Client will carry out measures to promote mobility	Teach client how to conserve energy and lessen stress on joints Explain importance of maintaining a balance between exercise and rest Assist with prioritizing activities and taking planned rests Encourage client to perform active or passive range-of-motion exercises for specific joints as prescribed by physician or therapist Teach proper positioning and support of affected joints Observe for complications of immobility: pressure sores, phlebitis, muscle atrophy, contractures, weakness Teach client to avoid clothing with buttons and instead select clothing with Velcro snaps or front zippers, or clothes that open down the front
Knowledge deficit: self-care management of RA; related to lack of previous experience	Client will incorporate knowledge into daily activity routine	Follow teaching/learning principles individualized to this client; instruct client about management measures: systemic and emotional rest, exercises, assistive devices, therapies, and drugs Involve client's family, if possible, in all aspects of teaching; the family can reinforce the information Teach client the name, dose, frequency, action, and side effects of prescribed drugs Teach correct use of any devices, as well as safety precautions

NURSING CARE PLAN: RHEUMATOID ARTHRITIS—cont'd

Nursing diagnoses	Expected client outcomes	Nursing strategies
Potential body image disturbance related to physical changes secondary to RA	Client will verbalize feelings about body changes and will contact support groups as needed	Assess the meaning of the physical changes to client and adaptive responses to the changes and deformities Encourage client to talk about the problems the disease and physical changes are causing her Explore with client remaining strengths and abilities and how they can be used to overcome perceived problems Encourage client to network with self-care and support groups
Potential social isolation related to discomfort and physical changes in body	Client will regularly engage in social interaction	Involve client and family in all aspects of therapy to preserve a sense of value and control Discuss with client the meaning of loss or change of her body; ascertain how she feels about these changes to her life-style and sexual functioning Inform client of local and national networks such as the Arthritis Foundation Encourage client to plan some type of social interaction each day; discuss how isolation and loneliness may aggravate or precipitate an acute attack of RA; encourage client to plan a social event such as meeting someone for lunch or coffee or just talking on a regular basis Encourage client to join a telephone network by which a phone call would be received each day to check on client's well-being; encourage client to make calls to friends and acquaintances Encourage client to join social clubs such as reading clubs, video clubs, bridge clubs, canasta clubs, poker clubs, or hobby clubs Give positive reinforcement for activities the client is already involved in
Activity intolerance related to immobility	Client will maintain present level of mobility	Help client plan activities with scheduled rest periods; instruct client that some pain may be experienced with activity Instruct client to take medication one-half hour before an activity Instruct client that if pain continues for 2-3 hours after the activity, then the activity may have been too rigorous Teach the client that during an acute attack, bed rest may be indicated for a limited time to rest the joints to help reduce articular inflammation Devices such as small pillows, rolls, and splints may be used to support affected joints Teach client always to use the largest muscle group for any activity, and show her how to do so (e.g., carrying a shoulder bag instead of a handbag, pushing doors open with shoulder instead of hand, and bending over at the knees instead of the back)

Continued.

NURSING CARE PLAN: RHEUMATOID ARTHRITIS—cont'd

Nursing diagnoses	Expected client outcomes	Nursing strategies
Potential self-care deficit: bathing, dressing/grooming, feeding; related to joint stiffness and immobility	Client will demonstrate optimal self-care ability	Teach client use of specially built utensils and devices for performing activities of daily living (e.g., Velcro on clothes, open-front shirts and blouses, large built-up handles on cookware, built-up utensils, long-handled devices to extend reach, walkers, and canes; grooming aids are available to help comb hair, brush teeth, shave and clip nails); refer to occupational therapist if indicated

NURSING ALERTS

1. Since rheumatoid arthritis is a systemic disease, the nurse cannot focus only on the involved joints but must also be alert for cardiovascular, respiratory, and ocular manifestations.
2. The nurse must remember that the amount of pain does not correlate with the amount of destruction in the joints. A small amount of destruction can cause excruciating pain, or great destruction can cause little pain.
3. Long-term drug therapies need to be periodically assessed for effectiveness and side effects. Also, dosage changes may be indicated over time.
4. Elderly clients who take long-term medication such as aspirin are at risk for side effects and complications, especially if their medication regimens are complex and they have a variety of chronic health problems. The absorption, distribution, metabolism, and excretion of drugs are altered as a result of the aging process. A client may have to alter the medication dose and frequency to eliminate side effects and complications (Remember that most drugs used for RA need to be taken with food because of the gastrointestinal side effects.)
5. Multiple doses of a variety of medications may be confusing to the elderly. Forgetting to take medicine and repeating doses are common problems. A timed or labeled container with multiple compartments for each medication may help the client remember when to take medicine.
6. Heat relaxes the muscles and relieves joint stiffness. When applied immediately before an activity, heat may also increase the effectiveness of exercise. A warm bath in the morning may relax muscles and decrease joint stiffness. Cold induces local anesthesia, thus decreasing pain. The relief derived from heat or cold therapies is highly individual.
7. Bed rest is the treatment of choice during an acute attack of rheumatoid arthritis. The bed should be firm and the client positioned to prevent footdrop or flexion contractures. Extension of joints (at least 10 hours a day) is important during the acute phase.
8. Using the largest muscle for any activity should increase the amount of activity a client can perform and should minimize discomfort.

EVALUATION

1. The client is pain free or experiences only slight discomfort most of the time.
2. The client reports an ability to comfortably perform daily activities.
3. The client adheres to her medication regimen.
4. The client regularly participates in an exercise routine.
5. The client recognizes when assistive devices are necessary and arranges for the purchase or making of these devices.
6. The client verbalizes acceptance of physical changes.
7. The client verbalizes feelings of control over her body.
8. The client networks with at least one person each day.
9. The client joins one club that has a purpose she enjoys.
10. The client has incorporated the use of appropriate adaptive devices into her daily routine.
11. The client demonstrates the ability to independently perform self-care tasks.

Bibliography

Brassell MP: Pharmacologic management of rheumatic diseases, Orthopaedic Nursing 7:43, March-April 1988.

Brietung JC: Caring for older adults, Philadelphia, 1987, WB Saunders Co.

Carpenito L: Nursing diagnosis: application to clinical practice, ed 2, Philadelphia, 1987, JB Lippincott Co.

Eliopoulos C: Gerontological nursing, ed 2, Philadelphia, 1987, JB Lippincott Co.

Gioiella EC and Bevil CW: Nursing care of the aging client, Norwalk, Conn, 1985, Appleton-Century-Crofts.

Lorig K, Konkol L, and Gonzalez V: Arthritis patient education: a review of the literature, Patient Education and Counseling 10:207, Dec 1987.

Loring K et al: A comparison of lay-taught and professional-taught arthritis self-management courses, The Journal of Rheumatology 13:763, August 1986.

Schoen DC: Assessment for arthritis, Orthopaedic Nursing 7:31, March-April 1988.

Van Deusen J and Harlowe D: The efficacy of the ROM dance program for adults with rheumatoid arthritis, The American Journal of Occupational Therapy 41:90, Jan 1987.

Van Deusen J and Harlowe D: Rheumatoid arthritis, Medical Times 116:45, Sept 1988.

Osteoarthritis

Janet T. Barrett

KNOWLEDGE BASE

1. Osteoarthritis, also known as degenerative joint disease (DJD), hypertrophic arthritis, and senescent arthritis, is considered a noninflammatory joint disease, as opposed to rheumatoid arthritis, which is inflammatory in nature.

2. Osteoarthritis is a nonsystemic, slow, progressive disease of the movable joints. Weight-bearing joints are most affected: hips, knees, ankles, cervical and lumbosacral joints, and distal interphalangeal joints of the fingers. The disease is asymetrical in its distribution and progress.

3. Osteoarthritis is the most common form of arthritis. Its cause is unknown, but aging, obesity, heredity, and trauma are contributing factors. The incidence of osteoarthritis is positively correlated with age. It increases in frequency after age 40; more than 80% of persons over age 60 are symptomatic.

4. Osteoarthritis involves destruction of the cartilage between the joints. Accumulated wear and tear causes the cartilage to lose its elasticity and eventually fray. In addition, a decrease in the water content of the cartilage creates narrowing of the joint spaces. As the cartilage thins, exposed bones rub together, thus producing the characteristic pain and swollen joints. Over time, the shape of the joint thickens because of osteophyte formation at the joint margins, resulting in limited joint movement.

5. Heberden's nodes on terminal interphalangeal finger joints are hypertrophic spurs (outgrowths of bone).

6. Osteoarthritis may be mild and cause only slight discomfort. Many older people experience stiffness and slight swelling of the joints, requiring no medication or other treatment. Symptoms usually develop gradually and progress slowly. Aching pain after motion and weight bearing and morning stiffness are the two most frequently reported symptoms. When pain is not relieved by drugs, rest, and physical therapy, hip or knee arthroplasty can be performed to provide greater mobility and comfort. Symptoms, severity, and degree of degeneration in the joint may not always be correlated.

7. Crepitation (grating in joints) is a common finding.

8. Some people with osteoarthritis tend to be chronically overweight, which places more stress on the joints over time.

9. Osteoarthritis cannot be cured. The discomfort can be treated, but the degeneration of the joint remains.

10. A change in atmospheric pressure and temperature may precipitate pain in the affected joints.

11. The pain pattern is variable. Joints may be more painful after a long period of inactivity or after overuse. Relief may occur after a period of limbering up.

12. The elderly with osteoarthritis experience morning stiffness, which increases discomfort and the risk of accidents. Heat relaxes the muscles, having an analgesic effect and relieving joint stiffness. A morning bath will help decrease joint stiffness. Moving the affected joint under warm water provides resistance and warmth to the joint.

13. The impact of osteoarthritis on self-concept and independence cannot be forgotten. Decreased ability to carry out routine activities can lead to a variety of psychosocial alterations.

14. X-ray film of the involved joint will show the destruction and help confirm the diagnosis of osteoarthritis.

15. Injections of corticosteroids into the affected intraarticular joint will temporarily relieve pain and increase function.

16. Medications for osteoarthritis include aspirin and nonsteroidal antiinflammatory drugs (NSAIDs) such as ibuprofen, fenoprofen, naproxen, tolmetin, sulindac, and piroxicam. These drugs help relieve the joint pain.

17. One quarter of all prescriptions are written for persons over 65 years of age. One half of all adverse drug reactions are experienced by the elderly. A client's knowledge of the drugs he or she takes may promote adherence to drug therapy.

18. A firm mattress and bedboard will add support to the joints and possibly decrease pain. Contractures of the hips can occur if pillows are placed under the knees for a prolonged time.

CASE STUDY

Mrs. Tidd, age 72, began experiencing slight morning joint stiffness 10 years ago. She noticed that it was at least 30 minutes to 1 hour after awakening before her fingers "would work right" and before she "could bend over and tie my shoes." Mrs. Tidd now notices an aching in her hips and knees after she has walked several blocks or after she has climbed stairs.

Her physician has prescribed ibuprofen (Motrin), 400 mg three times a day, which Mrs. Tidd says helps "the aches and pain of these old hips." Her physician has diagnosed osteoarthritis of the hips, knees, and fingers.

Mrs. Tidd has also noticed a slow, progressive thickening around the distal phalangeal joints, which her physician has diagnosed as Heberden's nodes. Other physical changes include a joint thickening around the knees and a decrease in height by 2 inches (she was 5'6" in 1950, now 5'4"). Her weight has ranged from 150 to 180 pounds over the years and now is stable at 162 pounds.

Mrs. Tidd's major symptom is a localized, dull, aching pain in the affected joints after she has walked for about 30 minutes. The Motrin taken throughout the day has decreased the pain greatly. She also notices knee swelling at the end of the day when she has been on her feet a lot.

Mrs. Tidd has enjoyed excellent health during her 72 years. She has four grown children, who were all delivered at home. She was hospitalized in 1962 for dilatation and curettage. Her husband died of heart disease in 1984 at the age of 68. She now lives alone and is able to maintain her home. She enjoys needlework such as sewing, embroidery, and crochet. She is active in church work, Eastern Star, and the area Senior Citizen's Center, where she regularly exercises and takes painting classes.

ASSESSMENT CRITERIA
Physical

Pain
  Location and radiation
  Character
  Quality
  Severity
  Duration
  Timing
  Associated symptoms (muscle aching, weakness, clumsiness, crepitation)
  Alleviating factors (rest, analgesics, position change, heat)

Affected joints
  Edema
  Redness
  Nodules or other deformities
  Crepitation
  Skin changes
Muscle strength
  Degree of active and/or passive range of motion
  Reflexes
  Activities of daily living (walking, cooking, etc.)
Dietary habits
Height and weight compared with previous years
Typical activity pattern and degree of functional ability
Complete head-to-toe assessment using inspection, palpation, percussion, and auscultation as appropriate for all body systems

Psychosocial

Description of typical day
Recreation/leisure profile
Occupational profile
Living environment profile
Family profile
Resources/support systems used
Adherence to medication regimen
Knowledge of drug action, dose, frequency, therapeutic and side effects

Spiritual

Religious practices/beliefs
Networking system with friends and family

Mrs. Tidd is probably experiencing a worsening of her symptoms of osteoarthritis because of advancing age. The morning joint stiffness is related to the extended period of inactivity during the night. The aching Mrs. Tidd is experiencing in her hips and knees after activity is typical of osteoarthritis in the major weight-bearing joints. Heberden's nodes are a characteristic sign of osteoarthritis and occur most often in women. Mrs. Tidd's shortened stature is probably indicative of vertebral degeneration associated with flattening of the intervertebral disks. The Motrin prescribed for Mrs. Tidd's pain is a frequently used analgesic. The activities in which she participates, when done in moderation, can help to maintain muscle strength and joint motion.

NURSING CARE PLAN: OSTEOARTHRITIS

Nursing diagnoses	Expected client outcome	Nursing strategies
Chronic pain related to loss of cartilage and irregular bone formation at joints	Client will be able to effectively manage pain	Carefully apply moist heat to affected joints, especially in the morning, for 10- to 15-minute periods Take medication as prescribed for chronic pain Plan rest periods during the day Plan most vigorous activity for the time when pain is least intense Help client plan a daily routine of active or passive exercise that will keep the joint as flexible as possible Suggest purchase of bed board and firm mattress that will keep the body in good alignment during the night Instruct client not to place pillows under the knees Teach client posture and positioning techniques
Activity intolerance related to joint pain and limitation of mobility	Client will maintain or increase activity	Develop a daily activity plan with client; consider strength, endurance, energy levels, and pain/discomfort Promote a positive attitude with sincere encouragement; convey that activity can be maintained Teach client to rest joints when increased pain is felt; resting can decrease pain, but bed rest is not usually required If osteoarthritis is severe, assistive devices such as canes, crutches, Ace bandages, or a walker may be necessary Teach correct use of these devices, as well as safety precautions Physiotherapy may be needed if osteoarthritis is severe; a planned therapy regimen could include heat, passive and active exercises, and assistive devices; consult with physician for orders
Knowledge deficit about osteoarthritis, related to lack of previous experience	Client will incorporate information into daily activity routine Client will verbalize knowledge of prescribed medication	Following teaching/learning principles individualized to this client, instruct regarding disease process, causes, factors contributing to symptoms, and methods for symptom control Teach client to make appropriate self-care decisions related to disease stage, activity toleranace, and pain tolerance Teach client the name, dose, frequency, action, and side effects of Motrin
Potential social isolation related to increased signs and symptoms of osteoarthritis	Client will plan social events and activities according to health status	Teach client to anticipate social interactions and plan rest and activity periods so that no discomfort will develop Plan participation in activities that do not cause exacerbation of symptoms Encourage client to join social clubs, such as reading clubs, bridge clubs, and hobby clubs, that are of personal interest
Impaired physical mobility related to stiffness and pain in joints	Client will maintain present level of mobility	Teach client the importance of regular exercise for joint motion and function; offer suggestions based on client-expressed desires and needs Teach use of adaptive devices and equipment for enhancing self-care ability (e.g., Velcro snaps, front zippers, clothes that open down the front); referral to occupational therapist may be indicated

Continued.

NURSING CARE PLAN: OSTEOARTHRITIS—cont'd

Nursing diagnoses	Expected client outcome	Nursing strategies
Potential body image disturbance related to physical changes secondary to osteoarthritis	Client will verbalize feelings regarding body changes	Assess with the client the meaning of the physical changes Encourage client to talk about the problems the disease is causing in her life Explore client's remaining strengths and abilities and how they can be used to overcome perceived problems
Potential self-care deficit: bathing, dressing, grooming; related to decreased joint function	Client will maintain present self-care functional ability as long as possible	Help client to establish realistic activity and medication regimen to maintain present level of function Referrals to occupational therapy and physical therapy may be indicated A social work referral, for any type of home assistance such as cleaning, cooking, or transportation, may become necessary; client should have name of referral agency.

EVALUATION

1. The client reports minimum discomfort from the osteoarthritis.
2. The client is able to perform daily activities with minimum joint discomfort.
3. The client verbalizes understanding of the disease process and methods for symptom control.
4. The client adheres to the medication regimen.
5. The client reports a satisfactory program of activity and socialization.
6. The client participates in a regular exercise program.
7. The client has incorporated the use of appropriate adaptive devices into her daily routine.
8. The client expresses confidence in her ability to cope with limitations imposed by the disease.

NURSING ALERTS

1. To be an effective teacher and observer, the nurse must be aware of the actions, side effects, and complications of the medications used for osteoarthritis. Common side effects of NSAIDs include eighth nerve damage (auditory), which causes dizziness, ringing of the ears, and vertigo, and gastrointestinal disturbances such as gastritis, peptic and duodenal ulcers, nausea, vomiting, dyspepsia, flatulence, diarrhea, constipation, and bloating. Other side effects may include fluid retention, confusion, weakness, disorientation, edema, blurred vision, nephrotoxicity, hemolytic anemias, and liver dysfunctions.
2. The elderly usually do not have only one medical problem. Osteoarthritis is very common, so one can expect the older adult to have other medical problems that may affect management of the osteoarthritis.
3. Chronic pain can lead to depression, so a thorough assessment regarding the pain is required. Osteoarthritic pain should be able to be relieved.

4. Elderly people who are taking long-term medications such as aspirin are at risk for side effects and complications. This is especially true if they are taking multiple medications. Absorption, metabolism, and excretion of certain drugs are altered with the aging process. The nurse needs to assess the effectiveness of drugs to determine if adjustment is needed. (The nurse would consult the physician if changes in medication are indicated.)
5. Treatment of osteoarthritis is highly variable, depending on symptomatology. The goals of treatment are relief of pain and prevention of additional damage. Drugs, a balance of rest and activity, psychosocial support, and surgery are the measures used.

Bibliography

Blechman WJ, Roth SR, and Wilske KR: Are you up-to-date on osteoarthritis? Patient Care 22:57, March 30, 1988.

Brassell MP: Pharmacologic management of rheumatic diseases, Orthopaedic Nursing, 7:43, March-April 1988.

Brieturg JC: Caring for older adults, Philadelphia, 1987, WB Saunders Co.

Carpenito L: Nursing diagnosis: application to clinical practice, ed 2, Philadelphia, 1987, JB Lippincott Co.

Eliopoulos C: Gerontological nursing, ed 2, Philadelphia, 1987, JB Lippincott Co.

Gioiella EC and Bevil CW: Nursing care of the aging client, Philadelphia, 1987, JB Lippincott Co.

Olivo JL: Developing an exercise program for the elderly with osteoarthritis, Orthopaedic Nursing 6:23, May-June, 1987.

Rippey RM et al: Computer-based patient education for older persons with osteoarthritis, Arthritis and Rheumatism 30:932, August 1987.

Rippey RM et al: Treatment of osteoarthritis, Patient Care 22:181, March 30, 1988.

Osteoporosis

Janet T. Barrett

KNOWLEDGE BASE

1. Osteoporosis is the most common metabolic bone disease in this country. It is characterized by a steady decrease in the amount of bone to a level where the structural integrity of the skeleton can no longer be maintained. Bone formation exceeds bone resorption until about age 30, when bone resorption begins to exceed bone formation. This phenomenon occurs particularly in trabecular bone, which is found in greatest amounts in the vertebral bodies, hips, and wrists. Consequently there is an increased risk of compression fractures, femoral neck fractures, and Colles fractures in older persons.

2. Osteoporosis is usually a primary disorder associated with a variety of etiologic factors; however, it may be produced secondarily by a number of disorders. The most commonly cited risk factors for primary disease include (a) female sex, (b), inactivity, (c) aging, (d) decreased levels of sex hormones, particularly estrogen, and (e) calcium deficiency. Causes of secondary osteoporosis include endocrine diseases such as hyperthyroidism, Cushing's disease, hyperparathyroidism, and acromegaly, or bone marrow disorders such as myeloma or leukemia.

3. The largest number of persons with osteoporosis are postmenopausal women. A relationship between estrogen deficiency and bone loss has been identified, but estrogen therapy for treatment of osteoporosis remains controversial. Benefits, risks, and side effects along with the woman's personal health history must be carefully explored by the physician prescribing therapy.

4. Insufficient calcium may be due to decreased dietary calcium intake, increased loss of calcium, or poor absorption of calcium. For example, diverticulitis interferes with the absorption of calcium and Cushing's syndrome inhibits formation of bone matrix as a result of excessive production of glucocorticosteroids. Prolonged use of heparin causes increased resorption of calcium and inhibits bone formation. Vitamin D is necessary in the diet for absorption of dietary calcium. Older persons who are institutionalized or spend most of their time indoors are frequently lacking in vitamin D.

5. Vitamins E, D, B_6, and zinc are important in maintaining good nutrition. Vitamin E aids in controlling hot flashes, and vitamin B_6 helps mental disturbances and insomnia. Zinc regulates hormonal changes. The minimum amount of vitamin D required for optimal absorption of calcium is 400 mg/day and sunlight.

6. Osteoporosis is very common in women over 45 and men over 55 years of age. Women are affected more than men. Eighty percent of white women over 65 have some form of osteoporosis.

7. Lack of exercise, which frequently accompanies advancing age, speeds osteoporotic activity. Exercise stresses the long bones, in turn stimulating bone formation. When bones are not stressed, bone resorption is accentuated.

8. Diets high in protein, consumption of coffee and alcohol, and cigarette smoking have been implicated in causing excessive calcium loss.

9. Significant loss of height can occur with osteoporosis as a result of collapse of the thoracic and lumbar vertebrae. Eventually the costal margins may come to rest on the iliac crests.

10. Many elderly people with osteoporosis are asymptomatic. The first symptom may be pain secondary to vertebral fractures. Early physical signs are kyphosis and decreased height.

11. Shortening of the body trunk caused by narrowing and flattening of the intervertebral spaces is another osteoporotic change. Discomfort in the lower back increases with walking and other spine-stressing activity because the shock-absorbing capability is now gone.

12. In addition to the hormone therapy with estrogen, flouride and calcitonin are sometimes prescribed.

CASE STUDY

Mrs. Willis, at age 50, went to her physician regarding symptoms of menopause, which included dry hair, dry skin, scanty or no monthly periods, and hot flashes. When the nurse measured her height, Mrs. Willis had lost 1 inch since her last visit 1 year ago. Mrs. Willis also reported experiencing mild lower backache. She was diagnosed as having osteoporosis and placed on low estrogen therapy.

Three months ago Mrs. Willis turned 79. At her birthday party she slipped on a rug at her daughter's home, causing her to fall and fracture her right hip. Physical findings on hospitalization revealed:

EENT: head, neck, eyes, ears, nose, and throat essentially normal; full dentures

Skin: dry/flaky, especially on her lower extremities; poor turgor

Vital signs: temperature, 37.1°, pulse rate, 96 beats/min; respiratory rate, 24 breaths/min; BP 142/86

Heart: Normal sinus rhythm, no murmurs, possible S_4

Lungs: Clear from anterior to posterior, increased anteroposterior diameter of chest, kyphosis present

Abdomen: soft, rounded; bowel sounds present; no hepatosplenomegaly; no tenderness or masses

CNS: intact, mentally alert to time, place, and person

Right hip: discolored from waist to mid thigh; top of femur out of socket; unable to move right leg; can move left leg, but doing so increases the pain in the right leg; x-ray film disclosed a pathological basilar fracture of the right hip, with the loss of internal bone matrix in the long bones consistent with long-term osteoporosis; chest x-ray film showed narrowing and flattening of the intervetebral spaces

Surgery was performed and the right hip was pinned. Mrs. Willis was able to sit in a chair several times a day without weight bearing on the right hip within 5 days after surgery. She was discharged from the hospital 3 weeks after surgery, at which time she was able to ambulate short distances with the use of a walker. Her medications included calcium tablets, vitamin D, and estrogen.

It is now 3 months since surgery, and Mrs. Willis is totally independent in her apartment. She still uses the support of the walker for extended periods of walking or standing. She has a planned set of exercises that she faithfully follows each day. She has increased her dietary intake of calcium by eating yogurt for lunch.

ASSESSMENT CRITERIA
Physical

Nutrition
  Dietary habits
  Intake of calcium and vitamin D
Musculoskeletal
  Stature, posture, body alignment, gait
  Mobility, flexibility, and strength
  Height and weight compared with previous years
  Typical exercise pattern
  Past history of fractures and falls
  Musculoskeletal-related pain/tenderness
Hormonal therapy: history of hormone supplement, use
Past/present history of endocrine disorders, prolonged heparin use, and smoking
Head-to-toe assessment using inspection, palpation, percussion, and auscultation as appropriate for all body systems

Psychosocial

Life-style
  Description of typical day
  Recreation/leisure profile
  Living environment profile
Family profile
Resources/support systems used
Knowledge of osteoporosis and specific treatment measures, planned surgical procedure, preoperative and postoperative care
Name of a responsible person in client's file for emergency
History of alcohol consumption and smoking

Spiritual

Religious practices/beliefs
Effect of hospitalization on belief system
Need for spiritual assistance

Mrs. Willis demonstrated changes at age 50 characteristic of menopause. Estrogen replacement therapy is frequently prescribed for treatment of the accompanying hot flashes as well as osteoporosis. The loss of height with advancing years is a result of collapse of the thoracic and lumbar vertebrae.

The risk of hip fracture is increased with osteoporosis because of the demineralizion process that weakens the bone. Mrs. Willis' otherwise good health contributed to her successful recovery. The musculoskeletal changes that have already occurred are not reversible, but progression may be halted with appropriate continuous therapy.

NURSING CARE PLAN: OSTEOPOROSIS

Nursing diagnoses	Expected client outcomes	Nursing strategies

Altered nutrition: less than body requirements for calcium and vitamin D; related to lack of knowledge	Client will verbalize understanding of relationship between increased calcium and vitamin D needs and osteoporosis
	Client will eat a balanced diet with adequate intake of calcium and vitamin D.
		Assess potential obstacles to adherence to recommended dietary changes, ethnic or cultural values affecting food intake, and current eating patterns; teach the following as needed:
		  Four food groups, including calcium and vitamin D requirements
		  Increase calcium intake to 1500 mg daily 1; if supplement prescribed, take a full glass of water to help begin absorption
		  Ensure intake of iron, zinc, magnesium, vitamin B_6, phosphorus, vitamins E and D; review foods rich in these nutrients

Impaired physical mobility related to decreased agility secondary to musculoskeletal changes and recent fracture	Client will safely perform a set of daily exercises	Plan with the client a set of exercises that can be incorporated into daily life-style and that are suitable in view of recent hip fracture; the range of possibilities include simple range-of-motion exercises to walking, swimming, and water exercises; depending on type of exercise, adhere to the following guidelines:
		  Allow a warm-up period to increase circulation and avoid sudden muscle or cardiopulmonary system strain
		  Plan the active portion of the exercise so that intensity and duration are slowly increased
		  Allow a cool-down period to promote gradual return to normal
		  Alert client to signs of muscle fatigue and respiratory and circulatory stress

Potential for injury related to recent fracture, skeletal deformities, use of walker	Client will correctly perform activities that reduce or avoid injury	Teach client to avoid heavy lifting, jumping, and other strenuous activities that could lead to fractures
		Teach client how to get in and out of automobiles without injuring back
		Teach client to bend from the knees rather than the waist when lifting objects
		Teach client to roll from side to side before sitting up in bed
		Explore ways of making the home safer and decreasing risk for falling:
		  Keeping floors clean and dry but not highly polished
		  Removing throw rugs
		  Providing adequate light without glare
		  Wearing good-fitting shoes

EVALUATION

1. The client maintains a well-balanced diet with adequate intake of calcium, vitamin D, and essential nutrients, as evidenced by a 7-day diet log.
2. The client participates in a daily exercise routine within established guidelines.
3. The client has taken measures in her home to reduce the chance of sustaining further musculoskeletal injury.
4. The client remains injury free.
5. The client demonstrates safe, proper use of the walker.

NURSING ALERTS

1. The client should be cautioned about excessive doses of vitamin D, since toxicity is likely to occur.
2. Many older clients do not have the opportunity to get adequate sunshine. Vitamin D supplements are important if no sunshine is obtained.
3. Clients should avoid taking aluminum-containing antacids as a regular source of calcium. Foods that are high in calcium, such as whole milk, may also be high in cholesterol. Low-fat products such as skim milk or yogurt are good sources of calcium.

4. If supplemental calcium is prescribed, the client should be monitored for side effects such as constipation, flatulence, hypercalcemia, hypercalcinuria, and urinary tract stones.
5. When a person with osteoporosis is hospitalized, the nurse should exercise great care in using proper turning and positioning methods. Fractures can result from both proper and improper turning if bone loss is severe.
6. Avoidance or elimination of risk factors for injury should be taught to clients with osteoporosis. Risk factors include inadequate heating, obstacles, low furniture, loose carpeting or rugs, inadequate lighting, complex pattern of rugs or wallpaper, slippery floors, and even pets. Personal environmental characteristics that increase the risk for falls include tight restrictive clothing, poorly adjusted glasses, high-heeled shoes, and floor-length skirts or pants.
7. The immobilization imposed by prescribed bed rest hastens bone demineralization, so limiting inactivity to the shortest time necessary is advised.

Bibliography

Aisenbrey JA: Exercise in the prevention and management of osteoporsis, Physical Therapy 67:1100, July 1987.
Breiturg JC: Caring for older adults, Philadelphia, 1987, WB Saunders Co.
Brockie J: Preventive treatment for bone loss, Nursing Times 83:56, May 13, 1987.
Carpenito L: Nursing diagnosis: application to clinical practice, ed 2, Philadelphia, 1987, JB Lippincott Co.
Chestnut CH et al: New options in osteoporosis, Patient Care 22:160, January 1988.
Eliopoulos, C: Gerontological nursing, ed 2, Philadelphia, 1987, JB Lippincott Co.
Gioiella EC and Bevil CW: Nursing care of the aging client, Philadelphia, 1987, JP Lippincott Co.
Hickox PG: Choosing evaluative techniques pinpointing types of bone loss, focusing therapy, Consultant 28:110, December, 1988.
Howie C: Sparing the flushes, Nursing Times 83:51, December 9 1987.
Mac Kinnon JL: Osteoporosis: a review, Physical Therapy 68:1533, October 1988.
Peck WA: Falls and hip fracture in the elderly, Hospital Practice 12:72A, December 15, 1986.
Perry GR: Living with osteoporosis, Geriatric Nursing 9:174, May-June, 1988.
Sagraves R and Van Tyle JH: Osteoporosis in women: the importance of calcium, The Journal of Practical Nursing 37:16, September 1987.

Colles' Fracture

Jo Eva Ziegler Blair

KNOWLEDGE BASE

1. Colles' fracture, one of the most common fractures, often is caused by a fall or by breaking a fall with the outstretched hand. This fracture is a transverse fracture of the distal end of the radius with displacement of the hand backward and outward. Colles' fractures usually heal normally.
2. There is a high incidence of fractures in the elderly because of disturbances of balance and fragile bones (osteoporosis).
3. Initial severe pain after a fracture is due to (a) ecchymosis and swelling at the fracture site, which compresses nerve endings in the periosteum of the bone and the surrounding soft tissues, and (b) muscle spasms. Immobilization of the extremity must be a priority to prevent further soft-tissue and nerve injury.
4. Pain and swelling of a casted extremity are increased by venous pooling when the extremity is dependent. Elevating the arm on pillows or with a sling will minimize venous pooling by increasing venous return.
5. The blanching (capillary refill) sign can be used to determine patency of blood flow in the affected arm. The thumbnail is compressed, and the return of blood to the nail is observed. Sluggishness of blood flow (greater than 3 seconds) should be reported immediately.
6. Immobilization of the arm and wrist for fracture healing results in decreased muscle strength. Connective tissue in the joints shortens and becomes less elastic, causing contractures. The shoulder joint is particularly prone to become stiff. Active and passive range-of-motion (ROM) exercise of the shoulder joint prevents contrac-

tures. Exercise for the rest of the body promotes healing and aids in the rehabilitation process after the cast is removed.

7. Any injury to the body that results in immobilization of a body part will interfere with the client's ability to manage activities of daily living.

8. Participation in activities of daily living (ADLs) helps maintain independence and strengthens the body for ambulation.

9. A full diagnosis and history are important in planning care.

10. Salicylates are effective in relieving pain resulting from the bone and tissue injury. If more severe pain is present because of muscle spasms, a narcotic may be necessary.

11. Elderly clients with fractures may suffer many complications: shock, pneumonia, thrombophlebitis, pulmonary embolism, bladder incontinence, disorientation, pressure wounds, renal calculi, bladder infections, and hypostatic lung congestion.

12. Nursing management of clients with fractures is complicated by chronic diseases that affect the elderly (diabetes mellitus, renal disorders, cardiovascular disease, hypertension, obstructive lung disease). Conditions that the client had before the injury must be identified.

13. Adequate nutrition is required for healing. Trauma from fractures and surgery increases the metabolic needs of the elderly client. The nutritional status of the client may have been compromised before the fracture as a result of inability to chew, altered sense of taste, depression, decreased finances, inability to procure food, or gastrointestinal problems.

14. Major goals for care include promotion of healing, prevention of further injury and complications, and promotion of self-care.

CASE STUDY

Flossie Jones is an 89-year-old widow who has been living alone for 20 years since the death of her husband. She has no family except for several nieces and nephews. After falling at home and suffering a right Colles' fracture, she was a hospital patient for 2 days and then was transferred to a skilled nursing facility with her arm in a cast and a swathe and sling to keep her arm positioned. While she was in the hospital, the following pain medication was ordered: aspirin, 5 grains every 4 hours as needed for pain, and meperidine (Demerol), 25 to 50 mg given intramuscularly every 6 hours as needed for severe pain only.

She does not appear visibly depressed, but has a lack of energy. This could be due to poor motivation to gain independence. She expects to be "taken care of," instead of assuming self-care. She does say that she is planning to go home when she is strong enough.

Flossie has a hearing loss but suffers no other sensory losses. She has osteoporosis. She is 5'5" and weighs 84 pounds. She states that she has never had a large appetite. A nutritional history was taken and reviewed by the dietitian. Dietary orders called for increased caloric intake and high protein intake. A high-protein supplement was ordered, to be taken three times a day.

ASSESSMENT CRITERIA
Physical

History of falls
Present and past mobility, gait, balance
ADLs performed independently and those requiring assistance; past and present
Signs and symptoms of complications following fracture
    Shock (within first 24 hours)
    Pneumonia
    Thrombophlebitis
    Pulmonary embolism
    Bladder infections
    Hypostatic lung congestion
Chronic health problems affecting healing, remobilization
    Osteoporosis
    Arthritis
    Parkinson's disease
    Diabetes mellitus
    Hypertension
    Cardiovascular conditions
Appetite and nutritional status
    Dietary history and practices
    Anthropometric measurements
    Condition of mouth and skin
Neurovascular impairment in fractured arm
    Capillary refilling
    Coldness
    Pallor
    Cyanosis of fingers
    Swelling in fingers
    Finger movement
    Pain in fingers
    Ability to feel light brushing/pinch
Pain; location, characteristics

Psychosocial

Degree of motivation for self-care
Mental status
Family involvement and support

Emotional states
  Depression
  Dependence
  Fear
  Anticipatory grief
Coping style and strengths

Spiritual

Life satisfaction
Importance of religious activities
Faith affiliation

Upon admission to the skilled nursing facility, Flossie is unable to perform any activities of daily living without a great deal of assistance and encouragement. She is right handed, so she is learning to brush her teeth and comb her hair with her left hand. After the pain diminishes, she may be able to use her right hand for these activities. She is given assistance with a sponge bath, and uses a bedside commode or walks to the bathroom with assistance.

She has slight swelling in the fingers on the right hand. The fingers feel cool to touch but are not cold, and she is able to move the fingers. She states that she has no pain in the fingers, but does complain of a slight aching at the fracture site.

Flossie has a poor appetite. She is unable to feed herself with her right hand and is self-conscious about being "clumsy and messy" while using her left hand. Her past dietary habits may contribute to her low weight and osteoporosis.

Upon admission to the skilled nursing facility, Flossie refuses to care for herself. She has two nieces, who are her main family support, and they will visit daily. A priest from her church has visited.

 NURSING CARE PLAN: COLLES' FRACTURE

Nursing diagnoses	Expected client outcomes	Nursing strategies

Pain after fracture related to bone/tissue injury, muscle spasm, or neurovascular impairment	Client will report increased comfort
	Client will have prompt treatment for complication
	Client will have decreased swelling
		Assess neurovascular status; report significant findings immediately
		Keep right arm elevated on pillow and apply ice packs at fracture site
		Assess skin integrity at cast edges; encourage movement of fingers
		Administer medications as ordered (give with food):
		  Aspirin, 5 grains every 4 hours as needed for pain
		  Demerol, 25-50 mg IM every 6 hours as needed for severe pain only
		Assist with shoulder ROM exercises three times a day
		Attend to any complaints of unrelieved pain

Altered tissue perfusion related to neurovascular impairment	Client will report symptoms of neurovascular impairment	Observe for coldness, skin color, capillary refill, swelling, pain, paresthesia of fingers; teach client to report any of the above symptoms; frequency of checks would depend on stage of recovery Report significant changes immediately
Impaired physical mobility related to Colles' fracture and cast, poor motivation, and generalized weakness	Client will maintain muscle strength and joint mobility	Perform passive ROM exercises of shoulder to begin, per physician's order; teach client active ROM exercises when tolerated Encourage self-care Request physical therapist's evaluation and treatment Assess activity tolerance, gait, and balance Establish an ambulation and exercise program in collaboration with physical therapist See care plan on impaired mobility, p. 50

NURSING CARE PLAN: COLLES' FRACTURE—cont'd

Nursing diagnoses	Expected client outcomes	Nursing strategies
Potential for injury related to improper care of cast, continued falling, and inadequate knowledge	Client will request assistance when needed	Protect cast with plastic bag when client bathes
	Client will experience a lessened potential for injury	Observe skin at cast edges for irritation, cast crumbs, or pressure When client is in bed, position arm with pillows for correct alignment of shoulder; when client is ambulating, apply sling and swathe Establish which activities the client needs assistance with to maintain safety
Altered thought processes related to fracture, pain medication, and strange environment	Client will express increased confidence in perception of time and place	Assess for orientation to time, place, and events Orient client to surroundings, treatment rationale, and safety practices on an ongoing basis Assist client to dining room and activities Explain all procedures to help alleviate anxiety Encourage family visits; teach family how to orient the client; recommend an activities plan to encourage conversation about past and current events Observe for mental confusion resulting from pain medications
Altered nutrition: less than body requirements; related to poor appetite and increased body requirements secondary to fracture	Client will maintain or increase weight	Keep dietary intake record Adhere to food preferences Serve three meals and three high-nutrient snacks per day Monitor all dietary intake; offer alternatives when food is not eaten Ensure that client takes milk or calcium supplement to equal 1500 mg of calcium Assist with feeding to the extent needed; set up food tray, and open packages; provide finger foods; request consultation with occupational therapist to help with assistive devices Continue to reinforce that adequate diet is necessary for healing Weigh twice a week, before first meal of the day Increase activity as tolerated
Partial self-care deficit related to immobility of right arm, decreased motivation, and generalized weakness	Client will be clean and well groomed Client will be able to assume ADLs with minimal assistance	Assess activities that can be done independently and those that require assistance Provide assistance only as needed, but do not allow client to become fatigued Use positive approach Praise efforts Teach use of assistive devices Arrange occupational therapist consultation for ADLs Arrange for activity director to develop a program to address problems Arrange for restorative aide to provide ROM exercise 5 days a week Assess for depression (e.g., poor eating; sleeping at frequent intervals)
Potential for altered health maintenance related to client's desire to return home prematurely	Client will be able to return home, when capable of performing her own ADLs	Assess and document mobility, motivation, and degree of family or agency support required to live at home
	Client will be able to maintain health on returning home	Include client and family in all aspects of planning for dismissal needs Provide information and/or referrals as indicated by needs Make referral to social worker to contact family regarding home care Make referral to home care or public health agency if needed

EVALUATION

1. The client has only minimal pain in the arm, which is relieved by nonnarcotic analgesics.
2. The client has adequate circulation in the right arm, is able to move her fingers, and has no coldness, pallor, cyanosis, swelling, or numbness.
3. The client maintains muscle strength and joint mobility.
4. The client's mental status is maintained.
5. The client consumes adequate nutrients as evidenced by body weight gain and bone healing.
6. The client is independent in ADLs and will be returning home (with minimal assistance from an agency).
7. The client will demonstrate safe practices.

NURSING ALERTS

1. A cast may cause ulceration or necrosis of the skin. Fragile skin of the elderly is especially susceptible.
2. Check frequently for continued pain in the casted arm and other signs or symptoms of impaired circulation or excessive pressure to bony prominences or soft tissue.

3. The environment for the elderly client should be assessed for hazards that might lead to falls and fractures.
4. In preparation for cast removal, the client should be told the following: It may be several months before the appearance of the arm returns to normal. The skin under the cast has been protected, so it is extremely tender; it should not be washed vigorously. There may be some loss of muscle strength and joint mobility, which can be regained through appropriate exercise.

Bibliography

Caliandro G and Judkins B: Primary nursing practice, Glenview, Ill. 1988, Scott, Foresman/Little, Brown College Division.

Carpenito, LJ: Nursing diagnosis: application to clinical practice, Philadelphia, 1987, JB Lippincott Co.

Long BC and Phipps WJ, editors: Medical-surgical nursing: a nursing process approach, ed 2, St Louis, 1989, The CV Mosby Co.

Potter, PA and Perry AG: Basic nursing: theory and practice: St Louis, 1987, The CV Mosby Co.

Open Reduction of a Hip Fracture

Shirley Moore

KNOWLEDGE BASE

1. Hip fractures that result from falls are one of the most common injuries experienced by elders.
2. Elders are prone to fractures because of these age-related changes:
   a. Collagen production is decreased and that being produced is less elastic, so the resiliency of tendons and ligaments is reduced, as is the buffering mechanism.
   b. Bone cell density is decreased, which decreases the bones' ability to withstand the force of a fall.
   c. Longer response time does not allow the elder to correct a fall.
   d. The amount of cushioning provided by muscle and adipose tissue decreases.
   e. There is a high incidence of osteoporosis, especially in elderly women.

3. Immobility following a fracture may cause permanent loss of independence in self-care and mobility if the care of the client is not well managed after surgery. Principles of management include the following:
   a. Stabilization of existing medical problems
   b. Early diagnosis and reduction of the fracture
   c. Attending to the overall health of the client
   d. Minimizing immobility
   e. Preventing complications
   f. Promoting independence and the elder's control of his or her own life
4. When a bone is fractured, bleeding occurs both within the bone and in the surrounding tissues. Ecchymosis may be present throughout the upper leg and hip. A considerable amount of blood may be lost—especially in elders, because of the loss of elasticity in tissues.

5. Pain is the result of increased fluid from the inflammatory response compressing the nerve fibers, muscle spasms as a response to the bone injury, and pressure from the internal bone bleeding on the nerve fibers contained in the periosteum of the bone.

6. Pain behaviors in elders may not be the same as in younger clients. Restlessness, increased disorientation, and denial of pain are common pain behaviors. Pain needs to be differentiated from hypoxia, since restlessness is a shared symptom. Pain management becomes a priority of care.

7. The elder with a femoral fracture requires a coordinated, collaborative treatment and care plan throughout acute, skilled, and home care.

8. The members of the health care team, consisting of the patient and family, physician, nurse, dietitian, physical therapist, social worker, and professionals from other disciplines, must combine their expertise in helping the client solve his or her problems.

9. Recovery depends on adequate nutrients. Bone healing requires calcium and vitamins C and B. Many elders are malnourished prior to the surgery, requiring a complete assessment and nutritional intervention.

10. After surgery, the affected leg should be kept abducted. Hip flexion is to be avoided. Either a supine or left side-lying position should be maintained. If skin integrity is threatened by limiting positioning to these two, tilting the client to the right is acceptable. The abducted position decreases the stress on the pin site and increases comfort.

11. Age-related changes predispose the elder to multiple-system problems when he or she is immobilized. Therefore early mobilization is very important in preventing complications.

12. Disorientation, agitation, and restlessness are common problems in elders who have had anesthesia, surgery, and narcotic analgesics.

13. The elderly immobilized client runs the risk of pneumonia because of decreased vital capacity. Breathing exercises, use of the incentive spirometer, and early ambulation with good posture decrease the risk of lung complications.

14. The elderly are at high risk for constipation as a result of the aging process and inactivity. Adequate fiber, bulk, and fluids in the diet help to decrease problems with bowel irregularity.

15. Hypercoagulability resulting from dehydration related to the surgery and bed rest can result in thrombophlebitis. Adequate fluid and blood replacement, with concurrent monitoring of vital signs and laboratory values, is essential. The use of elastic stockings, elevation of the legs, and range-of-motion (ROM) exercises, with routine turning, positioning, and early ambulation, can decrease the risk of the complication. The legs should be assessed frequently for increased warmth, edema, and pain related to phlebitis.

Some patients are placed on anticoagulants postoperatively because of the related bleeding precautions, to lessen the risk of this complication.

16. Pulmonary embolism can result from a clot that is dislodged from the lower extremities. Symptoms include respiratory distress and shock. Treatment of the symptoms of pulmonary embolism includes the use of intravenous fluids, oxygen, electrocardiographic monitoring with frequent vital signs, anticoagulants, a narcotic for pain, pressors for hypotension, and intravenous sodium bicarbonate for possible metabolic acidosis.

17. Another complication for orthopedic clients is fat embolism. Early symptoms include confusion, chest rash, skin petechiae with progression to heart-lung involvement, respiratory arrest, and coma. Treatment is similar to that for pulmonary emboli.

18. Urinary tract infections can occur with urinary stasis and decreased fluid intake in the elderly on bed rest. Frequent offering of the bedpan, increased fluid intake, accurate intake and output records, and fluids that promote urine acidity will discourage bacterial growth. Increased fluids for the elderly client will also decrease the risk of stone formation in the kidney. Urinary catheter placement increases the risk of infection and should be a last resort for the client who is incontinent or cannot void.

19. Wound infection can occur as a result of either internal or external causes. Through the use of antibiotics and aseptic technique with dressing changes, the likelihood of infection is diminished. Also, proper monitoring of the blood counts and signs and symptoms of impending infection is necessary. If drainage occurs, a culture would be done to indicate the appropriate medication to be ordered.

20. The elder's depressed immune system predisposes him or her to osteomyelitis after the open reduction. Local symptoms would include pain, redness, and edema of the fracture site. Systemic symptoms are not the same as those for a younger person. The blunted immune response results in little or no increase in white blood cells and the resultant fever. The more typical symptoms are lethargy, loss of appetite, and increased disorientation. Positive blood culture results confirm the diagnosis.

21. Osteoarthritis can complicate ambulation activities and prolong progress.

22. Absorption, metabolism, and excretion of drugs are altered in the elderly. This suggests that a lower dosage of a drug might be as effective as the regular dosage. The nurse monitors the elderly client's response to prescribed medications and documents the need for adjusted dosages.

23. Activity progresses from the wheelchair on the first postoperative day to the walker or crutches after approximately 1 week of healing. The client

can start toe-touch weight bearing and progress to total weight bearing when x-ray films demonstrate adequate bone healing. It is important to follow the orthopedic's surgeon's orders for weight bearing.

pain medications, and a return clinic appointment in 1 week. Future plans indicate that she will return to her apartment. Her son assisted the social worker and the nurse in discharge.

CASE STUDY

Mrs. May Ennis, a 78-year-old widow, lives alone in an apartment. She fell this afternoon off her couch, injuring her right hip. She did not lose consciousness, but was unable to move because of the hip pain. She denied nausea, dizziness, or incontinence at the time of the accident. She requested to see her priest on admission and talked to her son about financial affairs.

Her past medical history is insignificant; her past history includes the removal of cataracts. She is a nonsmoker and a nondrinker, without contributing familial diseases.

The review of systems was negative, except for the affected extremity: peripheral pulses intact in extremities; right leg shorter than left leg, adducted, painful; hip ecchymosis; externally rotated right foot; no cyanosis, clubbing, or edema. The x-ray film showed intertrochanteric fracture of the right femur. Laboratory results indicated an elevated white blood cell (WBC) count and alkaline phosphatase level and decreased calcium, hemoglobin, and hematocrit values.

Mrs. Ennis signed the surgical consent for open-reduction internal fixation of the right leg with pin and plate. Postoperatively, her laboratory values progressed to the normal limits, and her vital signs were within her admitting parameters. Mrs. Ennis received a parenteral antibiotic and parenteral narcotics, with progression to oral medication for pain every 3 to 4 hours as needed. Her diet was advanced to a regular diet, and Peri-Colace was added to her medications.

Initially, her hip wound was drained by a Hemovac and covered with a sterile dressing; both were removed within 3 days postoperatively. The stapled incision remained dry. She was taught how to transfer from bed to chair and use a walker with the assistance of one person. She began toe-touch weight bearing on the right leg as ordered by the orthopedic surgeon. Mrs. Ennis was discharged to a nursing facility with physical therapy instructions,

ASSESSMENT CRITERIA
Physical
Description of the trauma event
Preoperative assessment
  Open or closed wound of right hip
  Hip pain and ecchymosis
  Position of leg and foot
  Length of limbs
  Neurovascular checks below the injury to evaluate skin color and temperature, pulse, sensation, loss of normal function, edema, capillary refilling of toenails, ability to move toes
Additional preoperative assessment
  Past medical and surgical history
  Allergies
  Current medications
Cardiopulmonary
  Vital signs
  Chest pain or discomfort
  Lung sounds
  Heart sounds
  Peripheral pulses
  Presence of pulmonary symptoms (i.e., cough, sputum production)
  Edema
Neurological
  Pain characteristics, location, duration, exacerbating factors, and relief measures
  Sensation of unaffected extremity
  Movement of unaffected extremity
  Movement
  Tremors
  Paresis/paralysis
  Headache: frequency and characteristics
  Level of consciousness
Mobility
  Usual activity level and endurance
  History of falls
  Self-care abilities
  Gait, coordination, and balance
  Joint flexibility/pain
  Muscle strength, especially quadriceps
Nutritional assessment
  Height and weight: ideal, usual, current
  Food history
  Appetite
  Food intolerance and preferences
  Fluid intake/hydration
  Prescribed limitations
Elimination
  Urinary: patterns, dysuria, frequency, urgency
  Bowel: frequency, consistency, flatulence, constipation

Laxative, suppository, enema usage
Incontinence of bowel or bladder
Skin
    Turgor
    Integrity
    Pressure areas

Meaning of the trauma
Ability to learn
Support systems
Social affiliations
Life-style and presence of risk factors (e.g., inactivity,
    smoking, drinking, social isolation)

Psychosocial

Fear/anxiety
Memory
Orientation
Judgment and decision making

Spiritual

Source of strength and hope
Perception of God's relationship to the accident
Affiliation with a religious denomination
Need/desire for visit by spiritual leader or chaplain

 NURSING CARE PLAN: OPEN REDUCTION OF A HIP FRACTURE

Nursing diagnoses	Expected client outcomes	Nursing strategies
Potential for infection related to surgical interruption of skin, pulmonary insult from anesthesia, and immobility	Client will be able to verbalize symptoms indicative of incisional or bone infection	Assess incision every shift for redness, edema, drainage Monitor vital signs and WBC count
	Client will verbalize rationale for hand washing, sterile dressings, and hygiene	Check lung sounds Be alert to atypical symptoms of infection Teach client about hand washing, especially after toileting Explain dressings; later on when dressings are removed, explain importance of hygiene Maintain clean and dry environment for bed and chair Teach client and family pulmonary tolieting measures Monitor client for adequate hydration and nutrition Monitor IV antibiotics and be alert to allergic response
Activity intolerance related to immobility and generalized weakness secondary to hip fracture	Client will transfer to chair after dangling, observing weight bearing limitations	Assess tolerance of activity, vital signs, and fatigue level Schedule rest periods
	Client will ambulate the length of the parallel bars, with toe-touch weight bearing, within 1 week	Give pain medications before physical activities Verbally reward client for participation Progress activity from dangling to chair transfer without weight bearing on the affected extremity Encourage walking with the walker with assistance and increasing distance in accordance with physical therapist and physician's order Encourage use of upper extremities with the overhead trapeze and ROM exercises Monitor client's participation and responses
Impaired physical mobility related to altered musculoskeletal function secondary to fracture and pinning	Client will ambulate specified distance	Assess the physical therapy goals for ambulation and request recommendations for daily ambulation Schedule ambulation to avoid excessive fatigue Bed exercises including ROM; avoid hip flexion and adduction on right Enforce correct use of walker for ambulation Encourage client in self-care activities; assist only to the extent needed Encourage family to be supportive of client but to allow independence Assess for all complications of mobility (see care plan on impaired mobility, p. 50)

Continued.

NURSING CARE PLAN: OPEN REDUCTION OF A HIP FRACTURE—cont'd

Nursing diagnoses	Expected client outcomes	Nursing strategies
Potential for injury related to unfamiliar environment, altered mobility, pin breakage, and disorientation	Client will demonstrate safe practices Client will not experience preventable injury	Assess risk factors and plan compensation measures Provide adequate lighting Teach client and family about use of call light and why bed rails are up Remind client to use glasses, hearing aid, and proper shoes for ambulation Use a transfer belt for transfers and ambulations Avoid restraints unless all other measures have failed and the client demonstrates unsafe behaviors Keep room furniture in the same place and away from route to toilet Consider a bedside commode until ambulation improves Establish regular visits to assess needs, especially for toileting Assess compliance with the order for limited weight bearing by having client pivot on the unaffected foot with affected foot placed on top of staff member's foot Explain each step of the transfer process until client demonstrates correct transfers consistently Request that physical therapist demonstrate the transfer and ambulation being used with the client
Impaired skin integrity related to altered circulation and pressure secondary to bed rest and chair activity necessitated by fracture	Client will have skin intact Client will verbalize rationale for measures that prevent pressure ulcers	Assess pressure points every shift; report erythema or blistering immediately Consider a pressure-relieving device in both bed and chair Teach client to change positions from left side to back and tilted slightly to right; provide assistance to maintain scheduled turning until client demonstrates ability to turn self Avoid continuous headrest elevation; teach client to shift position while in chair Monitor fluid and nutrient intake; explain importance to client Teach client rationale for bed exercises and ambulation
Potential for altered nutrition: less than body requirements; related to increased metabolic needs, decreased appetite, and pain	Client will consume adequate nutrients	Assess nutritional status (current and prior to admission) Request consultation from dietitian for planning and teaching Assess food preferences and food intolerance Provide a pleasant environment at mealtime; request family participation to increase social atmosphere Assess need for medication for pain 45 minutes prior to the meal Avoid excessive fatigue, especially at mealtime; schedule a rest period before meals Provide supplemental high-nutrient snacks Ensure adequate fluid intake; explain reasons to patient and family
Pain related to surgical procedure, muscle spasms, and bone trauma	Client will report measures that increase comfort	Assess pain; location characteristics, and duration Develop pain management program Do not allow pain to become severe before medicating Assess mental status and evaluate possibility of self-medication

NURSING CARE PLAN: OPEN REDUCTION OF A HIP FRACTURE—cont'd

Nursing diagnoses	Expected client outcomes	Nursing strategies
		Reposition or assist client in repositioning; keep right hip flexion minimal and leg in abduction
		Be alert to analgesic side effects and overdosage
		Use comfort measures such as back rubs, music therapy, and diversion; teach client relaxation and guided imagery
Altered bowel elimination related to pain medication side effects, decreased activity level, and interruption in dietary intake	Client will have adequate bowel elimination	Assess current status of bowel elimination
	Client will report measures that improve altered elimination	Assess ususal pattern and establish a schedule for toileting
		Increase dietary fiber and fluid intake
		Provide hot lemon drink on an empty stomach, preferably early in the morning
		Consider hot prune juice as an alternative drink
		Assist client in sitting upright on bedside commode or toilet
		Administer Peri-Colace as ordered
		Ensure privacy
		See care plan on constipation, p. 23
Anxiety related to unfamiliar situation; lack of knowledge about treatment plans, own role in care, and plans to return home; and feelings of powerlessness	Client will be able to use positive coping strategies	Assess client's level of anxiety and feelings of powerlessness
		Allow client to participate in planning care and treatment; require decision making to the extent possible
		Inform client about procedures and care before starting; listen carefully and answer questions
		Have staff members introduce themselves each time when interacting
		Establish a schedule with the client for self-care activities, ambulation, and therapy
		Encourage client to express feelings, and provide active listening
		Discuss the need for support with family and available friends
		Respond to client's request for priest/chaplain visit
		Request consultation from social services on admission to assist in post-hospital planning; have client and family involved in all phases of the plan
		Help client to plan for her transition to a nursing facility; consider obtaining pictures of the facility if client is unfamiliar with it; assure her that the nursing staff will communicate about her needs and care

EVALUATION

1. The client has increased toleration of non–weight-bearing physical activities.
2. The client reports increased comfort.
3. The client is actively involved in transfer and non–weight-bearing activities.
4. The family has been instructed in safety precautions and the client's progress with ambulation.
5. The client wears glasses and shoes during transfers and use of the walker.
6. The client uses the call light and is aware of the need for side rails being up during the night.
7. The client has developed a trusting relationship with nurses and has become a participant in her care.
8. The client understands the rationale for her treatments and care.
9. The client knows about diet, medication, and exercises.
10. The client is doing her activities of daily living with modifications and is aware of her accomplishments and limitations.
11. The client and her family have discussed her discharge with the professional team.

12. The client knows how to use the pain medications according to her tolerance and physical activities.
13. The client can repeat the signs and symptoms of infection and understands the skin care necessary for healing of her hip wound.
14. The client is actively involved in her family or significant others throughout the healing process.
15. The client is aware of her follow-up care with the physician and untoward symptoms to report.

NURSING ALERTS

1. The client is at high risk for injury; thus, safety precautions are mandatory.
2. The client has a potential for infection. Be aware of the atypical symptoms common in elders.
3. The client has experienced a major physiological and psychological stressor. She may need assistance in coping. Avoid adding additional unnecessary stressors.

4. The limitations on weight bearing and leg position must be continued until the physician orders otherwise. Communication with the nursing facility must be clear about these limitations.

Bibliography

Beyers M: The clinical practice of medical-surgical nursing, ed 2, Boston, Little, Brown & Co.
Crenshaw AH, editor: Campbell's operative orthopaedics, ed 7, St Louis, 1987, The CV Mosby Co.
Kim, MJ, McFarland GK, and McLane AM: Pocket guide to nursing diagnoses, ed 3, St Louis, 1989, The CV Mosby Co.
Long, BC and Phipps, WJ, editors: Medical-surgical nursing: a nursing process approach, ed 2, St Louis, 1989, The CV Mosby Co.
Steinberg F: *Care of the geriatric patient*, ed 6, St Louis, 1983, The CV Mosby Co.

Total Knee Replacement

Susan A. Ruzicka

KNOWLEDGE BASE

1. Osteoarthritis affects joint articular cartilage and subchondral bone. The joints most often affected are the lumbar spine, knees, and hips.
2. Osteoarthritis is the most common form of joint disease among the elderly. Eighty percent of persons over age 60 have some signs of osteoarthritis.
3. Indications for total knee replacement (TKR) are severe pain and joint destruction with decreased range of motion.
4. Short-term management of acute pain can be enhanced by the use of propoxyphene or codeine. Morphine is the narcotic of choice for long-term pain management.
5. Bone mass is constantly undergoing cyclic reabsorption and renewal. Disequilibrium in this process, with greater reabsorption and less calcium deposition, is characteristic of aging bone.
6. It is necessary for those who care for the aged with chronic conditions to focus on improving or maintaining function, managing the existing illness, preventing secondary complications, and delaying deterioration and disability. Progress is measured in maintenance of a steady state rather than curing the illness.
7. Much emphasis is placed on postoperative exercises, which are very important for regaining maximum knee function.
8. After surgery, the client is usually placed in a continuous passive motion machine (CPMM). The machine permits much earlier return of knee motion.
9. A wound sump drain prevents premature clotting, which could lead to a large hematoma and hinder early range of motion. It is usually removed 24 to 48 hours after surgery.
10. The leg is elevated in the CPMM, which encourages maximum venous drainage. This prevents flexion contractures and adhesions and, with application of ice bags, minimizes edema.

11. Ambulation and activities of daily living require 105 to 110 degrees of flexion and full extension. Flexion is often the most difficult component to obtain postsurgically.

12. Clients with impaired oxygenation can improve their sense of well-being and short-term exercise tolerance through progressive exercise programs. The client should not attempt activities that result in dyspnea.

13. Incorporation of three 1-hour applications of continuous passive motion each day into the postoperative rehabilitative programs of clients with TKR has been shown to aid in decreasing length of hospital stay, frequency of postoperative complications, and number of postoperative days before discharge.

14. Physical therapy should begin on the second postoperative day. This includes quadriceps setting, straight leg raising and flexion-extension exercises and will progress to going up and down stairs according to TKR protocol.

15. A period of decreased physical activity has an impact on an already altered musculoskeletal system. Leg and back muscles have greater strength loss than arm muscles. The greatest loss occurs in the fast-twitch fibers; hence, strength is more affected than is endurance.

16. Increased heart rate and respiratory rate during activity constitute objective evidence of decreased endurance.

17. Constipation is a problem resulting from insufficient dietary bulk, inadequate fluid intake, laxative abuse, diminished muscle tone and motor function, blunting or loss of the defecation reflex, postponement of defecation, lack of food intake, and use of drugs that lower intestinal motility or increase excretion of body water.

18. Using analgesics in control of pain is important, but there is a narrow margin between effective management of pain and onset of adverse effects such as confusion, incontinence, hypotension, and loss of balance.

19. Confusion, disorientation, and/or misinterpretation of the environment may occur postoperatively in elderly clients in an acute care setting.

20. Health care team members consistently underestimate the amount of pain that a client experiences, so it is very important for the client to rate the pain.

CASE STUDY

Mrs. Holden, 79 years old, is admitted to the hospital for a right total knee replacement. Her knee has been treated with cortisone injections for 3 months without relief. The last treatment was 2 months ago. There is no history of bone trauma or bone infection. She ambulated with the assistance of a cane prior to admission.

She has a history of osteoarthritis and had a left knee replacement a year ago. She also has a history of atrial fibrillation and tuberculosis. She has hypertension, is hard of hearing in her left ear, and wears dentures.

Mrs. Holden has a right total knee replacement done under spinal anesthesia. Her postoperative medications include digoxin, 0.25 mg/day; bisacodyl, 1 tablet twice a day; hydrochlorothiazide, 50 mg twice a day; diltiazem, 10 mg three times a day; potassium chloride, 10 mEq twice a day; warfarin sodium as indicated by daily prothrombin time; cefazolin sodium, 1 g every 8 hours for 48 hours; and acetaminophen with codeine, 2 tablets every 3 to 4 hours as needed.

Two days after surgery the physician removes the Ace wrap, dressings, and Hemovac drain. The incision of the right knee is stapled and well approximated; it is reddened and edematous. There is minimal serosanguineous drainage from where the Hemovac was removed. Support stockings are in place on both legs. She can get up to a chair with assistance. She uses a continuous passive motion device or her right leg while she is in bed.

Mrs. Holden was alert and oriented to time, place, and person before surgery but has been confused about place and time postoperatively. The confusion worsens after physical therapy. She does reorient easily. Present vital signs are as follows: blood pressure, 160/70; pulse rate, 70 beats/min; respiratory rate, 14 breaths/min; temperature, 36° C.

Her skin is clean, dry, and warm. There is redness to the buttock area bilaterally with a pale area (5 cm) that has poor capillary refill. Upon auscultation, the lung fields on the left side are found to be diminished. Mrs. Holden is receiving 2 liters of oxygen by nasal prongs except when she ambulates with her walker. She complains of right knee pain every 3 to 5 hours and states that it is managed well with Tylenol #3, 2 tablets. Mrs. Holden eats 90% of her meals. Her pulse if 78 and slightly irregular. Pedal pulses are strong, and the toes are bilaterally warm with a quick capillary refill at the nailbeds. She is neurologically intact in the lower extremities.

She lives alone in an apartment complex. Her sister and brother-in-law live in the same building and provide transportation for her. Mrs. Holden is very active and has many social interests. A housekeeper cleans her apartment twice a month. She used Meals on Wheels, home care, and physical therapy when she was discharged from the hospital following her left total knee replacement. She intends to use these services again.

Psychosocial

Employment
Living arrangements
Home environment
Support person

Spiritual

Religious affiliation and pattern of use
Perception of illness

ASSESSMENT CRITERIA
Physical

Sensory assessment, including vision/hearing
Integument
    Poor skin turgor
    Bruises, petechiae
    Interrupted integrity
    Pale, dry membranes
    Stomatitis
    Furrows in tongue
    Wound: incision approximated; amount/odor/color of drainage
Respiratory
    Lung souds
    Presence of cough, sputum production
Circulatory
    Chest pain/palpitations
    Diminished tolerance for activity
    Capillary refill, clubbing of nails
    Numbness, tingling, peripheral pulses
Nutritional
    Diet components: protein, carbohydrate
    Lymphocyte, serum albumin levels
    Weight gain/loss
    Dentures
Elimination
    Constipation, hesitance, urgency
    Incontinence
    Use of medications
    Rituals
Activity/exercise
    Ability to perform self-care activities
    Range of motion
    Decreased strength; fatigue
    Exercise routines
    Assistive devices
Comfort
    Pain character; precipitating/relieving factors
    Sleep patterns
    Medications used
Neurological/cerebral
    Orientation, alertness
    Headache
    Difficulty expressing self
    Memory impairment
    Impaired attention span
    Inappropriate behavior
    Inaccurate interpretation of environment
    Numbness, lack of sensation

Mrs. Holden wears bifocal glasses for vision acuity. She is hard of hearing in her left ear. These deficits may potentiate misconception of her environment and increase her risk of confusion.

She has poor skin turgor but moist mucous membranes. She has a pale area resulting from sluggish capillary refill to the buttocks. This indicates a decrease in tissue perfusion and places her at high risk for pressure ulcer. She has no petechiae or bruising.

Mrs. Holden's lung fields are diminished on the left side. This decreases oxygenation of the blood. Cyanosis, restlessness, and confusion are early signs of hypoxia, especially in the elderly. Mrs. Holden did exhibit some restlessness and confusion.

Mrs. Holden's history of atrial fibrillation indicates that she should be closely evaluated for heart failure and pulmonary emboli.

Presently, Mrs. Holden needs assistance with bathing (sitting), ambulating (uses walker and standby assistance), and toileting (uses higher-seated toilet). She needs assistance in transferring positions and fatigues easily. She has limited flexion (60 degrees) of her right knee.

Mrs. Holden complains of discomfort localized at the right knee, with activity increasing the discomfort. She states that her knee aches at rest but that she achieves relief with Tylenol #3.

Mrs. Holden is confused, and this worsens after activity. She orients easily to reality with verbal cues.

She will need assistance with meal preparation upon discharge. She will need higher toilet seat in her bathroom.

NURSING CARE PLAN: TOTAL KNEE REPLACEMENT

Nursing diagnoses	Expected client outcomes	Nursing strategies
Impaired physical mobility related to limited use of lower limbs, pain, and limited weight bearing	Client will ambulate 50 feet with walker and standby assistance 5 days after surgery Client will participate actively in physical therapy sessions Client will do isometric exercises to quadriceps, hamstring, and gluteal muscles by self four times a day Client will have at least 90 degrees of right knee flexion by 15 days after surgery	Maintain continuous passive motion device in use when client in bed; Note order for increasing degree of flexion Reinforce and help client establish schedule for strengthening exercise done in physical therapy Encourage ankle exercises to be done often on right leg to prevent deep vein thrombosis; encourage exercises of left leg Give client positive reinforcement as she uses walker correctly and bears weight on right leg Schedule adequate rest periods between activity Instruct client on use of over-head trapeze Assist client with self-turning and movement in bed
Activity intolerance related to weakness, chronic decreased oxygenation capacity, and use of walker, which requires strength	Client will ambulate 50 feet with walker, maintaining blood pressure (within 6 beats) and pulse within baseline assessment 10 minutes after activity Client will increase time in chair and ambulating by 10 minutes each day after 3 days, with respiration maintained at baseline assessment Client will successfully pace her own activities throughout the day	Organize nursing care to activity tolerance Allow periods of rest between eating, physical therapy, visitors, and morning hygiene care Start ambulation for short distances and increase gradually Take resting pulse, blood pressure, and respiration; after exercise compare with baseline vital signs Encourage client in use of diaphragmatic breathing when performing activities Monitor client's respiratory status throughout activity
Altered thought process related to hearing loss, unfamiliar surroundings, surgical trauma, and pain medication	Client will be alert and oriented to time, place, and person on an ongoing basis by the fourth postoperative day Client will use the call light appropriately throughout hospitalization	Provide personal items of meaning and familiarity to the client in the room (pictures, sentimental items) Check on client frequently and always introduce yourself Talk to client from the right side Put client's dentures in and eyeglasses on early in the day, and keep them in place Explain hospital noises: public address system, vacuum, portable chest x-ray machine, ECG machine being moved in the hall Explain all procedures prior to implementation Use appropriate noise and light stimulation Position client near nurses' station when she is up in a chair Reorient client to call light function often Assess client's level of alertness every 4 hours
Altered bowel elimination related to decreased mobility, altered dietary intake, and use of codeine as analgesic	Client will identify the role fluids and fiber play in prevention of constipation Client will include two or three fiber-rich foods in daily diet Within 3 days client will have soft formed bowel movement without straining Client will reinstate own schedule and strategies for bowel elimination	Discuss with client the need for 6 to 8 glasses of water daily Provide a list of high-fiber foods, such as unpeeled fruits and slow-cooked oatmeal bran Discuss effective position for defecation Provide raised orthopedic toilet seat over toilet Provide privacy for client when toileting Assess client's laxative of choice and previous experience with laxatives If acceptable, offer senna tea (which increases colon peristalisis) in the morning and in the evening; hot lemonade on empty stomach in the morning and prune juice may also be offered

Continued.

NURSING CARE PLAN: TOTAL KNEE REPLACEMENT—cont'd

Nursing diagnoses	Expected client outcomes	Nursing strategies
Potential for injury related to intermittent confusion, unfamiliar surroundings, and limited mobility	Client will remain injury free throughout hospitalization	Monitor level of alertness every 4 hours Reorient client to environment and call light when interacting with her, and have client return demonstrate Keep side rails up when client is in bed Keep bed in low position Place familiar personal items (such as pictures) near the client's bed If client is confused, place her in sight of nursing division; if possible, place in geri-chair near nursing station Assist client in changing positions and ambulate client with use of walker Instruct in use of grab bars in bathroom Determine the need for night-lights Assist client with transferring and ambulating (transfer belt may be used) Instruct client to use shoes rather than slippers, to avoid slipping on floor
Impaired skin integrity related to sluggish capillary refill on buttocks area, secondary to limited mobility, hypertension, and cardiac disease	Skin will remain without interruption and have quick capillary refill at the buttocks area Client will verbalize need to reposition self Skin will remain without redness or interruption at bony prominences	Assess status of integument every shift Instruct client in need to reposition self frequently and assist her in doing so Maintain client's hydration and nutrition status Keep sheets soil-free and wrinkle-free under the client Assess bony prominences and heels every shift Gently massage bony prominences once a day Use pressure-relieving devices Keep skin dry and lubricated
Alteration in comfort related to trauma secondary to surgical intervention	Client will transfer position without facial grimacing or tightening muscles; client will verbalize that she is comfortable Client's vital signs will remain within her baseline	Identify client's specific pain behaviors Have client rate the pain on a scale of 0 (no pain) to 10 (intense pain) Have client move at her own speed when changing positions and when in physical therapy Gently cradle right knee in assisting client in repositioning Offer acetaminophen with codeine as prescribed and observe for ill effects Offer pain relief medications 30 minutes before activity Incorporate relaxation techniques and distraction techniques when caring for client Monitor for side effects of narcotics, particularly CNS changes, respiratory changes, depression, urinary hesitancy, nausea, vomiting, and constipation

EVALUATION

1. The client repositions herself in the bed with a reduced level of pain. The client has decreased facial grimacing when getting up to the chair or ambulating. The client's movements are less rigid when changing positions.
2. The client's blood pressure, pulse rate, and respiratory rate are maintained within her normal parameters.
3. The client states that she is more comfortable than the day or shift before.
4. The client ambulates 50 feet with proper use of walker and standby assistance.
5. The client actively participates in physical therapy.
6. The client performs isometric exercises for both legs by herself four times a day and active exercises for the left leg.
7. The client has increasing right-knee flexion each day.
8. The client's blood pressure, pulse rate, and respiratory rate are within her baseline parameters 10 minutes after activity.

9. The client increases the time spent in activities each day.
10. The client successfully plans her day, allotting adequate time for rest between activities.
11. The client is no longer confused but alert and oriented to time, place, and person on an ongoing basis.
12. The client appropriately uses the call light.
13. The client drinks eight glasses of water daily.
14. The client eats two or three fiber-rich foods daily.
15. The client has a bowel movement without straining.
16. The client remains injury free throughout the hospitalization.
17. The client's skin has quick capillary refill to all areas and is without interruption (except for the incision).
18. The client will verbalize the need to reposition herself frequently.

NURSING ALERTS

1. Selection of sites for injectable medications in elderly clients may present the nurse with a challenge. Muscle mass declines with age, so sites are fewer and more skill is required in detecting muscles of adequate body and size.
2. In many elderly clients, general loss of body weight may make it necessary to reevaluate the drug dosages used for them; the criterion for dosage should be weight. Central nervous system depressants produce intensified effects in the elderly. Sedatives and hypnotics tend to produce paradoxical effects of irritability, incontinence, confusion, and disorientation.
3. Merperidine should be avoided in the elderly population because of its potential for toxicity.
4. Pharmacokinetics are altered in the aged; reduced gastric acid and slowed gastric motility alter the absorption and dissolution rates. Decreased total body water, fat cell content, and serum albumin tend to increase blood levels of drugs to the point of toxicity.
5. Full-length side rails are very dangerous; a confused client may try to climb over them or fall from the end of the bed.

Bibliography

Carpenito LJ: Nursing diagnosis: application to clinical practice, Philadelphia, 1989, JB Lippincott Co.

Ebersole P and Hess P: Toward healthy aging: human needs and nursing response, ed 2, St Louis, 1990, The CV Mosby Co.

Eland JM: Pain management and comfort, Journal of Gerontological Nursing 14(4):10, 1988.

Gose J: Continuous passive motion in the postoperative treatment of patients with total knee replacement: a retrospective study, Physical Therapy, 1985, p. 39.

Hall GR: Alterations in thought process, Journal of Gerontological Nursing 14(3):30, 1988.

Jackson MF: High risk surgical patients, Journal of Gerontological Nursing 14(1):8, 1988.

McHutchion E and Morse J: Releasing restraints: a nursing dilemma, Journal of Gerontological Nursing 15(2):16, 1989.

McKenry LM and Salerno E: Mosby's pharmacology in nursing, ed 17, St Louis, 1989, The CV Mosby Co.

Milde FK: Impaired physical mobility, Journal of Gerontological Nursing 14(3):20, 1988.

Spellbring AM et. al: Improving safety for the hospitalized elderly, Journal of Gerontological Nursing 14(2):31, 1988.

Walsh C and Hess P: Total knee arthoplasty: biomechanical and nursing considerations, Orthopedic Nursing 4(1):29, 1985.

RESPIRATORY SYSTEM

Acute Respiratory Infection: Pneumonia

Virginia G. Levin

KNOWLEDGE BASE

1. Pneumonia is a leading cause of death in the elderly. Elders are especially prone to respiratory infections because of age-related changes. Decreased lung capacity, reduced functional reserve, decreased elasticity of the alveoli, diminished cough reflex, and an inefficient immune response predispose elders to respiratory infection.

2. A common cause of pneumonia in clients residing in nursing homes is *Klebsiella pneumoniae.* Pneumonia in elders not residing in nursing homes is usually caused by *Haemophilus influenzae* or *Streptococcus pneumoniae.*

3. Symptoms of pneumonia may be different for an elder than for a younger person. The diminished immune response commonly seen in elders may delay diagnosis and treatment. An elevated white blood cell count and resulting increase in body temperature frequently is not seen. The cough reflex is also diminished, requiring a higher level of irritant for initiation.

4. The early symptoms are disorientation, apathy, lack of appetite, poor fluid intake, and a general sense of "not feeling well." Chest sounds and x-ray films may be difficult to interpret because of lung scarring from a long history of respiratory insult.

5. Normal body temperature in the aged may be as low as 96° F, in which case a temperature of 98° F would be a significant elevation. This could delay diagnosis and treatment if not recognized.

6. A change in mentation could be evidence of hypoxia or elevated temperature. It is not uncommon for elderly clients to exhibit behavioral changes as a result of infections, without having changes in their vital signs.

7. Respiratory distress will deplete the oxygen reserve and can fatigue the client rapidly. Self-care activities must be spaced, with time being allowed for rest periods.

8. Cyanosis of the lips or nailbeds could indicate further respiratory compromise.

9. Preventive measures for respiratory infections include adequate nutrition and hydration, exercise, immunization for influenza and pneumonia, and avoidance of infectious people.

10. Inadequate nutrient intake is common in elders because of dental problems, depression, lack of exercise, and dietary restrictions. Poor nutrition increases the susceptibility to infection.

11. An exercise program is an important strategy for respiratory health. Lung expansion is increased, especially in the lower lobes, oxygen uptake is improved, and airway clearance becomes more effective. If an elder has a respiratory disorder, the exercise must be tailored to his or her tolerance.

12. Adequate fluid intake is critical for all body functions, especially to keep respiratory secretions liquid for more effective expectoration. Elders, because of the diminished thirst reflex, are at risk for dehydration.

13. Analgesics and hypnotics may cause confusion in elders. These clients must be monitored if these medications are being administered. Side rails must be up at night and precautions taken to minimize the potential for falls.

CASE STUDY

Mrs. Martin, 78 years old, has resided in a nursing home for 2 years. She has been brought to the emergency room with sudden onset of confusion, shortness of breath, diminished breath sounds, and cyanotic nailbeds. She is experiencing a productive, tenacious, incessant cough. The nursing home staff has reported that Mrs. Martin's family brought in a young grandchild with a cold to visit, approximately 1 week ago. Initial assessment reveals a frail elderly women in respiratory distress: temperature, 98.8° F, pulse rate, 110 beats/min; respiratory rate, 38 breaths/min; blood pressure, 104/60, breath sounds diminished bilaterally with rales and rhonchi present; skin turgor poor because of dehydrated state; client slightly disoriented to time and place.

Intravenous fluids are initiated immediately. Arterial blood gases determinations, chest x-ray films, complete blood count, urinalysis, and sputum for culture and sensitivity are ordered.

Musculoskeletal: movement of chest wall
General
    Activity/exercise habits
    Diet/nutritional status
    Fluids
    Medications
    Past medical conditions (e.g., chronic respiratory infections)
    Changes in weight
    Self-care abilities

Psychosocial

Mental status, orientation, memory
Anxiety level
Coping behaviors
Health maintenance behaviors
Knowledge of disease and treatment
Support system (e.g., client/family profile)
Risk factors (e.g., smoking, age)
Acceptance of nursing facility
Economic/insurance coverage profile

Spiritual

Sense of hope
Need to participate in religious practices
Feelings of social isolation

ASSESSMENT CRITERIA
Physical

Presenting symptoms
Onset and duration of symptoms
Temperature
Respiratory
    Dyspnea, shortness of breath, chest discomfort
    Presence of cough and sputum production
    Lung sounds
    Nostril flaring
    Pain
Cardiovascular
    Blood pressure, pulse
    Cyanosis
Neurological: mental alertness
Integument
    Color
    Skin turgor/integrity
    Temperature
Gastrointestinal
    Abdominal distension
    Bowel sounds

Mrs. Martin's sudden onset of confusion may indicate impaired gas exchange, possibly related to the tenacious mucus present in her airways. Her shortness of breath is symptomatic of her diminished breath sounds, which result from the increased production of secretions. Mrs. Martin's cyanotic nailbeds are indications of poor peripheral tissue perfusion.

Mrs. Martin's increased pulse rate and respiratory rate are related to her respiratory distress. Although the client's temperature is only 98.8° F, it is not uncommon for the elderly to have low normal temperatures. Therefore, 98.8° F may in fact be an elevation.

Mrs. Martin's poor skin turgor is evidence of fluid deficit. Even a slight temperature elevation or fluid intake alteration can result in dehydration in an elderly client.

The report of a recent contact with an ill child is consistent with the presenting symptoms of the client.

NURSING CARE PLAN: ACUTE RESPIRATORY INFECTION—PNEUMONIA

Nursing diagnoses	Expected client outcomes	Nursing strategies
Potential for ineffective airway clearance, related to secretions and ineffective cough	Client will have a minimum of dyspnea relative to condition; client will demonstrate proper coughing techniques	Assess the client's breath and lung sounds regularly Encourage fluid intake Request respiratory therapy intervention if appropriate Perform oropharyngeal or nasotracheal suctioning if necessary Teach client proper coughing techniques Ensure proper positioning in bed or chair to facilitate lung expansion
Potential for impaired gas exchange, related to obstructed airway secondary to pneumonia	Client will attain adequate oxygen–carbon dioxide exchange at the cellular level	Observe client for signs of cyanosis at lips or nail beds Request arterial blood gas sampling to determine oxygen and carbon dioxide levels if patient shows signs of hypoxia (e.g., sudden confusion, restlessness, combativeness, or altered level of consciousness) Follow physician's orders for oxygen administration (e.g., per nasal cannula at 3 liters/min continuously) Explain the treatment to the client Administer prescribed antibiotics and monitor for side effects and allergies Monitor patient's vital signs for changes in status Monitor client's level of orientation regularly
Pain related to pleuritic infection	Client will verbalize increased comfort	Monitor client's activity level; administer prescribed pain medication as ordered/necessary
Potential for alteration in nutrition, related to dyspnea, weakness, and increased metabolic needs secondary to pulmonary infection	Client will maintain nutrient intake adequate to meet metabolic needs	Assess nutrient intake on a daily basis Request dietary consultation to determine appropriate caloric requirements Determine client's ability to masticate (i.e., properly fitting dentures) Plan frequent small meals instead of three large meals Consider high-calorie between-meal supplements (e.g., milk shakes or Ensure) according to the dietary plan
Anxiety related to unfamiliar environment	Client will experience a reduction in fear and anxiety, as evidenced by relaxed facial expression and body movements and verbalization of feeling less anxious or fearful	Assess level of anxiety Orient client to new environment, including nurse call system telephone, bathrooms, and unit routine (e.g., meal times) Instruct staff members to introduce themselves before providing care Encourage verbalization of fears and anxiety
Activity intolerance related to weakness and shortness of breath secondary to pulmonary infection	Client will perform self-care activities to toleration level	Assess tolerance of activities (i.e., pulse, respiration, fatigue level) Plan client activities so as to conserve energy (e.g., place necessary articles nearby) Allow for rest periods between activities (e.g., after meals, after bath, after procedures) Plan for a gradual progression of activities as the pneumonia improves Help client to pace activities within toleration limits

Knowledge deficit related to the disease process	Client will verbalize understanding of the disease process and the need to maintain adequate caloric and fluid intake and to take medications, as well as precautions to prevent spread of the infection	Assess client's current level of knowledge; client knowledge should include:
		  Precautions necessary to prevent the spread of infection
		  Proper hand-washing techniques
		  The need to follow instructions on activity, diet, and prescribed medications after discharge
		  The importance of pacing activity to level of toleration

NURSING CARE PLAN: ACUTE RESPIRATORY INFECTION—PNEUMONIA—cont'd

Nursing diagnoses	Expected client outcomes	Nursing strategies
Potential for altered bowel elimination, related to decreased activity and alteration in medication	Client will have adequate bowel elimination	Assess the client's usual pattern of bowel elimination Encourage and monitor client's dietary and fluid intake Encourage physical activity in accordance with activity tolerance Assess bowel sounds Administer prescribed stool softeners, or request an order for one (see nursing care plan for constipation, p. 23)
Potential for impaired skin integrity, related to inactivity and alteration in nutrition	Client's skin will remain intact	Assess client's skin over pressure points every 5 hours Ensure client is turned every 2 hours if unable to reposition herself regularly Monitor client's nutritional status Observe client for urinary incontinence or wet bed resulting from diaphoresis Keep bed clean and dry Instruct client about the importance of pressure relief and symptoms to report
Potential for injury related to weakness and possibility of disorientation	Client will remain free of harm from preventable accidents	During every shift, assess for elements that pose risk for the client Keep side rails up when client is in bed Use safety belts when the client is up in a wheelchair only if needed Assess the client's strength and endurance before helping her to transfer or ambulate; additional assistance may be required Reorient the client on a regular basis Ensure availability of call light

EVALUATION

1. The client displays a decreased level of anxiety.
2. The client demonstrates increased activity and endurance after improved gas exchange.
3. The client demonstrates an ability to take in adequate nutrients and fluid.
4. The client reports having less difficulty clearing her airway of secretions unassisted.
5. The arterial blood gas values reflect an appropriate oxygen–carbon dioxide exchange after the disease process is being managed and nasal oxygen is removed.
6. The client verbalizes an increased knowledge of the disease process and infection control mechanisms (e.g., good hand-washing technique).
7. The client reports that a usual bowel pattern is being maintained.
8. The client's skin integrity is maintained.
9. The client is free from preventable injuries.

NURSING ALERTS

1. Be aware of the atypical symptoms of infection exhibited by elders. Symptoms most commonly seen are disorientation, loss of appetite, lethargy, and restlessness.
2. Since body temperature and white blood cell count may not be elevated, it is important for lung sounds to be auscultated on a regular basis.
3. Since thirst is a neurological mechanism, the client must be taught to drink water even when she is not thirsty.
4. Because the cough reflex is diminished in elders, the client needs to be taught pulmonary toileting.

Bibliography

Doenges ME et al: Nursing care plan: nursing diagnoses in planning patient care, Philadelphia, 1984, FA Davis Co.

Ebersole P and Hess P: Toward healthy aging: human needs and nursing response, ed 3, St Louis, 1990, The CV Mosby Co.

Eliopoulos C: Gerontological nursing, ed 2, Philadelphia, 1987, JB Lippincott Co.

Long BC and Phipps, WJ, editors: Medical-surgical nursing: a nursing process approach, ed 2, St Louis, 1989, The CV Mosby Co.

Pritchard V and Kerry C: Streptococcal outbreak, Journal of Gerontological Nursing 14:19, Feb 1988.

Tucker SM et al: Patient care standards: nursing process, diagnosis and outcome, ed 4, 1990, St Louis, 1988, The CV Mosby Co.

Ulrich SP et al: Nursing care planning guides: a nursing diagnoses approach, Philadelphia, 1986, WB Saunders Co.

Chronic Obstructive Pulmonary Disease

Virginia G. Levin

KNOWLEDGE BASE

1. Diseases that cause airflow obstruction, including asthma, chronic bronchitis, and pulmonary emphysema, are categorized as chronic obstructive pulmonary disease (COPD).
2. The diseases grouped under this diagnosis range from intermittent reversible conditions such as asthma to progressive terminal stages of emphysema, which leads to cardiopulmonary insufficiency. The symptoms vary according to the pathology of the specific condition. Emphysema is characterized by degenerative changes in alveolar walls and enlargement of the distal air spaces.
3. The incidence of COPD has risen dramatically in the last decade. In 1984, COPD was the sixth leading cause of death. It is known that ongoing exposure to various pollutants, including cigarette smoke, causes serious lung tissue damage. Over time the exposure to these substances may result in COPD. An older adult, if a long-term smoker, has added years of insult to the lungs.
4. In obstructive lung disease, there is an increase in airway resistance, resulting in incomplete exhalation and extended time for exhalation. Residual volume increases while the total lung capacity may remain the same. Pulmonary function tests are used to confirm the diagnosis.
5. Values for pulmonary function have not been well established for elders. Other methods of identifying pulmonary problems need to be added to the assessment protocol.
6. Pulmonary changes related to the aging process include decreased lung capacity and reduced functional respiratory reserve resulting from the chest wall musculature becoming weaker and less elastic and flexible. Ciliary function and the cough reflex also decline. Unless there is undue stress, infection, or other pathology, age-related changes do not produce symptoms.
7. Blood gas values differ for elders. The blood oxygen (PO_2) level is lower—90 mm Hg for younger persons versus 75 mm Hg for older persons. Blood carbon dioxide (PCO_2) levels remain the same for younger people and older people.
8. As an age-related change, the alveoli in elders become enlarged. This is due to a decrease in the elasticity of the sacs, which resembles emphysema. There may be an absence of symptoms unless there is undue stress or an infectious process is present.
9. Since age-related changes may mimic desease states, it is important to establish a baseline with each elder in order to identify significant changes.
10. Elders with COPD are susceptible to infection because of their inability to clear their lungs and bronchial tree of excess mucus as a result of the diminished cough reflex.
11. The major focus for prevention of COPD is education. Health risks arising from smoking and pollution require individual, community, and governmental action.
12. Nutrition is a major problem for the elder with COPD. He or she may have an underlying nutrition problem that is compounded by shortness of breath and low energy levels.
13. Care for elders with COPD focuses on the following:
    a. Preventing complications
    b. Adequate oxygen
    c. Pacing energy expenditure to toleration
    d. Maximum function and independence
    e. Comfort
14. Respiratory distress is anxiety producing; fear of death is ever present. During episodes of severe distress, the nurse should stay with the client to calm him or her. Measures must be instituted to improve airway clearance and minimize hyperventilation, which potentiates impaired gas exchange.
15. Symptoms of hypoxia include increased heart rate, increased respiratory rate, and circumoral pallor.
16. The medical treatment regimen for COPD depends upon the symptoms, pulmonary function test results, and blood gas findings. Treatment focuses on education, medications, respiratory therapy, physical conditioning and rehabilitation, breathing retraining, and assisting the client to decrease anxiety through positive coping strategies.

CASE STUDY

Mr. Jacobs, 70 years old, has been brought into the emergency room by paramedics in response to his sudden onset of dyspnea shortly after awakening this morning. Mr. Jacobs has experienced evident fatigue and is producing mucoid sputum resulting from violent coughing spasms. He has audible expiratory wheezes, diminished breath sounds bilaterally, and evidence of rales, rhonchi, and bronchospasm. Understandably, Mr. Jacobs is very anxious, restless, and diaphoretic. He has a history of heavy smoking—two to three packs a day for 55 years. Mr. Jacob was forced to take an early retirement 12 years ago because of his respiratory status and activity intolerance. With retirement have come boredom and depression, which have resulted in an increase in his smoking habit and a deterioration in his nutritional status and fluid intake. He has been divorced for 5 years and lives alone.

Arterial blood gas tests, a complete blood count, and a sputum culture were performed. Intermittent positive-pressure breathing (IPPB) treatment was initiated with a bronchodilator. Oxygen at 2 liters/min was administered by nasal cannula, and baseline vital signs were determined. An IV of 5.5% dextrose in normal saline with 30 mEq of potassium chloride was started at 60 ml/hr.

ASSESSMENT CRITERIA
Physical

Neurological
   Mental alertness
   Memory loss
Integument and extremities
   Edema
   Skin turgor/integrity
   Color
   Temperature
Cardiovascular
   Blood pressure, pulse, temperature
   Heart sounds
   Neck vein distension
   Dependent edema
Respiratory
   Dyspnea, shortness of breath, cyanosis
   Presence of cough and sputum
   Lung sounds/breath sounds (e.g., wheezes, rales, rhonchi)

   Orthopnea
   Activity tolerance
Gastrointestinal
   Presence of bowel sounds
   Nutritional status
   Bowel status/habits
Genitourinary
   Frequency, quantity, appearance of urine
   Nocturia
Musculoskeletal
   Muscle tone and strength
   Chest dimensions (barrel)
   Use of accessory muscles
General
   Onset and duration of symptoms
   Exacerbating events
   Relief measures used at home
   Activity/exercise habits
   Diet
   Medication
   Past medical condition
   Changes in weight
   Smoking habits
   Self-care abilities
   Sleep patterns

Psychosocial

Self-described life-style, health perception
Health maintenance behavior
Knowledge of disease and treatment
Support systems (e.g., family, friends, neighbors, community organizations [actual and potential])
Risk factors (e.g., smoking, drinking)
Coping patterns
Self-concept
Behaviors/feelings (e.g., reported boredom and depression)

Spiritual

Ability/desire to participate in religious practices
Feelings of social isolation
Faith affiliation

Mr. Jacobs is currently alert, oriented, and not experiencing symptoms of hypoxia. He is an elderly gentleman living alone and is in a poor nutritional state, which can contribute to skin integrity compromise. Although he currently has no edema or other skin integrity problems, his intolerance to activity, resulting from severe respiratory distress, can result in skin breakdown.

Mr. Jacobs' vital signs must be monitored often because respiratory distress could result in increased blood pressure and pulse rate, which would be especially detrimental to an elderly client. An elevated temperature could indicate an infectious process.

Mr. Jacobs is experiencing audible expiratory wheezing, indicating the narrowing of his bronchioles as a result of his bronchospasms and the production of tenacious secretions.

Mr. Jacobs' general nutritional status has been deteriorating, including his fluid intake.

Dehydration is a common problem of the elderly and can complicate respiratory problems by thickening the respiratory secretions. Decreased urinary output could result from the low fluid intake.

Mr. Jacobs is on a fixed income, which contributes to financial constraints. In addition, his documented depression has kept him socially isolated.

 NURSING CARE PLAN: CHRONIC OBSTRUCTIVE PULMONARY DISEASE

Nursing diagnoses	Expected client outcomes	Nursing strategies
Ineffective airway clearance related to excessive mucus production and tracheobronchial obstruction secondary to COPD	Client will experience improved airway clearance Client will demonstrate relief measures Client will report symptoms of respiratory distress	Monitor client for changes in respiratory status by auscultating lung sounds every 2 hours Encourage client to turn at least every 2 hours and have activity to toleration Encourage oral fluid intake and provide preferred fluids Monitor blood gas results and report abnormal values Provide postural support to improve respiratory status (e.g., place bed in semi-high Fowler's position, and position overbed table so client can lean on it) Instruct client about symptoms that require immediate intervention or indicate complications Maintain oxygen therapy as ordered, including IPPB treatments Provide adequate supply of tissue and disposal receptacles
Anxiety related to dyspnea and unfamiliar environment	Client will experience only a mild or moderate level of anxiety	Assess the client for signs and symptoms of anxiety (e.g., restlessness, diaphoresis, verbalization of fear/anxiety) Reduce anxiety by providing a quiet environment, adequate explanations, timely responses to requests, and empathetic listening Maintain a patent airway Stay with the client during acute distress episodes Orient the client to the new environment, including the nurse call system, telephone, bathroom and unit routine (e.g., mealtimes) Explain the nature and purpose of all treatment procedures and medications Instruct staff members to introduce themselves before providing care Encourage verbalization of fears and anxieties Arrange client's immediate environment to reduce dyspnea (e.g., place things within reach, open curtains to decrease the feeling of "being closed in," set temperature control as preferred by client, and provide for adequate ventilation) Allow client to participate in care planning and pacing of activities

NURSING CARE PLAN: CHRONIC OBSTRUCTIVE PULMONARY DISEASE—cont'd

Nursing diagnoses	Expected client outcomes	Nursing strategies
Activity intolerance related to dyspnea	Client will perform activities within toleration	Plan client's activities to conserve energy (e.g., place necessary articles nearby) Monitor client for activity tolerance and fatigue Teach client pursed-lip breathing Allow for rest periods between necessary activities, such as meals or procedures
Altered nutrition: less than body requirements; related to dyspnea, weakness, and living condition	Client will maintain adequate nutrient intake to meet metabolic needs	Determine the client's current nutritional status Have dietitian develop the client's dietary plan; evaluate need for more easily chewable food and pulmonary diet Identify the client's food preferences and ability to chew Provide supplemental small feedings on a frequent basis, ascending to the dietary plan Plan rest periods before and after meals Allow client adequate time to eat Consult social services to determine client's current living conditions and how meals are planned and prepared Consider contact with support services, such as Meals On Wheels or homemaker for shopping and meal preparation
Potential fluid volume deficit, related to diaphoresis, hyperventilation, and decreased oral intake resulting from dyspnea	Client will maintain adequate fluid volume	Monitor client for signs and symptoms of fluid volume deficit (skin turgor, mucous membranes, daily weight, intake and output) Encourage oral intake by providing fresh water and other fluids as preferred Teach client the importance of adequate fluid intake
Potential for impaired skin integrity, related to intolerance to activity and hypoxia secondary to COPD	Client will maintain skin integrity	Monitor client's skin status every 8 hours Provide routine skin care per client's needs Provide pressure-relieving devices Teach client the importance of changing positions to prevent skin breakdown Instruct client in skin inspection and which signs are significant Monitor nutritional intake, and educate client in the need for and maintenance of adequate nutrition for skin integrity
Self-care deficit related to dyspnea, fatigue, and activity intolerance	Client will demonstrate increased participation in self-care activities	Identify activities that can be done independently Develop a plan with the client for self-care activities Request consultation with occupational therapist for assistive devices and assistance in retraining for self-care Teach client energy-conserving ways of performing tasks Request social services to assist in dismissal planning Consider home health or possibly day care Plan and provide rest periods before and after activities; teach importance of activity and exercise to tolerance, avoiding excessive fatigue
Potential for trauma related to hypoxia and weakness	Client will state behaviors that decrease risk for falls or injury	Assess factors that increase risk for falls Implement measures to reduce risk factors (e.g., bed in low position, side rails, safety belt, call bell within reach), and maintain oxygen therapy Discuss with client observed behaviors that may decrease or increase risks

Continued.

NURSING CARE PLAN: CHRONIC OBSTRUCTIVE PULMONARY DISEASE—cont'd

Nursing diagnoses	Expected client outcomes	Nursing strategies

Knowledge deficit related to self-care after discharge	Client will identify ways to minimize respiratory problems	Assess current level of knowledge
		Instruct client in health practices such as adequate diet, adequate rest periods, stress reduction
		Teach client importance and methods of avoiding pollutants; for example:
		  Stop smoking (may be referred to stop-smoking group)
		  Remain indoors during times of heavy air pollution
		Educate the client about the importance and methods of avoiding risk factors such as crowds and very cold air
		Inform client as to the availability of influenza and pneumonia vaccines as preventive measures

Ineffective individual coping related to a sense of powerlessness, multiple stressors, and inadequate resources	Client will be able to identify and exhibit effective coping behaviors	Assist the client in identifying existing coping mechanisms
	Client will verbalize a realistic sense of confidence regarding respiratory status	Establish an environment of trust and acceptance Encourage client to verbalize his fears of respiratory distress, and teach methods to minimize dyspnea, such as pursed-lip breathing and energy-conserving techniques
	Client will express positive feelings regarding controlling his situation	Make efforts to encourage and incorporate the client's self-care decisions, such as time of bath, time for rest periods, degree of exertion Teach client new coping techniques and reinforce them Initiate social services referral for community resources and support Consider psychiatric consultation to rule out depression and to teach cognitive/behavioral strategies and techniques

EVALUATION

1. The client experiences optimal airway clearance.
2. The client experiences decreased levels of anxiety and fear.
3. The client demonstrates improved tolerance of activity.
4. The client demonstrates the ability to maintain adequate diet and fluid level.
5. The client demonstrates skin integrity.
6. The client exhibits increased knowledge of self-care and control of his medical condition.
7. The client participates in self-care activities.
8. The client sustains no preventable injury while in the hospital.
9. The client exhibits an understanding of ways to minimize respiratory problems through avoiding risk factors and through early intervention.
10. The client demonstrates positive coping strategies.
11. The client increases the resources available for post-hospital care.

NURSING ALERTS

1. Monitor mood, affect, and motivation as contributing factors to coping strategies: insight, self-confidence, and ability to set long-term goals may be elusive in the older COPD client.
2. Monitor arterial blood gas values at least weekly for 3 weeks. Then as signs begin to subside, monitor every 2 weeks for 3 weeks, then one time a month as needed for distress.
3. During episodes of severe distress, the nurse should stay with the client to calm him, thereby minimizing hyperventilation, which increases the hypoxia.
4. Be alert to the atypical symptoms of pneumonia seen in older clients (refer to the care plan on pneumonia, p. 188).

Bibliography

Doenges ME et al: Nursing care plans: nursing diagnoses in planning patient care, Philadelphia, 1984, FA Davis Co.
Ebersole P and Hess P: Toward healthy aging: human needs and nursing response, ed 3, St Louis, 1990. The CV Mosby Co.

Eliopoulos C: Gerontological nursing, ed 2, Philadelphia, 1987, JB Lippincott Co.

Long BC and Phipps, WJ, editors: Medical-surgical nursing: a nursing process approach, ed 2, St Louis, 1989, The CV Mosby Co.

Pritchard V and Kerry C: Streptococcal outbreak, Journal of Gerontological Nursing 14:19, Feb 1988.

Tucker SM et al: Patient care standards: nursing process, diagnosis and outcome, ed 4, St Louis, 1988, The CV Mosby Co.

Ulrich SP et al: Nursing care planning guides: a nursing diagnoses approach, Philadelphia, 1986, WB Saunders Co.

DIGESTIVE SYSTEM

Diverticular Disease

Roberta Purvis Bartee

KNOWLEDGE BASE

1. A diverticulum occurs when the intestinal mucosa prolapses through a weakened area of the muscle wall, forming a sac or pouch. The presence of multiple noninflamed diverticula is called diverticulosis.
2. The term diverticulitis is used to indicate inflammation of diverticula, which occurs when food or feces lodge in the pouch. Macroperforation or microperforation of the diverticula may occur with the inflammation.
3. Diverticulitis occurs primarily in the descending and sigmoid colon; however, a high incidence of right-sided occurrence has been documented among Oriental populations.
4. Diverticula occur in approximately 40% of the population by the age of 70. It is thought that age-related changes in the muscle wall and slowed peristalsis, aggravated by increased intraluminal pressure from constipation and insufficient dietary fiber, cause the majority of diverticula. However, some clients inherit the tendency and do not have the other etiological factors. Diverticular disease may be symptomatic or diagnosed incidental to another problem.
5. Colonic intraluminal pressure, which contributes to the formation of diverticula, is increased by insufficient dietary bulk because high pressures are required to propel low-volume masses.
6. Laxatives increase colonic pressure because high pressures are necessary to evacuate watery stools.
7. Colonic pressure is increased by obesity, constipation, coughing, sneezing, the Valsalva maneuver, and the cholinergic gut-stimulating effect of some emotions.
8. Drugs that may alter motility or induce constipation include analgesics, anticholinergics, tricyclic antidepressants, antiparkinson agents, diuretics, and hypotensive medications.
9. Constipation most frequently precedes episodes of diverticular symptoms. Some clients report alternating constipation and diarrhea. Bowel motility may be slow because of the insufficient fiber, leading to constipation, or fast because of the inflammation, leading to diarrhea.
10. The incidence of diverticulitis increases with age. Seventy-five to eighty-five percent of clients recover with conservative medical therapy. Age-related changes include the following:
    a. Slowing of the nervous system diminishes gastrointestinal motility.
    b. Abdominal muscle strength diminishes.
    c. Receptors for the urge to defecate have decreased sensitivity.
11. Constipation is a tendency, not a fact, of age.
12. Elders tend to increase laxative and enema use.
13. Older people may demonstrate diminished inflammatory responses of pain, temperature elevation, leukocytosis, and abdominal rigidity.
14. Stasis within diverticula may lead to inflammation and infection or cause a fecalith that may compromise blood supply and support bacterial invasion.
15. The most serious complication of diverticular disease is peritonitis, which is caused by intestinal perforation and leakage of contents into the peritoneal cavity. The symptoms are fever, chills, distensions, diffuse abdominal pain, and a rigid boardlike abdomen, progressing to sepsis and shock.
16. Inflammatory edema or accumulated fibrotic tissue from recurrent episodes may narrow or completely obstruct the colon.
17. Fistulas may occur. The most common are those that track from the colon to the bladder and manifest with pneumaturia or fecaluria. Associated frequent urinary tract infection and dysuria may be the first symptoms of diverticular disease.
18. Persistent leukocytosis, tenderness, and temperature spikes suggest abscess formation. Prompt antibiotic treatment may permit abscess resorption. Elders may manifest only a modest increase in white blood cell (WBC) count.
19. Diverticular bleeding is abrupt, brisk, massive, and self-limiting, whereas that of diverticulitis is slight, recurrent, and most likely coming from granulation tissue.
20. Diverticular disease may mimic gynecological problems, pyelonephritis, renal stones, irritable bowel syndrome, inflammatory bowel disease, Crohn's disease, ulcerative colitis, or carcinoma.

21. Nursing care should focus on bowel rest, managing infection, observing responses, preventing complications, and client teaching.
22. Pain management is important in maintaining intestinal motility and normal colonic intraluminal pressure. Morphine tends to cause colonic spasms; therefore meperidine hydrochloride is the preferred narcotic. Acetaminophen is preferred to aspirin, since aspirin increases bleeding time. Antispasmodics and anticholinergics relieve bowel spasms.
23. Enemas should be avoided because they threaten the integrity of the mucosa and risk perforation and entrapment of intestinal debris in the sacculations. Products that increase bulk facilitate passage of stool.
24. Colonoscopy, sigmoidoscopy and barium enema are not done during acute episodes, to avoid colonic trauma.
25. Dietary teaching is very important to the management of diverticular disease. The following facts should be integrated into the teaching plan:
    a. Dietary fiber increases motility and stool bulk, reduces intestinal gas and intraluminal pressures, and prevents lumen closure during contractions.
    b. Added fiber relieves the symptoms in 85% of clients with diverticular disease and may reduce the occurrence of diverticulitis and complications.
    c. Corn, peanuts, some fruit, and vegetable skins may be tolerated if they are finely chewed.

CASE STUDY

Gertrude Clifford is an active 82-old widow who enjoys gardening and golf. She considers her health to be good, although she takes medication for hypertension. Arthritis sometimes interferes with her activities.

Occasionally a vague lower left abdominal discomfort would occur when she overate or was constipated. Over the years, to prevent constipation, she began using laxatives more frequently. After an unusual period of alternating diarrhea and constipation, she noticed a bloody stool. Gertrude went to her physician when she became feverish and her abdomen became quite painful.

She was surprised to be admitted to the hospital for observation and management of the abdominal pain. A CT scan was scheduled. After laboratory specimens were drawn, an intravenous line was started and Gertrude was to take nothing by mouth. Parenteral broad-spectrum antibiotics were ordered. The diagnostic workup confirmed diverticulitis. Orders for analgesics and antipyretics to be taken as needed were written. That evening her diarrhea stopped. Days later, Gertrude's pain diminished and her white blood cell count steadily fell. The IV was discontinued when she tolerated clear liquids and began to eat. She expressed interest in the information provided by the nurse about diverticulitis. After 5 days in the hospital, Gertrude was discharged.

ASSESSMENT CRITERIA
Physical
Current and past health status
Over-the-counter and prescribed medications
Vital signs
Allergies
Nutrition
　Height, present and usual weight, ideal weight
　Nutrient intake and patterns of intake
　Restrictions and food intolerance
　Dentition
　Laboratory test results: complete blood count, creatinine
Hydration
Elimination
　Voiding patterns
　Dysuria, frequency, urgency
　Bowel elimination patterns and recent changes
　Consistency of stool, color, amount, presence of blood
　Client's definition of constipation and diarrhea
　Pain when eliminating; location and description
　Flatulence, distension
　Use of laxatives, enemas, suppositories
Abdomen
　Bowel sounds
　Distension
　Rebound tenderness
　Masses
　Pain; location and characteristics
Rectal bleeding, pain
Activity level and tolerance
Infection symptoms
　Lethargy
　Loss of appetite
　Presence of chills
Self-care ability

Psychosocial
Ability to discuss current health problems
Life-style and health beliefs
Anxiety, tension, stress
Use of alcohol, caffeine, tobacco

Impact of health problem on life
Coping mechanisms
Role in family, community

Spiritual

Religious practices and support systems
Beliefs regarding health problem

Gertrude's history suggests that diverticular disease has not been a problem until now. Gardening and golfing have provided her exercise. The degree that arthritis interferes with her activities may be a significant factor.

Her ability to follow health teaching is indicated by her taking of medication for hypertension. Gertrude's concern for health management is demonstrated by her going to her physician and by her expressed interest in health teachings pertinent to diverticular disease. In many cases, financial constraints or fear of surgery, colostomy, or cancer cause a client to delay seeking medical care.

Gertrude's increased laxative use contributed to increased colonic pressure. Before the present incident, constipation and overeating had caused vague symptoms. Both increase in-

---

traluminal pressures within the colon. Gertrude is slightly overweight from episodes of overeating, which increases intraabdominal pressures. She also complains of bloating and flatulence, which also are manifestations of diverticular disease.

Gertrude's history, lower left abdominal pain, and alternating diarrhea and constipation are typical of diverticulitis. Her episode was severe enough to cause bloody stools and fever and to disrupt her health status. The diarrhea compromised fluid and electrolyte and acid-base balance.

Gertrude was admitted for a clinical workup to rule out an abdominal emergency or malignancy. The intravenous line provided venous access for medication and hydration needs during the nothing-by-mouth period imposed for assessment, diagnostic tests, and bowel rest. Parenteral broad-spectrum antibiotics provide protection against possible bacterial peritonitis caused by bowel perforation, a complication of diverticulitis.

The cessation of diarrhea, diminishment of pain, and declining WBC count during hospitalization indicate resolution of Gertrude's acute episode of diverticulitis.

NURSING CARE PLAN: DIVERTICULAR DISEASE

Nursing diagnoses	Expected client outcomes	Nursing strategies
Pain related to inflammatory process, bowel spasms, possible peritoneal irritation, and stress	Client will experience decreased pain Client will, with assistance, use techniques of relaxaion, imagery, and distraction	Assess presence of pain: location, character, pattern Assess bowel sounds, distension, and rigidity Assess client's methods of pain control Assess vital signs Incorporate noninvasive methods of pain control: relaxation, imagery, distraction, and application of warmth to the nonacute abdomen
	Client will verbalize sources of stress	Assess level of stress Identify and reduce chronic tension, anxiety, guilt, resentment
	Client will identify helpful coping mechanisms and resources	Assist with coping mechanisms, and refer client to available resources Provide analgesia before pain becomes severe; evaluate whether narcotic or nonnarcotic most appropriate Provide anticholinergics, antispasmodics as ordered Evaluate and document effect of medications
	Client will define diverticulitis and state management techniques by time of discharge	Provide information about present health problem, management, course, and home care

NURSING CARE PLAN: DIVERTICULAR DISEASE—cont'd

Nursing diagnoses	Expected client outcomes	Nursing strategies
Potential for infection related to tissue destruction, trauma, inadequate immune response, and presence of intestinal contaminants	Client will verbalize understanding of ongoing assessments Client will state symptoms of peritoneal infections	Assess vital signs pattern indicative of infection Assess abdomen for peritoneal irritation: boardlike, absence of bowel sounds, distension, increased pain, rebound tenderness Assess client mentation and orientation Report and document client status and changes Evaluate WBC count elevations Obtain blood cultures as appropriate Teach client about diagnostic tests (CT scan, x-ray film, etc.)
	Client will experience antibiotic therapy safely	Safely administer and monitor effects (vital signs, WBC count, pain) of broad-spectrum antibiotics Observe, report, and document hypersensitivity, nephrotoxic and ototoxic effects Review available serial laboratory data for renal function, WBC count, culture and sensitivity
	Client will state signs of infection prior to discharge	Review manifestations of infection with client Document outcome of client teaching

Impaired tissue integrity related to increased colonic intraluminal pressure, saccular entrapment, and altered motility	Client's colon tissue will not be disrupted or compromised by controllable factors
	Client will verbalize rationale for decreased physical activity, nothing-by-mouth status, and adequate hydration
	Client will express understanding of the dietary plan, and its rationale
		Assess client's over-the-counter and prescribed medications that may alter motility
		Assess client's factors that may increase intraluminal pressure
		Assess for impaired tissue integrity: pain, abdominal distension, altered stool patterns, leukocytosis, blood in stool
		Teach client rationale for physician's orders—i.e., bowel rest, bed rest, nothing-by-mouth status, and:
		  Nasogastric intubation for nausea/vomiting/distension
		  Hydration with intravenous fluids until pain, elevated temperature, and WBC count decrease
		  Advancement of diet as tolerated when ordered, from a clear liquid to a high fiber diet
		  Assess change in bowel habits
		  Request consultation with dietitian for evaluation, planning, and teaching of diet therapy
		  Provide dietary information congruent with dietitian's teaching plan:
		  Avoid large meals
		  Encourage diet high in fiber
		  Gradually modify diet to include more bulk
		  Avoid foods that may become entrapped in sacculations: tiny hard seeds of figs, strawberries, raspberries, cucumbers, or tomatoes; poppy, sesame, caraway, or anise seeds; eggplant; green pepper
		Monitor nutritional status

	Client will thoroughly masticate all foods	Assess integrity of teeth and denture fit for ability to properly chew Instruct client to masticate thoroughly; large food chunks may provide the nidi for fecaliths Supplement diet with psyllium hydrophilic mucilloid as ordered Avoid dehydration

Continued.

NURSING CARE PLAN: DIVERTICULAR DISEASE—cont'd

Nursing diagnoses	Expected client outcomes	Nursing strategies
	Client will state circumstances known to increase colonic pressure	Avoid situations that increase colonic pressure (e.g., stress, constipation, valsalva maneuver
	Client will relate plans for weight maintenance within normal range	Teach effect of obesity on intraluminal pressure; encourage and assist with a dietary plan for optimal weight
		Document outcome of client teaching
Potential fluid volume deficit related to diarrhea, elevated temperature, and bleeding	Client will remain adequately hydrated	Diarrhea:
		Assess stool frequency, assist client to quantify diarrhea episodes per day, identify pattern
		Record number of episodes
		Assess level of hydration
		Provide fluid and electrolytes (oral, parenteral)
		Evaluate input and output record
		Administer medication as ordered, noting effect on diarrhea episodes
		Note effect of diarrhea on laboratory results: hydration status, acid-base balance, electrolytes
		Provide available, private, safe toileting facilities
		Assess skin; keep clean, dry
	Client will be able to verbalize rationale for assessments	Elevated temperature:
		Monitor, record temperature; identify patterns
		Provide antimicrobials and antipyretics as ordered
		Provide comfort measures; keep client dry
		Evaluate intake, output, hydration status
		Provide hydration and electrolytes
		Observe time and document episodes of chills, diaphoresis
		Secure blood cultures as appropriate
		Protect during chills, providing warmth without overheating
		Bleeding:
		Assess stool for frank and occult bleeding
		Obtain history of prior episodes
		Inspect laboratory data for compromise of oxygen-carrying cells: complete blood count, hemoglobin, hematocrit
		Administer iron preparations as prescribed, observing for constipation and stool color changes
		Assess, document, report vital signs during and after bleeding episodes, and calm the client
		Assess neurological status and cardiovascular status for indications of compromise (stroke, myocardial infarct)
	Client will state management for diarrhea, fever, and bleeding episodes	Instruct for home care: observation and management of episodes of diarrhea, fever, bleeding
	Client will list reportable symptoms	Teach the client reportable symptoms
		Document outcome of client teaching
Constipation related to lack of bulk, hydration, response to urge, and adequate musculature and probable overuse of enemas, laxatives	Client will maintain bowel elimination and be free from constipation	Assess client's perception of constipation by assisting to quantify stooling
		Assess expectations or changes in regard to bowel habits
		Assess client's knowledge about diet and bowel retraining
		Assess client's usual schedule for elimination; frequency and time of day

NURSING CARE PLAN: DIVERTICULAR DISEASE—cont'd

Nursing diagnoses	Expected client outcomes	Nursing strategies
	Client will identify medication that may contribute to constipation	Assist the client in evaluating the propensity of over-the-counter and prescribed medications to cause constipation
	Client will verbalize plan for prevention of constipation	Help client to plan the addition of fiber to meals: Increase bran intake, with adequate hydration Teach client to gradually increase fiber over 4-6 weeks and to expect initial bloating and mild discomfort before improving; advise client to notify health care provider of problems Teach client about the fiber and water ratio of foods and that larger quantities of high-water-content foods (apples, lettuce, potatoes) need to be taken to obtain adequate fiber value Supplement diet as appropriate with psyllium hydrophylic mucilloid (as ordered) and sufficient water Oil retention enema (90-180 ml) gently done may be required for obstipation
	Client will state plans for meeting hydration needs	Assess and instruct about meeting hydration needs without compromising renal or cardiac status Assess activity level, suggesting methods of increasing mobility within capability Provide available, safe, private toileting facilities Teach enema and laxative avoidance and that psyllium hydrophylic mucilloid provides bulk, making it the laxative of choice
	Client will establish a bowel training program and establish regularity	Encourage and assist the client with a bowel retraining program Establish a toileting schedule Instruct client to assume the following position on the toilet: leaning forward with thighs flexed, feet elevated on a small stool (see care plan on constipation, p. 23) Evaluate and document quality of stool Document outcome of client teaching

EVALUATION

1. The client describes the pain and identifies methods of pain control.
2. The client rates the pain lower on a scale of 1 to 10 after utilizing methods of pain control.
3. The client identifies stressors and their effect on diverticular disease.
4. The client lists effective management techniques and available resources to assist with current stressors.
5. The client reports any adverse effects of antimicrobial therapy.
6. The client reports any manifestations of infection.
7. The client states reasons why increased intraluminal pressure exacerbates health problems.
8. The client recalls factors that increase intraluminal pressure.
9. The client relates diet to intraluminal pressure, pain, and motility.
10. The client restates her dietary instructions.
11. The client's skin remains intact.
12. The client identifies the salient points of home care and names reportable symptoms.
13. The client names drugs that may cause constipation.
14. The client explains how to meet her hydration needs daily.
15. The client names activities that she plans to start or maintain.
16. The client explains the management of constipation without the use of laxatives or enemas.

NURSING ALERTS

1. Assess the abdomen with care because indiscriminant or rigorous palpation or percussion increases pain and risks perforation, leakage of intestinal contents, and extension of inflammation.
2. Anticholinergics are contraindicated for clients with glaucoma or obstructive urinary problems.
3. Diets high in vegetable fiber have been found to reduce protein and carbohydrate absorption and increase fecal loss of calcium, magnesium, and zinc.

Bibliography

Altman DF: The effect of age on gastrointestinal function. In Sleisenger MH and Fordtran JS: Gastrointestinal disease: pathophysiology, diagnosis, management, vol 1, ed 4, Philadelphia, 1989, WB Saunders Co, pp 162-169.

Bowers AC and Thompson JM: Clinical manual of health assessment, ed 3, St Louis, 1988, The CV Mosby Co.

Boyer MJ: Management of patients with intestinal disorders. In Brunner LS and Suddarth DS: Textbook of medical-surgical nursing, ed 6, Philadelphia, 1988, JB Lippincott Co, pp 799:848.

Brandt LJ: Gastrointestinal disorders of the elderly, New York, 1984, Raven Press.

Carpenito LJ: Handbook of nursing diagnosis 1989-1990, Philadelphia, 1989, JB Lippincott Co.

Corder A: Steroids, nonsteroidal anti-inflammatory drugs, and serious septic complications of diverticular disease, British Medical Journal 295:1238, 1987.

Devroede G: Constipation. In Sleisenger MH and Fordtran JS: Gastrointestinal disease: pathophysiology, diagnosis, management, vol 1, ed 4, Philadelphia, 1989, WB Saunders Co, pp 331-368.

Gioiella EC and Bevil CW: Nursing care of the aging client: promoting healthy adaptation, Norwalk, Conn, 1985, Appleton-Century-Crofts.

Given BA and Simmons SJ: Gastroenterology in clinical nursing, ed 4, St Louis, 1984, The CV Mosby Co.

Gordon M: Manual of nursing diagnosis, 1988-1989, St Louis, 1989, The CV Mosby Co.

Greenberger NJ: Gastrointestinal disorders: a pathophysiologic approach, ed 4, Chicago, 1989, Year Book Medical Publishers.

Haubrich WS, editor: Diverticula and diverticular disease of the colon. In Berk JE, editor-in-chief: Bockus gastroenterology, vol 4, part 2, ed 4, Philadelphia, 1985, WB Saunders Co, pp 2445-2473.

Heitkemper M and Bartol MA: Gastrointestinal problems. In Carnevali DL and Patrick M: Nursing management for the elderly, ed 2, Philadelphia, 1986, JB Lippincott Co, pp 423-446.

Hines C, Rogers A, and Weakly FL: When colonic diverticula cause trouble, Patient Care, 21(1):38, 1987.

Ismail-Beigi F et al: Effects of cellulose added to diets of low and high fiber content upon the metabolism of calcium, magnesium, zinc and phosphorus by man, Journal of Nutrition, 107:510, 1977.

Kelsay JL, Behall KM, and Prather ES: Effect of fiber from fruits and vegetables on metabolic responses of human subjects, American Journal of Clinical Nutrition 31:1149, 1978.

Kim MJ, McFarland GK, and McLane AM: Pocket guide to nursing diagnoses, ed 3, St Louis, 1989, The CV Mosby Co.

Malasanos L et al: Health assessment, ed 4, St Louis, 1990, The CV Mosby Co.

Matteson MA: Age related changes in the gastrointestinal system. In Matteson MA and McConnell ES: Gerontological nursing: concepts and practice, Philadelphia, 1988, WB Saunders Co, pp 265-277.

Morrissey K and Schein CJ: Surgical problems of the aged. In Rossman, I, editor: Clinical geriatrics, ed 3, Philadelphia, 1986, JB Lippincott Co, pp 472-493.

Munro A: Large bowel emergencies. In Imrie CW and Moossa, AR, editors: Gastrointestinal emergencies, Edinburgh, 1987, Churchill Livingstone, pp 150-175.

Naitove A and Almy TP: Diverticular disease of the colon. In Sleisenger MH and Fordtran JH: Gastrointestinal disease: pathophysiology, diagnosis, management, vol 2, ed 4, Philadelphia, 1989, WB Saunders Co, pp 1419-1434.

White EH: Nursing role in management: problems of absorption and elimination. In Lewis SM and Collier IC: Medical-surgical nursing: assessment and management of clinical problems, ed 2, New York, 1987, McGraw-Hill Book Co, pp 1045-1088.

Colon Resection and Colostomy

Lois Robinson

KNOWLEDGE BASE

1. The incidence of malignancies of the bowel tends to increase as people age.
2. Because of the recovery rates of elders who have an early diagnosis, increased education and screening should be part of health care.
3. Excessive fat intake and insufficient dietary fiber may contribute to the development of large-bowel cancer. There are also genetic links in colorectal cancer.
4. Most rectal cancers can be detected with a digital examination, while colonoscopy can diagnose up to 70% of cancer of the colon. Sigmoidoscopy, colonoscopy, and barium enema are used for diagnosis. An x-ray film of the upper gastrointestinal (GI) tract is necessary for higher colon lesions.
5. Symptoms vary according to the area of the colon involved and the degree of obstruction and penetration. Common symptoms are as follows: bleeding, change in bowel habits (constipation to diarrhea), abdominal pain, anemia, anorexia, nausea and vomiting.
6. Tumors of the colon spread by direct extension to nearby organs by lymphatic and hematogenic channels and by seeding and implanting of cells.
7. Treatment of cancer of the colon is always surgical. The tumorous area and associated lymph nodes are removed, with an anastomosis of the remaining segments. When the tumor is near the anus or the terminal portion of the rectum, an abdominoperineal resection is done, with the formation of a permanent colostomy.
8. The prognosis after surgery depends on the stage and location of the growth. Low-lying colorectal cancer with lymphatic involvement has a lower survival rate.
9. The major concern with bowel surgery is fecal contamination. Preoperative preparations focus on minimizing the contamination. The client eats a low-residue diet and takes laxatives and enemas. Antibiotics such as neomycin or kanamycin are given to decrease the intestinal bacteria.
10. The extensive cleansing and purging to prepare the bowel for surgery are poorly tolerated by older people. Elders are at risk for fluid and electrolyte imbalance, hypotension, and malnourishment. These and other chronic conditions may be present when the client is admitted, but the surgical preparation makes them worse.
11. During the preoperative period, the client should be encouraged to be as mobile as possible. This maintains musculoskeletal strength and flexibility, enhances circulation, and enhances the sense of normalcy.
12. Nutritional status must be carefully assessed on admission. An early request for a dietary consultation helps the health care team to identify the nutrient need throughout the acute episode. If the client is malnourished before surgery for wound infection, wound dehiscence and delayed recovery are very likely. Malnourishment increases mortality rates, especially in elders. Both enteral and parenteral feeding should be considered both before and after surgery for the malnourished elderly client.
13. Preoperative evaluation and management of co-existing medical problems can improve operative risk. Clients with chronic obstructive pulmonary disease, hypertension, cardiac problems, or diabetes are especially prone to complications during the perioperative time.
14. Preoperative teaching is extremely important. The client's knowing what to expect and what is expected of him or her decreases anxiety and increases the ability to cooperate. Elders are able to learn if caregivers will allow sufficient time, compensate for vision and hearing problems, and use multiple teaching techniques. The client who is to have a colostomy needs information about the ostomy, the need for mobility, aeration of the lungs, hydration, nutrition, and safety and pain management.
15. The most common response of the client to the need for extensive surgery and a colostomy is shock and disbelief. Being told that the procedure is lifesaving is a strong influence in the client's decision to have the surgery. The short time from diagnosis to surgery does not give the client adequate time to adjust, which results in an increased surgical risk because of stress overload.

16. After assessing the client information obtained by the physician, the nurse provides as much information as the client indicates he or she wishes to have. It is desirable for the client to know at least what is meant by ostomy surgery and the planned management (use of pouches) it will require. The following should be considered in the teaching plan:
    a. Simple anatomy of the gastrointestinal tract
    b. Explanation of the surgical removal, how the stoma will be formed, and where it will be located
    c. Appearance of the stoma and the type of bowel elimination expected
    d. Management of the stoma and bowel elimination

17. When an abdominoperineal resection is done, two incisions are made:
    a. An abdominal incision is made, in which the tumor and sigmoid colon are freed and the proximal end of the bowel brought out to the surface through a separate incision
    b. A perineal incision is made and the rectum and anus are excised and then, along with the sigmoid colon, are removed via the perineal incision

18. A colostomy is performed; it is usually placed in the left side of the abdomen so that the client can work with it more easily. The abdominal incision and perineal incision are closed with sutures or staples. A drain is placed in the perineal area, since it is in a dependent position and serosanguineous drainage is profuse during the first 48 hours postoperatively, decreasing gradually thereafter.

19. Marking of the stoma site preoperatively is commonly very traumatic for clients. The reality of the surgery and the threat to body image may be overwhelming. Emotional support is needed through this time.

20. Several factors are considered in the selection of the stoma site:
    a. Visible to the client when sitting or standing
    b. Within the rectus muscle
    c. Avoids scars, bony prominences, and skin folds
    d. Avoids the belt line

21. Postoperatively the elder is especially at risk because of age related changes to the cardiopulmonary systems. The older heart has a decreased ability to respond to increased demands quickly. As a result the combination of the stress response which retains body fluids and IV therapy may cause fluid overload. The pulmonary capacity and reserve is decreased. Elders who have a smoking history have further damage.

22. Postoperative care is focused on prevention of infection, oxygenation, fluid and electrolyte balance, comfort, nutrition, elimination, self-care needs, and change in body image.

23. The stoma is observed for redness, edema, intactness of the suture line, and function. The stoma drainage initially consists of mucus and serosanguineous secretion. Flatus and fecal drainage usually begin within 4 to 7 days, depending on diet progression.

24. Removal of any body part results in a sense of loss. Grief, shock, denial, anger, and depression are expected. The expelling of fecal contents through the abdomen may cause feelings of disgust or embarrassment. Clients may need counseling to adjust. Learning to care for the ostomy has been shown to help in the adjustment. Having support from a person with an ostomy has proved to be very helpful.

CASE STUDY

Mr. Baker, a 75-year-old black male, is admitted to the hospital with acute rectal bleeding. He states that he has been very tired and weak and has had no appetite for the past 2 weeks. He denies any rectal bleeding prior to admission. When asked about his stools, he relates that he has had some constipation and dark-colored stools. Laboratory findings are as follows: hemoglobin, 7.9 g/dl; hematocrit, 30%; white blood cell count, 18,000/mm³; erythrocyte sedimentation rate, 18 mm/hr. The urinalysis shows the following: color, dark amber; specific gravity, 1.031; pH, 7. The remainder of urine findings are negative. Mr. Baker states that he has been very well; although he has a family history of heart disease, he has never had any indications that he has problems. Mr. Baker has been a longtime smoker: "I started smoking when I was still in knee pants." He states that he never takes medication, not even aspirin. Dr. Brown orders the following: a colonoscopy this afternoon; nothing to be taken by mouth; type and cross match for 2 units packed red blood cells to give immediately; start IV of 1000 ml of 5% dextrose in 0.5 normal saline, plus 20 mEq of potassium chloride. After the diagnostic studies Dr. Brown schedules Mr. Baker for an abdominoperineal resection, to be done in 2 days.

Mr. Baker reports that his wife died 3 years ago and that his only family is a niece who lives in another state.

ASSESSMENT CRITERIA
Physical

Past medical and surgical history
Current medications
Gastrointestinal
  Nausea
    Time of day
    Frequency and duration
    Relationship to food intake
    Exacerbating factors
    Relief measures
  Vomiting
    Type
    Color
    Amount
    Relation to food intake
    Time
    Frequency and duration
  Discomfort/pain
    Location
    Characteristics
    Intensity
    Duration
    Exacerbating factors
    Relief measures
  Bowel/elimination
    Bowel sounds
    Distension
    Pattern of elimination
    Color of stool
    Consistency
    Flatulence
    Use of laxatives
    Blood in stool
Nutritional status
  Height
  Weight
  Usual and ideal weight
  Food history
  Appetite and recent change
  Food intolerances
Cardiovascular
  Blood pressure, pulse
  Edema
  Shortness of breath
  Heart sounds
  Peripheral pulses
Respiratory
  Respiratory rate and depth
  Temperature
  Cough
  Lung sounds

Neurological
  Sensation and pain
  Mental alertness
  Cognitive function
  Memory
Integument
  Skin turgor
  Color
  Integrity, especially over pressure areas
  Oral mucosa/tongue
Musculoskeletal
  Condition of joints, muscles, and bone
  Ability for self-care
  Activity and exercise levels
  Activity tolerance
  Functional ability; activities of daily living
  Pain/discomfort

Psychosocial

Mental status and attitude toward the surgery
Knowledge level related to:
  Diagnostic tests (procedures)
  Surgical procedure
  Colostomy
  Drainage system
  Health practices
Support systems
Current life-style
Risk factors (e.g., smoking, alcohol consumption)
Coping style and skills
Anxiety level
Feelings about loss of body part
Concerns about impact on sexuality

> Mr. Baker's age and his lack of family and support systems indicated the need for dismissal planning starting with admission. A health care team was organized for Mr. Baker. The social services department found in its evaluation that Mr. Baker had strong ties in his immediate neighborhood and with his church. Contacting key people in those groups rallied continued visits and offers for post-hospital care. Mr. Baker, after his initial shock and grief, began to show a willingness to learn his colostomy management. He was discharged to his home with home health care, Meals on Wheels, and a schedule for friends to assist and visit.

NURSING CARE PLAN: COLON RESECTION AND COLOSTOMY

Nursing diagnoses	Expected client outcomes	Nursing strategies
Knowledge deficit related to diagnosis of cancer, preparation for surgery, and establishment and care of a colostomy	Client will demonstrate understanding of diagnostic tests and preparation for surgery and postoperative care by verbal explanation	Assess current understanding of diagnostic tests and surgical procedure Explain each diagnostic test prior to its occurrence Explain surgical procedure, including both abdominal and perineal incisions and the establishment of the colostomy Evaluate understanding of explanations related to diagnostic tests and surgery; repeat as necessary Provide instruction about IVs, nasogastric tube, Foley catheter, turning, coughing, and deep breathing; have client practice turning, coughing, splinting incision, and using spirometer
	Client will identify alterations in the GI tract requiring a colostomy	Provide explanations, charts, pictures, and equipment used with colostomy prior to surgery; evaluate client's understanding of why a colostomy is done and what it is
	Client will be able to define terms related to diagnostic procedures and surgery	Explain terms and abbreviations such as NPO, IV, Foley, abdominoperineal, colostomy, and colonoscopy Provide daily opportunity to review and reinforce teaching
	Client will be able to care for own colostomy when dismissed	Explain to client the equipment and supplies used for colostomy Request person from ostomy support group to visit Demonstrate application and changing of the pouch; demonstrate cleansing of pouch and skin around pouch Teach client the assessment procedure for determining whether the blood supply is compromised in the stoma Have client demonstrate the assembly of the supplies Have client demonstrate application of pouch Teach client how to irrigate the colostomy Have client describe and demonstrate irrigation procedure prior to dismissal Provide client with specific dietary teaching Provide client with list of necessary supplies and equipment
	Client is able to list available resources and support services	Provide list of community ostomy services with names and numbers Allow time for client to assimilate all instructions and then ask questions
Ineffective breathing pattern resulting from anesthetic agents, postoperative medications, and surgical procedure	Client will maintain respiration sufficient for tissue oxygenation	Monitor and record respiratory rate and depth every 15 minutes while client is in recovery room and every 4 hours on the nursing unit Insert an oral or nasal mechanical airway in recovery room as needed; use a finger oximeter in recovery room to measure oxygen saturation Administer oxygen by mask per physician's order Position client with head of bed at approximately 45 degrees, if tolerated, to help breathing Request respiratory therapy order
Altered tissue perfusion resulting from blood loss during surgery and low blood counts before surgery	Client will modify activities within activity tolerance	Assess activity tolerance Monitor dressings and drainage devices every 4 hours Record in chart and mark areas of bleeding as to time and amount Monitor hemoglobin findings Replace blood loss with blood or IV fluid within the cardiac tolerance Monitor for possible fluid overload in elderly clients Teach client symptoms of fluid overload and activity intolerance

NURSING CARE PLAN: COLON RESECTION AND COLOSTOMY—cont'd

Nursing diagnoses	Expected client outcomes	Nursing strategies
Impaired skin integrity related to abdominal and perineal incision and establishment of a colostomy	Client is able to demonstrate measures for aseptic practice	Assess incisions every shift and document Maintain aseptic technique with dressing changes Monitor nutrient intake, especially protein and vitamin C Teach client good hand-washing technique and which dressings he can handle Encourage turning and early ambulation Provide pressure-relieving device Assess pressure points
	Client will be able to describe the expected appearance of the stoma Client can explain the purpose of the perineal drain and expected drainage	Monitor color, edema, suture line, and temperature of stoma every shift Keep colostomy bag on to prevent contamination of incision Monitor color and odor and measure amount of drainage every 8 hours (more often if necessary at first) Record color, odor, and amount of drainage every shift Reassure client about the amount and appearance of drainage Encourage activity and ambulation Keep the bed clean and dry
Altered patterns of urinary elimination resulting from potential infection related to perineal incision and presence of drain	Client will report any symptoms of urinary infection	Frequent care around Foley catheter (every shift) Monitor patency of Foley catheter Record urine output every 8 hours Encourage high fluid intake unless contraindicated because of cardiovascular status Encourage acidic fluids (e.g., cranberry juice) Maintain intake and output record on a shift basis
Potential fluid volume deficit related to nothing-by-mouth status, loss of fluid during surgery, nasogastric tube following surgery, and colostomy	Client will maintain adequate fluid status in relation to output	Assess skin turgor, vital signs, and weight daily Maintain intake and output record every shift Maintain IV fluid infusion at prescribed rate while client is taking nothing by mouth; use caution during stress response: regulate infusion rate according to output to avoid overload Monitor vital signs and document every 2 hours or as indicated Monitor laboratory values such as hematocrit and electrolytes
Pain related to surgical incisions	Client's pain will be reduced and maintained at a tolerable level	Monitor and document occurrence of pain: location, characteristics Reposition frequently Administer pain medication as ordered Encourage diversional activities Document effects of medication given for pain; monitor for overdose
Body image disturbance related to incisions and establishment of colostomy	Client will express feelings about his altered body image	Assess coping behaviors Assess acceptance of ostomy Encourage discussion of colostomy by client and friends Encourage client to look at colostomy Encourage client to observe you as you care for colostomy Teach client daily observation of stoma
	Client demonstrates coping behaviors	Demonstrate correct measuring and application of pouch Encourage client to apply pouch Teach how to cleanse the skin and about products to toughen the skin Discuss activities of daily living Encourage client to visit with other individuals with an ostomy

Continued.

NURSING CARE PLAN: COLON RESECTION AND COLOSTOMY—cont'd

Nursing diagnoses	Expected client outcomes	Nursing strategies
Sexual dysfunction related to abdominoperineal resection and establishment of colostomy	Client will express fears or feelings about possible changes in sexual function	Assess fears about sexual function If client indicates, share information about effect of colostomy on sexual function Discuss alternate means to obtain sexual satisfaction Encourage discussion with physician and other ostomy clients

EVALUATION

1. The client demonstrates understanding of diagnosis, treatment, and care.
2. The client verbalizes feelings about changes in body function and body image.
3. The client demonstrates a beginning of adaptation to the colostomy and the change in health status.
4. The client demonstrates the ability to care for the colostomy.
5. The client regains skin integrity in the areas of the surgical incisions and maintains skin integrity on the rest of the body.
6. Any complications are promptly detected and reported for timely intervention.
7. Dismissal planning is done beginning on admission.

NURSING ALERTS

1. Caution should be taken in administering parenteral fluids, because of the aging client's decrease in cardiac output. Increased subendocardial fat and connective tissue and thickening of vessel walls and valves cause the aged heart to require additional adaptation time.
2. Monitor fluid balance postoperatively; distended neck veins and peripheral edema indicate fluid overload.

3. Monitor drainage from the perineal drain for amount and character.
4. Monitor the stoma; it should be red but not dark or dusky.
5. Monitor the client's response to pain medications, taking into consideration his age and his previous drug-free status.
6. Monitor the client preoperatively for exhaustion (i.e., fatigue and weakness plus the physical and emotional stress of admission tests and impending surgery).

Bibliography

Albanese JA and Nutz PA: Mosby's Nursing Drug Cards, ed 2, St Louis, 1991, Mosby–Year Book, Inc.

Carpentito LJ: Nursing diagnosis: application to clinical practice, ed 2, Philadelphia, 1987, JB Lippincott Co.

Doenges ME, Jeffries MF, and Moorhouse MF: Nursing Care Plans: nursing diagnoses in planning patient care, Philadelphia, 1984, FA Davis Co.

McKenry LM and Salerno E: Mosby's Pharmacology in Nursing, ed 17, St Louis, 1989, The CV Mosby Co.

Phipps WJ, Long BC, and Woods NF, editors: Medical-surgical nursing: concepts and clinical practice, ed 3, St Louis, 1987, The CV Mosby Co.

Taylor CM and Cress SS: Nursing diagnosis cards, Springhouse, Pa, 1987, Springhouse Corp.

Yurick AG, et al: The aged person and the nursing process, ed 3, Norwalk, Conn, 1989, Appleton & Lange.

Cholecystectomy

Lois Robinson

KNOWLEDGE BASE

1. Disorders of the gallbladder and ducts are very common. The two most common conditions are cholelithiasis and cholecystitis.
2. The treatment of choice for symptomatic cholelithiasis and cholecystitis is surgery. Cholecystectomies are among the most common surgical procedures.
3. Symptoms of cholelithiasis and cholecystitis vary in each client. They tend to mimic a number of other conditions. Other conditions to be ruled out are renal stones, pancreatitis, hiatal hernia, angina or myocardial infarction, peptic ulcer, irritable colon, cancer, pulmonary inflammation, acute hepatitis, liver disease, and acute appendicitis.
4. Pain, nausea and vomiting, jaundice, chills, and fever are the most common symptoms. The pain is a colic type if the stone becomes lodged in one of the ducts.
5. There may be no symptoms of gallstones until a stone becomes lodged in a biliary duct. Biliary colic is a very severe pain caused by spasms of the duct in an attempt to dislodge the stone. The pain radiates to the back under the scapula and to the right shoulder.
6. The most frequent diagnostic test for the biliary tract is an oral cholecystogram. If the client is unable to take the oral dye, a CT scan or magnetic resonance imaging may be used. Intravenous dye is sometimes used, but the possibility of an allergic response exists.
7. New technologies are now being developed that may provide alternatives to surgical removal of the gallbladder.
8. Preoperative treatment for clients who are dehydrated and acutely ill on admission include the following:
   a. Analgesic for colic pain. Meperidine hydrochloride is the drug of choice.
   b. Allowing nothing by mouth, with nasogastric suction if needed
   c. Intravenous fluids to replace fluids and electrolytes
   d. Antibiotics if infection is present
   e. Vitamin K if jaundice is present and prothrombin time is increased
9. Preoperative care is focused on improving the health status of the client. Respiratory function is a priority, since the incision is high in the right upper quadrant with pain restricting deep respiratory excursions.
10. Preoperative client teaching should include information about the following:
    a. Dressings, drains, and tubes
    b. Respiratory toileting
    c. Nutrition
    d. Moving about in bed; early ambulation
11. A cholecystectomy consists of excising the gallbladder from the posterior liver wall and ligating the cystic duct, vein, and artery.
12. In addition to the usual postoperative complications, the following may occur with cholecystectomy:
    a. Subhepatic abscess
    b. Bile leakage
    c. Duct stricture
    d. Jaundice
    e. Pancreatitis
    f. Disruption of the ducts
13. Interactions and side effects of medications and anesthetic agents are essential to assess, since the physiological changes in the elderly client may cause changes in the absorption, metabolism, and excretion of drugs.
14. Normal physiological changes that occur in the elderly client, such as decreased cardiac output and reserve and decreased pulmonary function, jeopardize the client's ability to endure surgery.
15. Even the most common surgical procedures may have an adverse impact on the elderly client because of the presence of other disease processes and the client's reduced ability to handle the stress of surgery.
16. Anesthesia presents a special risk in the elderly because of their decreased metabolic rate and possibly compromised cardiovascular, respiratory, and renal systems.
17. Whenever emergency surgery is necessary, there is less time for an in-depth evaluation of the client and preparation for surgery, thus increasing the risk.
18. Since clients are sent home with dressings and drains still in place, dismissal planning on admission is important. Referrals to home health care services will provide for needed dressing changes. Referrals for home-delivered meals and housekeeping services allow the client to continue his or her recovery with minimal problems.

CASE STUDY

Mrs. Green, an obese 72-year-old widow of 3 months, is admitted with acute spasmodic pain in the right upper quadrant radiating to the right shoulder area. She tells you that she has not been able to eat fried foods for years and has had lots of belching and bloating, but last week she started vomiting and has not been able to keep anything down since then. Mrs. Green states that she has taken Mylanta for years but that it hasn't helped the nausea and vomiting. She also reports that she is having yellow diarrhea and that her urine is very dark. Upon admission Mrs. Green appears slightly jaundiced and diaphoretic and has a temperature of 99.8° F, blood pressure of 160/100, pulse rate of 120 beats/min, and respiratory rate of 30 breaths/min. Laboratory findings demonstrate a white blood cell count within normal limits; values for bilirubin, alkaline phosphatase, cholesterol, phospholipids, and prothrombin time are elevated. Potassium, sodium, chloride, hemoglobin, and hematocrit values are found to be low. The remaining laboratory findings are within normal ranges. Further assessment reveals that Mrs. Green takes piroxicam (Feldene) and aspirin for arthritis and propranolol (Inderal) for hypertension.

Mrs. Green's history of intolerance of fatty foods, belching, abdominal distension, and clay- or light-colored stools are indications of gallbladder disease. Since she has been vomiting and unable to eat for a week, she has a fluid deficit as well as electrolyte deficits, especially potassium, cloride, and sodium.

A CT scan of the gallbladder reveals multiple stones. Because of her debilitation, she is admitted to the hospital for supportive care in anticipation of a cholecystectomy.

Mrs. Green has been working part-time as a teacher's aide. She has seven children who live within an hour's drive. Her brother and his wife live close to Mrs. Green, and she is active in her church. Her major concern is losing her independence if she cannot care for herself. She has Medicare health insurance and a supplementary health plan.

ASSESSMENT CRITERIA
Physical

Past medical/surgical history
Current medications

Gastrointestinal
  Nausea
    Time of day
    Frequency and duration
    Relationship to food intake
    Factors exacerbating and relieving
  Vomiting
    Type
    Color
    Amount
    Relationship to food intake
    Time
    Frequency and duration
  Pain/discomfort
    Location
    Characteristics
    Intensity
    Duration
    Factors exacerbating and relieving
  Abdomen/elimination
    Bowel sounds
    Distension
    Tenderness, guarding
    Pattern of elimination
    Color of stool
    Consistency
    Flatulence
    Use of laxative
    Blood in stool
  Nutritional status
    Height
    Weight: current, ideal, usual
    Food history for prior day
    Appetite and recent change
    Food intolerance, especially fat
Cardiovascular
  Vital signs
  Heart sounds
  Peripheral pulses
  Varicosities
  Edema
  Angina
Respiratory
  Lung sounds
  Shortness of breath
  Cough
  Sputum production
Neurological
  Sensation in periphery
  Mental status
  Memory
  Reflexes
Skin
  Turgor
  Color; jaundice
  Integrity
  Rashes, scars
Musculoskeletal
  Functioning of joints, muscles
  Ability for self-care
  Activity and exercise levels

Activity tolerance
Pain/discomfort
Genitourinary
Patterns of elimination
Urine characteristics (i.e., color, pH)
Symptoms of infection (i.e., dysuria, urgency, frequency)

Psychosocial

Knowledge level related to:
Symptoms of gallbladder disease
Diagnostic tests
Surgical intervention
Nutrition
Other medical conditions (arthritis and hypertension)
Current medications, side effects, and food interactions
Recent loss of husband and existing support systems
Meaning of illness and anticipated surgery
Financial and health insurance resources
Anxiety level
Coping skills
Effect of recent loss on coping ability
Memory
Decision-making style
Family dynamics and identification of family leader

Spiritual

Meaning of illness in relation to religious beliefs
Source of strength and hope
Degree of limitation in participating in a faith community
Impact of recent losses on spirituality and religious beliefs

Mrs. Green has been admitted to the hospital in an acutely ill state. Her vital signs demonstrate an overlay of dehydration on her hypertension and infectious process. A temperature of 99° F represents a significant elevation, given that her baseline is 97° F. The normal white cell count in the presence of indicators of infection demonstrates the inefficient immune response commonly seen in elders. The elevated body temperature also warns of dehydration.

The physician orders intravenous fluids and parenteral nutrition to ready the client for surgery.

Mrs. Green's dark urine is an indication of possible obstruction of the biliary tract.

Since Mrs. Green's blood pressure is elevated and she has a history of hypertension, she is to be evaluated for possible heart damage or failure.

The fact that Mrs. Green is obese and has suffered from gastrointestinal (GI) symptoms for several years demonstrates some knowledge deficit. Her knowledge of gallbladder disease, its diagnostic tests, and home care needs to be evaluated. She is taking medication for her hypertension and arthritis; thus knowledge of medications and their interactions and side effects must be evaluated before she is dismissed for home care.

The recent loss of her husband and the resultant stress and grief may increase her risk for surgery. Her strengths that have been identified are continued involvement with others (part-time work, family, church) and continued physical and social activity.

She wishes to return to home care. The social services department has discussed the possibility of home health services, Meals on Wheels, and a housekeeping service with her.

NURSING CARE PLAN: CHOLECYSTECTOMY

Nursing diagnoses	Expected client outcomes	Nursing strategies
Knowledge deficit related to unfamiliar situation secondary to gallbladder disease and surgery and need for home care	Client will demonstrate increased knowledge about gallbladder disease and surgery Client will verbalize understanding of laboratory and diagnostic tests Client will demonstrate understanding of preoperative and postoperative care Before dismissal, client will be able to verbalize and demonstrate care of wound Before dismissal, client will be able to verbalize and demonstrate care of her T tube Client will be able to verbalize medication action, side effects, and interactions	Assess present knowledge level Assess readiness and ability to learn Provide simple explanations about gallbladder disease Explain surgical procedure Provide pictures to enhance explanations Evaluate effectiveness of teaching by having client repeat information Determine extent of present knowledge of laboratory and diagnostic tests Provide simple explanations Ascertain understanding of laboratory tests and diagnostic procedures from client verbalization Give simple explanation of terms such as cholecystectomy, cholangiogram, IVs, NPO, nasogastric (NG) tube, T tube Provide explanations about type and location of incision Provide explanations about dress of operating room staff and equipment and supplies used Explain about T tube and NG tube that may be used Explain postoperative care and the importance of splinting the incision; turning, coughing, and deep breathing (TCDB); use of incentive spirometer; and early ambulation Before surgery, have client practice TCDB, using the incentive spirometer, and splinting the incision Instruct client and family in care of the wound Teach aseptic practices such as hand washing and care of dressings Allow client and family to perform wound care and apply dressing Provide printed instructions on wound care and dressing change Provide special home instruction about T tube care Provide a printed copy of instructions for T tube care Allow client to participate in caring for T tube Refer to home health care service for daily visits Explain that Feldene is an antiinflammatory agent Instruct client taking aspirin and Feldene to report any blurred vision or ringing in the ears Teach client taking aspirin and Feldene to monitor urination and report any changes in pattern or the presence of blood; also report weight gain and edema Teach client to take Feldene and aspirin on a full stomach for better absorption and fewer GI symptoms Instruct client taking Inderal to report headache or dizziness, since it may indicate a need to decrease dosage Instruct client taking Inderal not to get up quickly or fainting may result Instruct client not to stop taking Inderal except under the physician's direction Instruct client to take Inderal with an 8-ounce glass of water Instruct client to take Feldene with food or milk Teach client that Feldene is excreted via the kidneys, so any urinary symptoms should be reported to physician immediately

NURSING CARE PLAN: CHOLECYSTECTOMY—cont'd

Nursing diagnoses	Expected client outcomes	Nursing strategies
Potential for infection related to surgical procedure, age, and poor hand-washing practices	Client will promptly report signs of wound infection Client will explain rationale for diet high in protein, carbohydrates, vitamins A, B, and C Client will practice good hand-washing techniques	Assess for complaints indicative of infection Monitor vital signs every 8 hours Monitor wound daily for drainage, redness, edema, approximation of edges Use aseptic technique with wound care Encourage ambulation every 2 hours while client is awake Request consultation of dietitian for evaluation, planning and teaching Provide diet high in protein, carbohydrates, vitamins A, B, and C when NG tube removed Instruct client in correct hand-washing procedures prior to wound care

Ineffective airway clearance related to anesthetic agents and surgical procedure	Client will maintain a respiratory rate between 16 and 22 to maintain normal arterial blood gas values	Recovery room care:
		  Maintain patient airway with jaw lift, nasal or oral mechanical airway
		  Monitor respiratory rate and depth closely
		  Maintain pulse oximetry rate above 90%
		  Administer oxygen by mask at 8-10 L/min
		Nursing unit care:
		  Monitor respiratory rate and depth every 15 minutes until client is stable; then every 4 hours
		  Have client turn, cough, and deep breathe every 2 hours; splint incision site
		  Have client use incentive spirometer every hour while awake
		  Monitor temperature and pulse rate every 4 hours
		  Evaluate restlessness to determine if pain or hypoxia is the cause
		  Evaluate increased disorientation as a sign of pulmonary infection

Altered tissue perfusion related to blood loss resulting from surgery	Client will have adequate blood volume	Monitor for lowered blood pressure, rapid, shallow respiration, and dusky and cool skin every 15 minutes until client is stable; then every 4 hours Monitor dressings Report blood loss Monitor fluid replacement closely to prevent fluid overload in the elderly client Provide oxygen by nasal cannula as ordered
Impaired skin integrity related to surgical incision, age, and nutritional status	Client will report expected observations in a healing wound	Assess incision daily and document Assess pressure points on body Provide pressure-relief mattress Use aseptic technique when changing dressings When removing tape, use special techniques to protect fragile skin Use Montgomery tapes with ties for daily dressing changes Encourage bed exercises and early ambulation Provide teaching to reinforce importance of nutrition and ambulation
Pain related to surgical incision and arthritis	Client will report increased comfort	Assess pain: frequency, location, and characteristics Instruct client about splinting the incision Offer pain medication before pain becomes severe or as directed Teach methods of distraction to reduce pain Encourage use of various positions to reduce pain Encourage use of heat with arthritis, but caution against sleeping with heating pad

Continued.

NURSING CARE PLAN: CHOLECYSTECTOMY—cont'd

Nursing diagnoses	Expected client outcomes	Nursing strategies
Altered urinary elimination patterns related to medications, pain, decreased mobility, and age	Client will describe measures that prevent urinary problems	Monitor output closely, and record every 8 hours Observe color and consistency of urine Determine whether symptoms of urinary infection are present Provide bedside commode until mobility improves Provide preferred fluids to 2500 ml/day Assist client in assuming an upright position for voiding Assess the ability to completely empty the bladder Teach client to observe for symptoms of urinary tract infection

EVALUATION

1. The client demonstrates understanding of gallbladder disease and preoperative and postoperative diagnostic tests and treatment.
2. The client reports increased comfort.
3. The client demonstrates knowledge of the medications prescribed.
4. The client explains the rationales for good hand washing, aseptic techniques, early ambulation, and good nutrition.
5. The client is able to report early signs and symptoms of infection and other complications.
6. The client demonstrates the ability to perform her own wound care and to care for the T tube.

NURSE ALERTS

1. Instruct clients taking Feldene and aspirin to report any blurred vision or ringing in the ears and to monitor urine output and report any increase or decrease or the presence of blood.
2. Clients taking Inderal may be hypotensive after surgery. They are at risk for orthostatic hypotension.
3. Caution clients not to stop taking Inderal without the knowledge of the physician.
4. Typical signs of infection may not be present in elders. Disorientation or restlessness may indicate an infectious process.
5. Caution clients not to take any over-the-counter medications without consulting their physicians, because of the possible drug interactions with prescription medications.

Bibliography

Albanese JA and Nutz PA: Mosby's Nursing Drug Cards, ed 2, St Louis, 1991, Mosby–Year Book, Inc.

Carpentito LJ: Nursing diagnosis: application to clinical practice, ed 2, Philadelphia, 1987, JB Lippincott Co.

Phipps WJ, Long BC and Woods NF, editors: Medical-surgical nursing, concepts and clinical practice, ed 3, St Louis, 1987, The CV Mosby Co.

Skidmore-Roth, L: Mosby's 1990 nursing drug reference, St Louis, 1990, The CV Mosby Co.

Taylor CM and Cress SS: Nursing diagnosis cards, Springhouse, Pa, 1987, Springhouse Corp.

Yurick AG et al: The Aged Person and the Nursing Process, ed 3, Norwalk, Conn, 1989, Appleton & Lange.

NERVOUS SYSTEM AND SENSE ORGANS

Alzheimer's Disease and Related Dementias

Mary E. Allen

KNOWLEDGE BASE

1. Alzheimer's disease is a neurological disease that is the most common cause of severe progressive loss of recent memory and thinking ability in previously well middle-aged and older persons.
2. Currently, there is no cure for Alzheimer's disease.
3. Because there is no single test for Alzheimer's disease, it is diagnosed by ruling out all other causes of memory loss, both reversible and irreversible.
4. Pathophysiological changes in Alzheimer's disease include atrophy of the cortex of the brain, with enlargement of ventricles and development of nerve cell changes called neuritic plaques and neurofibrillary tangles. The nerve cell changes can be detected only after death at autopsy.
5. Alzheimer's disease is a progressive disorder in which the rate of progression varies from person to person. The course of the disease may take 1 to 15 years, with death being caused not by the disease directly but by a secondary infection, usually pulmonary.
6. Many conditions mimic the symptoms of Alzheimer's disease. Malnourishment, hypothyroidism, and medication side effects are but a few. It is critical to rule out reversible causes and to initiate prompt treatment.
7. Following is a summary of typical symptoms in each phase of the disease.
   Phase 1 may last from 2 to 4 years, leading up to and including a diagnosis. This phase is characterized by loss of recent memory, impaired judgment, loss of initiative, quickness to anger, and reduction in risk-taking. Usu-

ally the client realizes that something is wrong but has the cognitive ability to compensate for the losses. The symptoms are very subtle and are explained away as normal behavior. At some time during this phase, the person loses the ability to name people or objects (anomia). He or she becomes very adept at substituting "thingamajig" types of names.

Phase 2 may last from 2 to 10 years after the diagnosis, with symptoms of increasing memory loss and confusion coupled with a shorter attention span. Friends and family members cannot help but notice that something is obviously wrong. The client may get lost even in familiar surroundings. Possessions are lost, and others are blamed for the loss. Suspiciousness and hostility are common behaviors. Diagnostic testing reveals an inability to calculate. The client becomes increasingly self-absorbed. All ability to compensate is lost.

Phase 3 is the terminal phase, lasting 1 to 3 years, with symptoms of the neurological damage that has occurred in the brain. The affect is flat, and there is long-term memory loss. The client has Parkinson's-like symptoms of tremor, rigidity, and gait and coordination problems. Bladder and bowel control is lost, as is the ability for self-care. Aphasia is present, along with apraxia. If motor control is still present, wandering behavior is common. The client is unable to recognize spouse or relatives. Seizures, hallucinations, and delusions are common.

8. Once the diagnosis has been made, a comprehensive multidisciplinary team develops a plan to address the problems being experienced by the client and the family, identify strengths, and determine how to improve the quality of life for the client and the family.
9. For the family or caregiver, difficult decisions about care must be made. In the early stages, home care is usually attempted. Later, as the symptoms progress, institutional placement may become necessary.
10. Early diagnosis is important. The client may still be able to participate in financial planning, sign legal papers, and make his or her wishes known about the planning of care.
11. Caregivers may find little time or opportunity to look after their own needs. As a result, many caregivers experience physical and emotional health problems and social isolation. Support groups and respite care may delay the need for institutionalization of the client.
12. Each phase or stage has its own challenges and needs. The following suggestions are organized according to the stage of the disease:

Phase 1

Give information to the client and family if and when they request it. Keep the information as factual as possible, and give it both verbally and in written form.

Reassurance is needed by the client and family.

Encourage the family to accept the client's level of functioning. Discourage scolding or pressing the client to "try harder." Have reasonable expectations.

Instruct the family to avoid situations in which failure is predictable.

Keep the environment and schedules stable.

Expect the unexpected. Expect fluctuations in mood and performance.

Establish and use memory cues.

Address safety issues.

The family needs to maintain or develop support systems and to ask for help.

Help client and family arrange for legal and financial planning.

Refer the family to a support group.

Phase 2

Provide written information and discuss the situation in more depth. If a prognosis is asked for, be honest. Resource planning and realistic goal setting are critical.

The caregiver needs recognition for his or her efforts.

A carefully designed stress management program is needed, including respite care for the caregiver.

A support system is needed to provide for the caregiver's needs, including emotional comfort, stimulation, and intimacy.

The family should establish an opportunity and time to vent feelings, including those of both the client and the caregiver.

An opportunity is needed to discuss shared experiences and strategies for the caregiver.

Reinforce to the caregiver and the family the fact that the client's disease is causing his or her behaviors.

Discuss blaming behavior of the client with the caregiver and the family.

Encourage the family to use reminiscence to enhance long-term memory.

Aphasia and apraxia need to be identified, and the family needs help in planning strategies to cope with them.

Education about medications is important.

The caregiver and the family need to be informed about danger signals that require decisions to be made about the possibility of institutional care or arranging for a constant companion.

Phase 3

The caregiver assumes responsibility for all activities of daily living and should consider a home health aide.

Short-term memory and remote memory are lost. Avoid anger toward the client, do not expect memory.

Strategies for the caregiver are needed in handling disruptive behaviors, agitation, and combativeness.

Resource people and agencies to assist in making decisions about care are important for the survival of the caregiver.

Help the caregiver and family verbalize that they have done everything possible.

Help the caregiver and family verbalize feelings associated with the client and the disease.

Help the caregiver and family extract meaning from the experience.

CASE STUDY

Mrs. Smith, a 70-year-old widow, was diagnosed as having Alzheimer's disease approximately 6 months ago. She has been living with her oldest daughter, who is a 52-year-old housewife, her son-in-law, who is a 54-year-old lawyer, and two grandchildren, a boy and girl ages 16 and 14, respectively. The family has been able to care for Mrs. Smith at home, mainly because of the efforts of the oldest daughter.

Mrs. Smith's other two adult children, who live close by, refuse to become involved with her care. The family has contacted the local home health agency to arrange for visits by a community health nurse.

During a home visit by the nurse and an initial nursing assessment, the following data were collected: Mrs. Smith made a score of 9.7 on the Folstein Mini-Mental Status Examination, with severe impairment in the areas of orientation, registration, attention and calculation, recall, and language. She was unaware of and indifferent to her environmental surroundings and family during the visit. Her motor functions were generally normal in regard to speech, psychomotor speed, and posture. She did periodically exhibit a shuffling gait and other poorly coordinated movements.

The family reported needing to monitor and assist Mrs. Smith with feeding, bathing, dressing, and toileting. For the last 2 years the family had provided needed transportation for her because she no longer drove a car. Recently, the oldest daughter had been feeling very "burdened" and the entire family was extremely anxious and concerned about Mrs. Smith's wandering behavior. Mrs. Smith no longer recognizes her family members and often treats them like "strangers."

The following medications had been prescribed for Mrs. Smith by the family physician: thioridazine (Mellaril), 5 mg taken orally four times a day; dihydroergotoxine mesylate (Hydergine), 4 mg taken orally each day; and chloral hydrate, two 500-mg capsules taken orally at bedtime as needed. Mrs. Smith received her bedtime medication from her daughter every night. Mrs. Smith is frequently oversedated upon awakening and has difficulty engaging in morning self-care activities.

ASSESSMENT CRITERIA
Physical

General appearance
Daily activity patterns, including:
    Nutrition
    Elimination
    Exercise
    Hygiene
    Substance use
    Sleep and rest
    Sexual activity

Past biophysical health
    Medical and surgical experience
    Apparent physical dysfunction or limitations
    Allergies
    Medications
    Family health history
Ability/inability to perform activities of daily living
Mobility
    Gait
    Coordination
    Balance
    Flexibility
    Activity tolerance
Sensory
    Vision
    Hearing
    Tactile
    Smell

Psychosocial

Coping patterns
Interaction patterns
Cognitive patterns
    Orientation
    Registration
    Attention and calculation
    Recall
    Language
Self-concept
Emotional patterns
Life-style and health practices
Family coping patterns
Cultural patterns
Significant relationships
Recreation patterns
Environment

Spiritual

Religious beliefs and practices
Values and valuing

The physical assessment reveals problems that require the family to monitor and assist Mrs. Smith with activities of daily living. A potential for injury exists as a result of Mrs. Smith's inability to perform activities of daily living, coupled with her periodic shuffling gait and other poorly coordinated movements. The wandering behavior also poses a safety risk.

The potential for substance misuse exists because of the daughter's practice of giving Mrs. Smith her prescribed medication on a "regular" basis rather than as needed.

The psychosocial assessment reveals problems of coping for the family, including an older daughter who is feeling burdened as the primary caregiver.

NURSING CARE PLAN: ALZHEIMER'S DISEASE AND RELATED DEMENTIAS

Nursing diagnoses	Expected client outcomes	Nursing strategies
Impaired verbal communication related to inability of family system to cope with person who cannot communicate needs	Client and family will be able to work together to meet needs that cannot be communicated verbally	Identify with the family system the probable needs of the client Engage the family members in health teaching to facilitate their understanding of the disease Encourage the verbalization of family members' feelings Use active listening techniques Identify with the family a mechanism for "reading" the nonverbal cues of the client Teach the family to take advantage of the client's lucid periods Model and role play facilitative communication techniques: 　Communicate with gestures 　Limit the conversation to short discussions 　Offer feedback to communicated messages 　Provide objects related to message 　Refrain from saying anything not intended for the client 　Refrain from shouting messages to the client 　Repeat the message in a calm manner until it is received 　Terminate emotionally threatening conversations with the client 　Use client's name frequently 　Wait for a response to one message before delivering another 　Face the client and talk distinctly when delivering a verbal message
Self-care deficit related to altered thought processes	Client will maximize her abilities in feeding, bathing, grooming, dressing, and toileting herself	Teach the family to assist the client with only those activities she finds difficult to perform, and allow the client to do as much as possible for herself Work with the family to set up a consistent schedule of feeding, bathing, grooming, dressing, and toileting Teach the family the necessary skills for assisting with activities of daily living as appropriate
Sleep pattern disturbance related to misuse of hypnotic drugs	Client will be able to sleep after taking the minimum dosage of the prescribed hypnotic drug	Teach the family to provide comfort measures to induce rest and sleep: 　Reduce environmental stimuli 　Identify sleep/relaxation techniques 　Identify an appropriate level of activity during daytime hours Encourage the family to consult with the physician on the monitoring of the medication regimen
Potential for injury related to wandering behavior	Client will not wander outside of her home unaccompanied by family members or significant others Family will verbalize an understanding of the causes of wandering behavior	Discuss with the family the benefits of having the client wear an identification bracelet Work with the family on the creation of a safe, secure home environment to minimize the probability that wandering outside of the home will occur Collaborate with the family on setting up a schedule of regular outings for the client Refer the family to the appropriate agency for respite care
Potential for combative behavior related to altered thought processes	Client will exhibit minimal combative behavior Family will express an understanding of the potential for combative behavior by a person with Alzheimer's disease	Discuss with the family why the potential for combative behavior exists in Alzheimer's disease Identify with the family verbal and non-verbal cues indicative of potentially combative behavior Explore with the family the behavioral cues of the client that are indicative of agitation Discuss with the family ways to prevent and manage the client's agitated states and combativeness if necessary

EVALUATION

1. The family reports being able to work together to meet the needs of the client that cannot be communicated verbally.
2. The family members are able to express their feelings about the difficulties of caring for a person with Alzheimer's disease.
3. The client maximizes her abilities in regard to feeding, bathing, grooming, dressing, and toileting, as reported by the family.
4. The client is able to sleep after taking the minimum dosage of prescribed hypnotic drug, as reported by the family.
5. The client does not wander outside of her home unaccompanied, as reported by the family.
6. The family verbalizes an understanding of the causes of wandering behavior.
7. The client exhibits minimal combative behavior.
8. The family expresses an understanding of the potential for combative behavior by a person with Alzheimer's disease.

NURSING ALERTS

1. There is a great potential for altered family processes and some potential for violence if the oldest daughter, the primary caregiver, does not receive more support in her role.
2. A referral to an Alzheimer's Disease and Related Disorders Association family support group would be appropriate.

Bibliography

Abrahams PA, Wallach HF, and Diven S: Behavioral improvement in long-term geriatric patients during an age-integrated psychosocial rehabilitation program, Journal of the American Geriatrics Society, 27(5):218, 1979.

Drahman DA and Sahakian BJ: Memory and cognitive function in the elderly, Archives of Neurology, 37:674, 1980.

Folstein MF, Folstein SE and McHugh PR: "Mini-Mental State": a practical method for grading the cognitive state of patients for the clinician, Journal of Psychiatric Research 12:189, 1975.

Gallo JJ, Reichel W, and Andersen L: Handbook of geriatric assessment, Rockville, Md, 1988, Aspen Publishers, Inc.

Gwyther LP: Care of Alzheimer's patients, Chicago, 1985, Alzheimer's Disease and Related Disorders Association and American Health Care Association.

Heim KM: Wandering behavior, Journal of Gerontological Nursing 12(11):4, 1986.

Jacoby RJ and Levy R: Computed tomography in the elderly/senile dementia: diagnosis and functional impairment, British Journal of Psychiatry 136:256, 1980.

Johnson CL and Johnson F: A micro-analysis of "senility": the responses of the family and the health professionals, Culture, Medicine and Psychiatry 7(1):77, 1983.

LaBarge E and Danziger W: Dementia in the elderly: an educational model including information, management, and counselling, Patient Counselling and Health Education 4(4):182, 1983.

McCartney J and Palmateer L: Dementia and delirium: detection in the general hospital, Rhode Island Medical Journal 66:361, 1983.

National program to conquer Alzheimer's disease, Chicago, 1987, Alzheimer's Disease and Related Disorders Association.

Norberg A, Melin M and Asplund K: Reactions to music, touch and objective presentation in the final stage of dementia: an exploratory study, International Journal of Nursing Studies 23(4):315, 1986.

Pavkov J & Walsh J: Mental impairment of the elderly: three perspectives, The Journal of Long-Term Care Administration 13(4):120, 1985.

Reifler B: Clinical aspects of Alzheimer's disease, Modern Medicine of Canada 38(10):19, 1983.

Reifler BV and Wu S: Managing families of the demented elderly, Journal of Family Practice 14(6):1051, 1982.

Sandman PO, et al: Morning care of patients with Alzheimer-type dementia: a theoretical model based on direct observations, Journal of Advanced Nursing 11:369, 1986.

Wolanin M: Confusion: scope of the problem and its diagnosis, Geriatric Nursing 4(4):227, 1983.

Yanchick VA: Drug therapy. In Dye CA: Assessment and intervention in geropsychiatric nursing, New York, 1985, Grune & Stratton, pp. 246-269.

Parkinson's Disease

Dorothy E. Booth
Carolyn L. Morris

KNOWLEDGE BASE

1. Parkinson's disease is a degenerative neurologic disorder involving the basal ganglia and the extrapyramidal motor system.
2. The two major functions of the basal ganglia are to control muscle tone and to provide smooth voluntary movements.
3. Smooth voluntary movements and normal muscle tone are the result of a balance between the excitatory effects of acetylcholine and the reticular system and the inhibitory action of dopamine. When dopamine is deficient or is inactivated, the basal ganglia are overactive, causing the symptoms of Parkinson's disease.
4. In Parkinson's disease, loss of cells in the substantia nigra correlates with the degree of dopamine deficiency. The underlying cause is unknown. Parkinson's disease cannot be cured at this time; only symptomatic treatment can be used.
5. Parkinson's disease is a complex clinical syndrome. Although the main feature is movement disorder, all organ systems are eventually involved.
6. Most cases of Parkinson's disease are considered idiopathic. Encephalitis, manganese, carbon monoxide, hypoxia, trauma, neurosyphilis, and drug therapy may be contributing factors.
7. More people suffer from Parkinson's disease than from multiple sclerosis, muscular dystrophy, and amyotrophic lateral sclerosis combined.
8. Parkinson's disease is the number one neurological disease of the elderly. It affects 1 of every 100 people over 50 years of age. Approximately 50,000 new cases are diagnosed annually. Half of the people with Parkinson's disease are over 70 years of age.
9. The disease begins with subtle symptoms, often affecting a single finger or one hand.
10. The rate of progression and the degree of involvement are variable among individuals. Age at onset, cause (if known), and life-style may be influencing factors in this variability. A person who has Parkinson's disease may live months, years, or decades.
11. Treatment with levodopa may decrease the symptoms, but with time drug effectiveness diminishes, causing increased problems with motor control. Recent research has shown that controlled release or intravenous infusion of levodopa can stabilize the motor fluctuations by stimulating the dopamine-producing system at a constant level.
12. The "wearing-off" phenomenon is thought to be related to the gradual loss of dopamine receptors as the disease progresses.
13. There are no definitive tests for Parkinson's disease, but diagnostic tests are used to eliminate other possible diseases.
14. A diagnosis of Parkinson's disease is made on the basis of four major clinical features:
    a. Bradykinesia—a delay in the starting of all movements, an abnormal slowness of all voluntary activities, including speech, and the arrest of ongoing movements
    b. Rigidity—increased muscle tone present at rest and increasing with movement
    c. Loss of postural mechanisms—the inability to maintain equilibrium or to react to abrupt changes in position
    d. Tremor
15. Major symptoms include the following:
    a. Loss of joint range of motion as a result of muscle rigidity and increased muscle tone
    b. Flexion of neck, hip, knees, and elbows, giving a stooped body posture
    c. Shuffling gait with either propulsive or retropulsive movement
    d. Absent arm-swing
    e. Cogwheeling type of movement when flexing extremity
    f. Rigidity of pharyngeal muscles, causing chewing, swallowing, and articulation problems
    g. Very slow movement (bradykinesia)
    h. Decreased eye blinking
    i. Inability to start (akinesia) and stop movement
    j. Masked facies
    k. Drooling
    l. Micrographia
    m. Decreased pulmonary vital capacity
    n. Decreased thoracic excursion
    o. Low voice volume; monotone

222

p. Decreased endurance (deconditioning)

q. Decreased righting reaction, increasing falls

r. Tremors; disease starts with resting tremor (pill-rolling type) but may progress to action and static tremor

s. Decreased peristalsis, causing constipation and flatulence; predisposes person to ileus

t. Excessive perspiration

u. Seborrhea and psoriasis

v. Orthostatic hypotension

w. Thermal paresthesia

x. Bowel and bladder retention or incontinence

y. Cognitive disorders; commonly occur in the later stages of the disease, beginning as a sleep disorder and visual hallucinations and progressing to paranoia and disorientation

16. Because of its chronic and degenerative nature, Parkinson's disease is best managed by a health care team consisting of attending physician, neurologist, physical therapist, occupational therapist, speech therapist, nurse, dietitian, and social worker.

17. A thorough assessment is critical for planning care, since the symptoms are individualistic, the progression rate varies, and the response to drug therapy varies.

18. A client's ability to regain or maintain mobility varies according to level of motivation, stage of the disease, and mental status.

19. Realistic goal setting protects the client and the caregiver and identifies mutually derived priorities relating to all aspects of the client's life.

20. General goals of care include the following:

a. Assisting the client to maintain or regain optimal mobility, independence, and health

b. Helping client and family achieve or maintain role activity and a sense of well-being

c. Assisting the client to maintain control over his or her life

d. Helping client and family cope with an altered life-style and activity limitations

21. Although self-care is a desirable goal, providing assistance may be an appropriate priority for the use of the client's time and energy.

22. Mobility problems, altered self-concept, and altered social interactions often diminish life satisfaction.

23. Drug therapy includes the use of one or more of the following: carbidopa-levodopa (Sinemet), bromocriptine mesylate (Parlodel), amantadine hydrochloride (Symmetrel), selegiline (Eldepryl), trihexyphenidyl hydrochloride (Artane), procyclidine hydrochloride (Kemadrin), cycrimine (Pagitane), benztropine mesylate (Cogentin), and diphenhydramine hydrochloride (Benadryl).

24. Each drug involves major side effects and precautions. Education of staff, client, and family is critical to the efficacy of drug therapy.

25. It has been shown that an improved response to levodopa occurs when protein intake is lowered to minimum daily requirements.

CASE STUDY

Mr. Adam Brad, a 66-year-old single Caucasian, was diagnosed 4 years ago with Parkinson's disease. For 2 years, absence of voluntary movement, left-sided tremors, and rigidity were controlled by amantadine (Symmetrel). The medication was discontinued when Mr. Brad experienced a severe fall and it was noted that he had developed bilateral tremors, impaired postural reflexes, and a rigid, flexed posture. He began taking carbidopa-levodopa (Sinemet), with partial relief of these symptoms. Mr. Brad has small, illegible handwriting; infrequent blinking; slurred, low, monotone speech; masked facies; oily skin; and excessive perspiration. He also reports fatigue, musculoskeletal ache and stiffness, numbness and tingling of his extremities, hourly toileting to "prevent wetting," and bilateral foot edema when the feet have been in a dependent position for a short time. He experiences difficulty in swallowing some foods, has episodic constipation, and has a depressed affect. Six months ago, he moved to his widowed sister's home because he needed help in managing some of his activities of daily living (ADLs). Although denying memory problems, Mr. Brad had a low score on his mental status examination, suggesting deficits in both recent recall and orientation.

ASSESSMENT CRITERIA
Physical

Medical, surgical, and trauma history

Medication history and present drugs

Ability to perform ADLs
　　Bathing
　　Dressing
　　Feeding
　　Toileting
　　Transferring
　　Ambulation
　　Using the telephone
　　Managing personal accounts
　　Carrying out household chores

Mobility
　　Ability to ambulate/change positions
　　Muscle coordination and strength
　　Stiffness or slowness of movement
　　Signs of joint contracture
　　Extent of bradykinesia and cogwheeling
　　Nature, location, and types of tremors
　　Gait, posture, and balance

Fall history
Need to use ambulatory assistive devices
Activity level
Daily exercise patterns
Activity tolerance
Neurological
    Sensation in extremities
    Reflexes
Nutrition
    Weight: usual, current, ideal
    Height
    Dietary intake (foods and fluids); nutrients and
        calories
    Usual meal patterns; amount tolerated each meal
    Food preferences
    Foods tolerated in chewing/swallowing
    Need for nutritional supplements; type
    Signs of dehydration
    Ability to chew/swallow
    Incidence of choking/aspiration
    Degree of drooling and impact on nutrition
    Fatigue when eating
    Frequency of oral hygiene
Respiratory
    Difficulty in clearing mucus/fluids
    Abnormal breath sounds
    Increased sputum production
    Coughing episodes
    Shortness of breath
    Signs of respiratory infection
Circulatory
    Peripheral pulses
    Edema
    Warmth
    Activity tolerance
    Skin integrity
Urinary elimination
    Incontinence
    Retention
    Toileting patterns
    Assistance needed with toileting
    Frequency
    Ability to sense need to urinate
    Ability to get to toilet in time
    Ability to manipulate clothing

Bowel elimination
    Bowel sounds
    Toileting patterns
    Ability to sense need to defecate
    Constipation/diarrhea
Communication
    Slurred words
    Stammering
    Voice volume
    Ability to have voice inflection
Sleep and rest patterns
    Usual bedtime and arising time
    Bedtime rituals
    Sleep problems; description
    Amount of daytime napping
    Exercise; amount and time
    Caffeine and alcohol use; amount and time
    Environmental factors (noise, temperature)
Sensory: vision, touch, hearing, smell

Psychosocial

Cognitive status
    Orientation to place, time
    Memory
    Judgment
Coping mechanisms
Degree of adjustment to disabilities
Flexibility
Degree of motivation for self-care and learning
Self-esteem; self-concept
Anxiety
Depression
Supportive relationships/potential caregivers
Environmental barriers and hazards
Knowledge of and willingness to use support services
Financial status/insurance coverage
Presence of advance directives (living wills, resus-
    citation)

Spiritual

Spiritual beliefs and preferences
Ability to achieve spiritual satisfaction
Sources of strength/hope
Perceptions/concerns about client's own life
Limitation in participation in faith community be-
    cause of disability

NURSING CARE PLAN: PARKINSON'S DISEASE

Nursing diagnoses	Expected client outcomes	Nursing strategies
Impaired physical mobility related to muscle rigidity, altered posture, slowed movements, and tremors	Client will demonstrate exercises for joint mobility and muscle strengthening Client will maintain or increase mobility to his maximum potential	Teach client to put joints through normal range of motion daily Request consultation with physical therapist to establish an exercise, gait-training, postural-control, and ambulation program Teach client to do arm and leg lifts Educate about expected outcomes from levodopa therapy Teach family how to massage tense muscles Teach strategies for initiating movement (i.e., counting, rocking, diversion) Assess activity tolerance; establish rest periods within schedule of activity Explore possible access to heated pool for swimming Encourage tub baths; assess tolerance for temperature Teach relaxation; consider music therapy
Self-care deficit	Client will identify functional limitations Client will do self-care to the extent of his potential Client will direct assistance in self-care activities to the extent of his ability Client/family will demonstrate their ability to gain access to community services	Assist client and family in identifying abilities and disabilities in ADLs Request consultation with occupational therapist for evaluation of needs and establishment of a collaborative program Help client and family to set and prioritize realistic goals Encourage family to support client in carrying out those ADLs in which he is capable Teach family to give client adequate time to complete his ADLs Help family to develop a plan and learn skills to assist in client's self-care deficits; schedule and pace are based on activity tolerance Teach client to bathe frequently enough to prevent buildup of secretions and to dry thoroughly in skin fold areas and between toes to prevent maceration and/or candidiasis Listen to the client and family's anger and frustration related to self-care problems Help family to gain access to community services for home care, respite care, transportation, and social interactions
Potential alteration in nutrition: less than body requirements; related to chewing and swallowing difficulties and need for prolonged time for eating	Client's weight will be appropriate for height and age Client and family will verbalize kind, amount, and schedule for nutrient intake	Ask client and family to keep a nutrient diary Ask family to weigh client weekly and report any loss Request consultation with dietitian to evaluate needs and establish nutritional plan Instruct client to consume a low-protein diet for breakfast and lunch to enhance the absorption and therapeutic effect of Sinemet Evaluate chewing and swallowing ability on a weekly basis Provide foods that are tolerated and preferred Serve hot foods hot; cold foods cold Establish method for rewarming foods; consider small, frequent meals Have family assist during meal if cutting up food is too fatiguing Instruct in methods of using Heimlich's maneuver or suction machine for choking Suggest allowing client privacy during meals; protect clothing from spills (a shirt front backed with terry cloth) Encourage client's presence at meals with others, even if he eats most of his meal elsewhere

Continued.

NURSING CARE PLAN: PARKINSON'S DISEASE—cont'd

Nursing diagnoses	Expected client outcomes	Nursing strategies
Alteration in bowel elimination: constipation; related to slowed peristalsis, poor nutritional intake of fiber, and decreased hydration	Client will have soft bowel evacuation every 1-3 days	Assess usual pattern of bowel elimination Request consultation with dietitian to assist client and family with meal planning to increase fiber Teach client to add 1 to 2 tablespoons of raw bran to soft foods and drink 8 glasses of water daily Use a glycerin suppository as needed to stimulate rectal muscle contraction Have client drink hot lemonade (1 ounce of lemonade to 4 ounces of hot water and a sweetener to taste) or 4 ounces of hot prune juice Develop method with client and family for providing toileting with privacy and safety Teach client how to complete evacuation with a rocking motion Consider requesting a prescription for a stool softener Use laxatives and enemas only as a last resort
Alteration in urinary elimination; related to autonomic system involvement causing detrusor dysfunction, infection, or depression	Client will experience an increase in control of voluntary urinary elimination	Assess current patterns of toileting, urgency, and frequency Request that a diary be kept of fluid intake and urinary output Assess client's ability to empty bladder Report findings to attending physician for evaluation and drug review Establish bladder training program based on identified causes Assist the family in obtaining protective items until problem is alleviated
Impaired verbal and written communication; related to muscle rigidity of throat, tongue, and face and decreased air flow	Client will improve his ability to communicate his needs and preferences to others Client and family will demonstrate strategies or techniques that enhance verbal communication between client and others Client and family will use various forms of nonverbal communication effectively	Teach client to take a deep breath before speaking, to use a slower speed in conversing with others, and to enunciate words, especially those at beginning and end of long sentences Teach client and family to use short sentences and nonverbal messages (pointing to objects, head shaking, etc.) Refer client for speech evaluation and therapy, and establish a collaborative program; consider using a speaking aid (e.g., microphone) Teach family the use of touch, eye contact, and longer response time to provide adequate stimulation and enhance interactions with client; demonstrate communication techniques to family Teach client to enhance speech by singing scales to a metronome, reciting poetry, or holding vowel sounds Teach client to do facial and tongue exercises Massage face, neck, and throat Establish a general exercise program in collaboration with physical therapist Provide electric typewriter or word board if client is unable to be understood
Activity intolerance related to muscle disuse	Client will increase activity without experiencing extreme fatigue	Assess present level of tolerance Maintain established exercise and ambulation program Teach family to monitor pulse of client before and after a walk (distance and speed should be reduced if pulse is greater than 100 beats/min or does not return to baseline in 2-3 minutes) Assist client and family in planning periods of activity with periods of rest Instruct client to elevate lower extremities during rest Teach client and family to arrange an environment conducive to restful sleep Teach client to keep a urinal at the bedside to limit sleep interruption resulting from nocturia

NURSING CARE PLAN: PARKINSON'S DISEASE—cont'd

Nursing diagnoses	Expected client outcomes	Nursing strategies
Alteration in thought processes; related to side effects of Sinemet and secondary to disease process	Client will use remaining cognitive abilities Client and family will demonstrate only mild levels of anxiety related to altered thought processes	Encourage family to maintain client's mental stimulation by observing time and date, encouraging him to read the newspaper, and following current news Help family to view client's behavior as communication of an unmet need or as a fear Teach family members to help client in accurately interpreting stimuli Reassess each aspect of mental functioning each month; recognize and support intact functions; help client to compensate for lost function Report change of mental status to the physician for drug review Encourage family to engage client in reminiscence Teach family to remove distractions when client is trying to complete a task and offer suggestions when he seems to be unsure of himself or to be making faulty decisions
Potential for injury: falls, choking	Client and family will verbalize preventive measures Client and family will institute home safety measures Client will use measures to compensate for neuromuscular and cognitive changes Client and family will use precautions to prevent choking and food or fluid aspiration by the client	Teach client and family fall-prevention measures Avoid full cups of hot liquids if client has tremors Monitor client for orthostatic blood pressure changes Encourage use of a night-light, and encourage client to request assistance during the night Teach home-environment safety in terms of lighting, elimination of throw rugs, use of rails, and bathing aids Request physical therapist's evaluation of need for assistive devices Assess activity tolerance and fatigue level with each activity Assist client and family to decide which ADLs and IADLs (instrumental activities of daily living) the client can continue to do safely Help client and family to develop strategies to avoid hazards from fire, drug, and chemical poisoning and car accidents Suggest that client dangle feet before arising and avoid hurrying, fatigue, and drugs that cause drowsiness or dizziness Remind client to wear corrective lenses and well-fitting shoes and to use assistive walking aids at all times Request consultation with speech therapist, and establish a collaborative feeding/swallowing program Instruct client and family to prepare soft, easily chewable foods Assess ability to handle thin liquids; if problematic, add thickening agent Instruct family to supervise client during meals and to assist if choking occurs (teach Heimlich maneuver) Have suction equipment available Instruct client to maintain an upright position during the ingestion of any food or liquid and to avoid eating or drinking 2 hours before bedtime Teach symptoms of pulmonary infection and inadequate airway clearance; encourage prompt treatment

Continued.

NURSING CARE PLAN: PARKINSON'S DISEASE—cont'd

Nursing diagnoses	Expected client outcomes	Nursing strategies
Chronic pain related to muscle rigidity and decreased joint movement	Client will report a decrease in pain	Teach client muscle relaxation techniques and the use of mental imagery Teach family to promote relaxation with a back rub Teach client importance of using daily range of motion movements and other exercises (e.g., walking) to stretch muscles and maintain joint strength Teach client and family use of hot and cold applications for the control of pain Consider pool exercises or exercises during tub bath Help client and family to manage pain relief with careful use of nonprescription or prescription medication
Alteration in self-esteem; related to change in body image, decreased function, increased dependence, and social isolation	Client will increase positive verbalizations about self Client will verbalize a purpose for his life Client will have social interaction with others of his choice	Assess client's feelings about self and current situation Encourage family to listen to him when he talks about his feelings Teach family communication skills to allow expression of feelings Encourage talk about source of strength and hope Help client and family to identify roles and tasks within the family Encourage family reminiscence Encourage the family to allow the client autonomy and to make decisions within his capabilities Encourage good hygiene and grooming and properly fitted clothing Protect clothing from drooling (terry cloth–backed shirt front) Assess for unmet sexual needs; assist client in problem solving Assist in developing ways client can interact with others outside the home Assist in maintaining or regaining spiritual resources Refer client and family to a support group

EVALUATION

1. The client is able to communicate with others.
2. Client and family acknowledge needs and perceptions.
3. The client states that with daily use of muscle relaxation techniques, range-of-motion stretching exercises, back rubs, and other measures, the chronic pain and stiffness are lessened. The client participates in physical activities and has fewer signs of pain or stiffness.
4. The client has not experienced falls or other injuries or accidents.
5. Client and family have taken the appropriate actions to ensure safety in the home and know how to use the Heimlich maneuver.
6. Client and family report that the client performs ADLs and IADLs and that he seeks assistance with activities that he cannot safely manage independently.
7. Client and family indicate that the client has established a 1- to 3-day pattern of bowel elimination of soft stool and that the frequency of urinary incontinence has decreased.

8. Client and family report that the client has established a pattern of daily physical activities.
9. The client demonstrates deep breathing and coughing exercises and reports no recent upper respiratory tract infections. Lung sounds are normal.
10. The client's face, body, and feet are free of odor, lesions, buildup of sebaceous or other secretions, redness, and edema.
11. A 2-week diet diary reflects that client is taking in adequate nutrients to maintain optimal weight. Foods high in protein are recorded as being consumed with evening meals. The daily intake of fluids (i.e., water, juices, and other beverages) is 2000 ml/day.
12. Client and family report client participation in daily activities providing mental stimulation and that they are tolerated well by the client.
13. A written record kept by client and family reflects that the client is accurately taking prescribed medications (dosage, time, etc.). Client and family verbalize the use of necessary precautions with each drug (prescribed and over-

the-counter) consumed by the client, the expected benefits, potential and actual side effects, and any adverse effects that should be reported.

14. The client states that he actively participates in and enjoys activities that are known to enhance self-esteem (e.g., Parkinson's disease self-help support group, reminiscence therapy, hobbies selected by client).

15. The client reports involvement in self-selected activities that enhance his sense of spiritual well-being.

16. Client and family seek assistive devices and community resources as needed.

NURSING ALERTS

1. Atropine-like drugs such as Artane, Kemadrin, Pagitane, and Cogentin may precipitate an acute glaucoma.

2. Urinary retention is a common side-effect of the atropine-like drugs. Men with enlarged prostates are especially susceptible.

3. Pyridoxine (vitamin B_6) is contraindicated with levodopa or Sinemet.

4. Alcohol in large amounts is an antagonist to Sinemet.

Bibliography

Arminoff JJ: Nervous system. In Schroeder SA, Krupp MA, Tierney LM, editors: Current medical diagnosis and treatment, Norwalk, Conn, 1988, Appleton & Lange, pp 571-620.

Carpenito LJ: Nursing diagnosis: application to clinical practice, ed 2, Philadelphia, 1987, JB Lippincott Co.

Folstein MF, Folstein SE, and McHugh PR: Mini-Mental State: a practical method for grading the cognitive state of patients for the clinician, Journal of Psychiatric Research 12:189, 1975.

Friedenberg DL and Cummings JL: Parkinson's disease, depression and the on-off phenomenon, Psychosomatics 30(1):94, 1989.

Gerald MC and O'Bannon FV: Drug treatment of Parkinson's disease. In Nursing pharmacology and therapeutics, ed 2, Norwalk, Conn, 1988. Appleton & Lange, pp 212-224.

Guilliland BC: Degenerative joint disease. In Braunwald E et al, editors: Harrison's principles of internal medicine, New York, 1987, McGraw-Hill Book Co, pp 1456-1458.

Hazzard WR: The biology of aging. In Braunwald E et al, editors: Harrison's principles of internal medicine, New York, 1987, McGraw-Hill Book Co, pp 447-450.

Matteson MA: Age-related changes in the neurological system. In Matteson MA and McConnell ES, editors: Gerontological nursing: concepts and practice, Philadelphia, 1988, WB Saunders Co, pp 255-263.

McLane AM, editor: Classification of nursing diagnoses: proceedings of the Seventh Conference, North American Nursing Diagnosis Association, St Louis, 1987, The CV Mosby Co.

Orkin LA: Bladder problems in Parkinson's disease, Parkinson Report 10(3):6, 1989.

Pincus JH and Barry K: Influence of dietary protein on motor fluctuations in Parkinson's disease, Archives of Neurology 44(3):270, 1987.

Sziegti E: Nursing care of patients with Parkinson's disease, Neuroscience Behavior Review 12(3-4): 307, 1988.

Weiner WJ: Non-motor symptoms in Parkinson's disease. Parkinson Report 10(1):1, 1989.

Weiner WJ and Singer C: Parkinson's disease and nonpharmacologic treatment programs, Journal of American Geriatric Society 37:359, 1989.

Yesavage JA et al: Development and validation of a geriatric depression screening scale: a preliminary report, Journal of Psychiatric Research 17:37, 1983.

Cataract

Joan D. Nelson

KNOWLEDGE BASE

1. Cataracts are the most frequent cause of reduced vision in the elderly. The presence of cataracts presents a twofold problem for the client. First, depending on the degree of cataract development, significant amounts of light cannot reach the retina, which reduces the ability of the individual to see detail. Second, the opacity of the lens scatters light, causing ocular glare and thus reducing the visibility of objects. Adjustment between light and dark environments is difficult, and too much or too little light often makes it difficult to distinguish objects and faces. Effects of glare are exaggerated if the client is too close to reading lights or windows. Dimly lit rooms, wet streets at night, and poorly lit stairs can become very dangerous.

2. Shadow interpretation is difficult, and adaptation from light to dark and vice versa is a major problem.

3. Cataracts can be classified by location (nuclear, cortical, subcapsular) and by stage of development:
   a. Immature: opacities are separated by areas of clear lens
   b. Mature: total opacification of lens
   c. Intumescent: swollen, enlarged lens encroaches on anterior chamber
   d. Hypermature: wrinkling of anterior lens occurs, usually representing progression of mature cataract to liquefaction of lens cortex, leakage of fluid through lens capsule, and, finally, shrinkage of capsule
   e. Morgagnian: total liquefaction of lens cortex occurs; nucleus sinks in the fluid in lens capsule
4. Retinal detachment, senile macular degeneration, therapeutic agents (e.g., corticosteroids and miotics, both of which are cataractogenic), diabetes, tetany, galactosemia, myotonic dystrophy, and dermatologic conditions (e.g., atopic dermatitis) can be contributing factors to cataracts.
5. Special tests for diagnosis of cataracts include the following:
   a. Ophthalmoscopy with dilation of pupils
   b. Visual acuity testing with refraction: determines whether the cornea, aqueous, lens, and vitreous are clear and retina is healthy
   c. Slit-lamp and fundus examination: performed for confirmation of cataracts and evaluation of maturation stage
   d. Guyton-Minkowski Potential Acuity Meter (PAM): estimates if the retina is intact
   e. Glare tester: provides information on the client's ability to see in presence of glare
   f. Contrast sensitivity test: assesses discrimination of low- and medium-contrast images
   g. Ruling out of underlying macular disease or retinal detachment as part of attempt to determine degree to which cataract surgery will improve vision
   h. Color vision testing: in early cataract, can determine function of macula
   i. Interferometry: a laser or achromatic light is used to determine postoperative acuity and health of retina
6. Sensory-motor deficits (e.g., presbyopia, presbyacusis, senile macular degeneration, glaucoma, decreased depth of focus, loss of contrast and visual acuity, loss of accommodation, diminished taste, touch, and smell) can increase the risk of confusion, social isolation, injury, and anxiety and may decrease mobility.
7. The elderly's delayed response to stress, followed by a delayed return to normal, can increase the potential for injury.
8. Musculoskeletal deficits (e.g., arthritis, osteoporosis, gait instability, decreased mobility and flexibility) increase the potential for injury and impair social interaction.
9. Neurologic deficits (e.g., parkinsonism, Alzheimer's disease, decreased blood supply to the central nervous system, slowed sensory and motor impulses, dulled sensation to heat and cold, impaired memory) increase the risk of injury.
10. Major life adjustments (e.g., outliving family and friends, accepting increasing dependency, loss of employment and friends through retirement, loss of social status, financial instability) can produce depression and anxiety.
11. The developmental issue of ego integrity versus despair needs to be explored to assess feelings of self-worth, self-respect, and life satisfaction.
12. Elderly people who have an increased susceptibility to glare are more prone to falls.
13. The treatment for cataracts is removal of the opaque lens through surgical intervention. Light can then enter the eye freely, but the eye cannot focus without a lens. Three methods are used to compensate for the removed lens: cataract glasses, contact lenses, and implanted lens. Well over 90% of cataract clients are enjoying full restoration of vision following surgery.
14. The most common surgical procedure for cataract extraction is the extracapsular approach—that is, removal of the lens and anterior capsule, leaving the posterior capsule intact. The lens may be removed by breaking the lens into small pieces and flushing the pieces out (phacoemulsification).

CASE STUDY

Seventy-eight-year-old Mr. Marconi is seeing his ophthalmologist for diminishing visual acuity in his right eye. He describes his problem as "trying to see through a dirty, greasy window." Night driving has become difficult because of glare from headlights, and he suffers from fatigue and tearing of the right eye when reading or watching television for long periods of time.

After extensive testing, the ophthalmologist informs Mr. and Mrs. Marconi that Mr. Marconi has cataracts in both eyes but that the cataract in the right eye is more advanced. The ophthalmologist recommends surgical removal of the right cataract when the left cataract begins to cause problems in the performance of activities of daily living.

Mr. Marconi expresses anxiety about "going blind" and his loss of independence. He is irritable and restless and naps during the day from "boredom." Mr. Marconi worries about "going out socially and spilling things or, worse, falling and breaking an arm or leg." Yet he has grave concerns about his eye "being cut into." He is advised to talk to the nurse educator at the hospital for assistance in assessing his problems and seeking solutions.

ASSESSMENT CRITERIA
Physical

Visual
  Sensitivity to light, glare, contrasts; reaction
    to dark
  Visual acuity
  Visual accommodation
  Visual fields
  Color discrimination
  Visual-spatial ability
  Ocular structures and movement
  Other visual disorders or pathology
  Corrective devices (e.g., glasses, bifocals)
  Lumination needs
Other sensory deficits (e.g., hearing, taste, touch,
  smell)
Musculoskeletal
  Functional limitations
  Deformities
  Gait instability
  Muscle tone and strength
Neurological
  Chronic organic brain syndrome
  Acute organic brain syndrome
  Mental status testing
General
  Activity/exercise habits
  Sleep habits
  Prescription and over-the-counter medications
  Health history, chronic disorders
  Coping patterns
  Self-care abilities
  Immediate environment (e.g., stairs, lighting,
    throw rugs, terrain)
  Use of aids (hearing aids, canes, etc.)

Psychosocial

Health perceptions, self-described life-style
Health maintenance behaviors
Knowledge of disease and treatment
Support systems
Risk factors (e.g., smoking, drinking)
Reality orientation
Cognitive ability
History of falling

Spiritual

Ability to participate in religious activities
Feelings of social isolation
Cultural influences
Depression, anxiety; presence or history of unre-
  solved conflicts or grief

Mr. Marconi was well-groomed, but his facial expression was grim, eye contact was in-
consistent, and he fidgeted with his fingers and
shifted position frequently. He appeared uncomfortable, anxious, and ill at ease.

The client stated that the only medication
he took was aspirin occasionally (maybe four
or five a week) for "arthritis" and his "artificial
tears" for dryness and itching of both eyes,
which is a normal aging change. Mr. Marconi
had been told by his family physician that he
had arthritic changes in both knees, hips, and
wrists, but mobility was not noticeably limited
and he used no aids for walking. He liked to
walk and garden and "just be outside," but was
anxious about being anywhere alone in case he
fell or could not see an obstacle in his way.

Mr. Marconi's weight was in proportion to
his height, he did not add salt to his food, and
he ate three meals a day and rarely snacked. He
had a physical examination every year and revealed that he had a slightly enlarged heart and
some arteriosclerosis but that his physician
was not concerned and did not recommend any
treatment. The client had no peripheral edema,
and vital signs were within normal limits.
There is no history of diabetes or other chronic
diseases, with the exception of those already
mentioned.

The client was able to hear questions and to
answer appropriately and stated that other senses were not creating a problem. Mr. Marconi
was alert and oriented and performed well on
the mental status test. There were no overt
signs of acute or organic brain syndrome.

The client was able to read newspaper print
quite easily with his bifocals, but his eyes tired
quickly and the right eye "became teary" if he
read for more than 30 minutes. Mr. Marconi's
lenses in his glasses had been changed since his
visit to the ophthalmologist, and visual accommodation was adequate for reading and distance, with some presbyopia noted. Mr. Marconi stated that he could not read with just the
right eye, "that the left eye is doing most of
the work." Visual field and visual spatial ability seemed adequate, peripheral vision was
good, and it was noted that Mr. Marconi's cataract in the right eye was centrally located.
Color discrimination testing showed that Mr.
Marconi had changes in color value, particularly some loss of blues and yellows.

The eyelashes were evenly distributed, the
eyebrows sagged, and there was moderate lid
ptosis, but these findings did not seem to obstruct the visual field. There was no sign of
conjunctivitis or pathology in the sclera, but
Mr. Marconi did have photophobia, saw halos
around lights, had difficulty adjusting to dark-
ness, and was sensitive to glare, especially in
the right eye. Visual acuity was reduced, es-

pecially in the right eye, upon Snellen testing in a well-lit room, but the new eyeglasses were compensating for low vision at the time of the examination. Mr. Marconi also stated that night driving was becoming more difficult and also very anxiety producing. Penlight examination revealed a visible white area behind the right pupil. Mr. Marconi's problem of itching and dryness in both eyes was being treated with "artificial tears." Eye muscle functioning was within normal limits. The ophthalmologist's report showed that there were no signs of vitreous or retinal detachment, macular degeneration, glaucoma, diabetic retinopathy, hemianopia, or corneal pathology.

Mr. Marconi perceived himself as a relatively healthy "old" man who was "going blind." He tended to eliminate activities that emphasized his visual deficit, such as reading or night driving, and even social activities that involved crowds or unfamiliar terrain. The client indicated that he felt that he was losing control over his life and his independence. His degree of acceptance of his disability was low, and his anxiety was high.

Mr. Marconi stated that he knew death was not too far off and "statistically I'm living on borrowed time," and he hoped he would die before becoming helpless and unable to care for himself. He still went to church and his children's homes (son and daughter) but had eliminated other trips outside of his home. He had been active with the Veterans of Foreign Wars and formerly "shot pool with some of the guys," but he did not enjoy these activities any more because of embarrassment about his visual deficit. His wife and family were supportive and caring. He spoke lovingly of his five grandchildren but demonstrated symptoms of depression and anxiety through self-deprecating remarks and doubt that life was "really worth living any more."

A review of the treatment for cataracts revealed that because of his anxiety, he had not retained or processed much information given to him by the ophthalmologist. He had not read the booklets on cataracts and focused on the image of someone "cutting up his eye." He was surprised to learn that his ophthalmologist was planning to perform surgery under local anesthesia, in the outpatient surgical unit, and was recommending a permanent implant. Further education and reinforcement of information were planned.

NURSING CARE PLAN: CATARACT

Nursing diagnoses	Expected client outcomes	Nursing strategies
Potential for injury related to impaired vision in right eye	Client will identify household safety measures that prevent injury	Ensure adequate indoor and outdoor lighting: Should be soft, nonglare, and incandescent Adequate night-lights at night; window shades or blinds during the day Avoid glossy surfaces such as highly polished floors and glass-top tables Turn head away when switching on lamps All inside and outside steps must be well lighted Adequate lighting in task areas such as stove, telephone and reading areas, closets Eliminate household hazards: Throw rugs, litter, footstools Objects that protrude from the wall, such as hooks, shelves Utilize safety measures: Nonslip surfaces in tub and showers Hand rails in bathroom Railings in hallways and stairways Color-code edge of steps Avoid clear glasses and dishes, chrome utensils Use bright color contrasts for visual discrimination

NURSING CARE PLAN: CATARACT—cont'd

Nursing diagnoses	Expected client outcomes	Nursing strategies
	Client will demonstrate personal health measures that prevent injury	Encourage client to wear sunglasses and/or hats with brims or use umbrellas to reduce outside glare
		Instruct client to avoid looking directly into headlights
		Review prescription drugs, their purposes and side-effects:
		Know interactions with other drugs, food, and alcohol
		Stress importance of taking drugs at right times and never discontinuing them abruptly
		Review commonly used over-the-counter drugs, side effects, and interactions with prescription drugs
		Instruct client to avoid driving when sun is glaring into windshield (e.g., dusk, early morning)
		Instruct client to avoid rush-hour traffic
		Institute an exercise and nutrition program to maintain fitness
		Instruct client to allow sufficient time for eyes to adapt when moving between extreme light and dark areas
Anxiety related to actual and perceived threat to visual integrity	Mr. Marconi will identify symptoms of his anxiety	Assess and document level of anxiety
		Encourage client to verbalize thoughts and feelings to externalize anxiety
		Help client to identify behavior that is connected with these feelings and to focus on present situation
	Mr. Marconi will verbalize a reduction in anxiety	Explore with client coping mechanisms that have been effective in the past for him
		Provide reassurance and comfort in a calm and level voice, and encourage expressions of irritability and frustration
		Suggest methods of reducing anxiety, such as relaxation techniques, deep breathing, and progressive relaxation
		Discuss with client his concern about social functions and "spilling things," and explore solutions
	Mr. Marconi will state ways in which he is functioning independently inside and outside of his home now	Review self-care activities and how he has adapted to compensate for visual loss
		Discuss garden and his success there
Knowledge deficit related to inadequate understanding of cataracts and treatment	Client and wife will identify need for additional information concerning cataracts and treatment	Assess and document client and wife's level of understanding of cataracts and surgery
	Client and wife will be able to state function of the lens, define cataracts, and describe two possible choices for lens replacement	Assess and document readiness to learn
		Offer an audio-visual or film presentation on cataracts to enhance learning
		Invite family to attend a cataract support group, if available
		Present a hotline phone list of persons who have had cataract surgery
		Review and reinforce specific cataract information and postoperative instructions with family; elicit verbal feedback and encourage discussion
		Discuss the high success rate of phacoemulsification and permanent lens implant and the increased freedom that will follow surgery

EVALUATION

1. Mr. Marconi and his wife make the following household safety improvements:
   a. Increase the number of lamps with frosted bulbs to decrease glare
   b. Provide night-lights of adequate wattage and use mini-blinds during the day to deflect glare
   c. Continue to ensure that inside and outside steps are well lit
   d. Provide lighting by the telephone that would allow for message taking and proficient dialing
   e. Purchase a magnifying glass with a light and stand so that reading is easier and less frustrating
2. Mr. Marconi purchases a jaunty hat with a wide brim and very stylish sunglasses with prescription lenses as a special treat and to help prevent glare.
3. The client states that he avoids night driving, rush-hour traffic, and dusk and early-morning driving.
4. Mr. Marconi takes great interest in discussions about anxiety and reiterates how he has overcome the previous stresses in his life. He cites several coping patterns that he has used successfully, such as a brisk walk with his wife when he feels overwhelmed or playing pool with his son (he feels less embarrassed about his "bad shots" now).
5. Since Mr. Marconi is not a very verbal person, he has been making lists of the things that annoy him every day and has attempted to problem solve when his frustration level ebbs. He has also listed ways in which he has been functioning independently and has figured out solutions to some of the previous obstacles to functioning.
6. The client's knowledge improves concerning cataracts and treatments, and his family also becomes educated about the disease. He expresses the desire to talk to people who have had cataract surgery and permanent implants.
7. Mr. Marconi still has reservations about surgery, since he has never had any previous surgery and has nothing to relate the experience to. However, it is hoped that by the time surgery is required, he will have had sufficient input from former cataract surgical clients to alleviate much of this anxiety. Focusing on the positives in his life has decreased some of his depressive symptoms.

NURSING ALERTS

1. The potential for suicide is extremely high in elderly Caucasian males.
2. Intraocular lens implants have not been in use long enough for a complete assessment of long-term complications.
3. Review the technique for giving eyedrops as a required skill postoperatively.
4. An untreated cataract can cause the lens to swell, resulting in glaucoma, or, more rarely, an infection in the iris.

Bibliography

Brink TL et al: Screening tests for geriatric depression, Clinical Gerontologist 1(1):37, 1982.

Brown B: Preoperative evaluation of cataract patients, Journal of Ophthalmic Nursing and Technology 7(6):204, 1988.

Capino D and Liebowitz HM: The elderly patient with cataract, Hospital Practice 22(3A):19, March 30, 1987.

Carpenito J: Nursing diagnosis: application to clinical practice, Philadelphia, 1987, JB Lippincott Co.

Folstein MF et al: Mini-Mental State: a practical method of grading the cognitive state of patients for the clinician, Journal of Psychiatric Research 12:189, 1975.

Gordon M: Manual of nursing diagnosis, 1988-1989, St Louis, 1989, The CV Mosby Co.

Kim MJ, McFarland GK, and McLane AM: Pocket guide to nursing diagnoses, ed 3, St Louis, 1989, The CV Mosby Co.

Mahoney F and Barthel D: Functional evaluation: the Barthel index, Maryland Medical Journal 14(2):61, 1965.

Robinson B: Validation of a caregiver strain index, Journal of the American Geriatrics Society 38(3):344, 1983.

West K: ABCs of cataract surgery preparation, Journal of Ophthalmic Nursing and Technology 6(4):156, 1987.

Yurick A et al: The aged person and the nursing process, Norwalk, Conn, 1984, Appleton-Century-Crofts.

Lens Extraction with Implant

Jean Nelson

KNOWLEDGE BASE

1. A cataract is an opacity (loss of transparency) of the ocular lens. Most cataracts are associated with normal aging. The cause is structural changes in the lens proteins, leading to liquification and swelling within the lens capsule. The result is progressively blurred vision.

2. The early symptoms of cataracts are caused by swelling of the lens before the formation of a visible opacity. Frequent prescription changes in glasses are associated with cataract development because the lens swelling changes the refraction error. Symptoms of cataract formation include poor vision, eye fatigue, headaches, increased light sensitivity, and blurred or multiple vision.

3. The treatment of choice for cataracts is surgical removal of the lens by intracapsular or extracapsular extraction. The procedure is usually done under local anesthesia on an outpatient basis. Surgery is recommended when visual deterioration causes significant changes in the client's life-style.

4. After lens extraction the operated-on eye is aphakic. Correction of the aphakia may be achieved with eyeglasses, contact lenses, or an intraocular lens implant. The lens implant is the method of choice, since it is most convenient for the client and achieves the best visual results. Since the implanted lens represents a foreign body in the eye, problems may occur after several years. Consequently, the procedure is most useful for people over 70 years of age.

5. Medications administered before and after cataract surgery include the following:
   a. Preoperative
      (1) Facial scrub with an antibacterial soap
      (2) Prophylactic antibiotics administered orally and by ophthalmic instillation
      (3) Mydriatic/cycloplegic agents to dilate the pupil and place the eye at rest prior to surgery. These drops must be administered at frequent intervals on the morning of surgery.
   b. Postoperative
      (1) Oral and ophthalmic antibiotics
      (2) An ophthalmic steroid to decrease the inflammatory response. A nonsteroidal antiinflammatory agent may be substituted when steroid use is undesirable in certain clients.

6. Since cataract surgery is usually performed on an outpatient basis, preoperative and postoperative care will be performed by the client and/or a significant other. Adequate teaching of the client or significant other is essential to ensure that care is administered safely and effectively.

7. Most elderly people have good cognitive function; however, certain age-related factors may influence the learning process: sensory impairments, mental status changes, tendency to fatigue easily, increase in the time required to respond to new stimuli, difficulty separating meaningful stimuli from distractors, variations in capacity to remember new information, and tendency to become anxious in learning situations.

8. Most persons contemplating eye surgery express apprehension about the possibility of blindness. Apprehension is increased by misconceptions about surgery. Elderly people often recall the drastic activity restrictions that were imposed on postoperative cataract clients many years ago. There is a common belief that a cataract is a growth on the eye that must be peeled off or cut out; some people think that cataract surgery entails removal of the entire eyeball.

9. Opportunity for open verbalization of specific fears allows the client to deal with fears constructively on a conscious level and allows the nurse to respond to the client's individual needs.

10. Fear may be internalized in the form of subconscious anxiety. This tends to be more maladaptive than fear that is openly expressed.

11. Correct knowledge about surgery and the events surrounding the procedure helps the client gain a sense of control.

12. Although the insertion of an intraocular lens produces immediate visual improvement, fluctuations in clarity of sight are common during the healing process. In addition, the operated-on eye must be covered at specific times: with an eye patch for the first 24 hours postoperatively and with an eye shield at night for 4 to 6 weeks thereafter. These alterations in vision place the client at risk for injury.

13. Surgery of any kind creates a risk for infection because of tissue trauma associated with the operative procedure. The eye structures are very delicate and highly vulnerable to infection.

235

14. Prevention of infection after cataract surgery requires that the client or significant other implement basic medical aseptic measures during postoperative care.

15. It is normal to observe slight redness and edema surrounding the operated-on eye for about 48 to 72 hours postoperatively. Clear drainage that forms crusts on the eyelids is also common.

16. Signs and symptoms that indicate postoperative infection include increased redness and swelling, severe pain, fever, purulent drainage, and a marked decrease in vision.

17. Pain following cataract surgery is normally mild to moderate and should be adequately relieved by a nonnarcotic analgesic. Clients often describe the discomfort as an aching, itching, scratchy sensation, or sensitivity to light. Severe pain is abnormal.

18. Clients who are in good health should be able to perform personal care and light housework after cataract surgery. Strenuous activity is restricted for 4 to 6 weeks.

19. Since cataract surgery is done on an elective basis, advance planning can be done to minimize household maintenance problems.

CASE STUDY

Mary Quick is a 75-year-old widow who lives alone and has no close relatives. Her general health is good, and she is active in various church and community organizations. Several years ago her ophthalmologist diagnosed bilateral cataracts during a routine eye examination. Since her vision was minimally impaired at that time, no immediate treatment was recommended. Recently Mrs. Quick experienced significant visual deterioration, especially in her right eye. Favorite activities such as reading, sewing, and writing letters became difficult; attendance at church and other activities was curtailed because she was afraid to drive her car, and she became dependent on friends to assist with shopping and other errands. The ophthalmologist recommended right lens extraction with implant. Despite many fears associated with "horror stories" she had heard about eye surgery, Mrs. Quick consented to have the operation. Preoperative teaching took place in an eye clinic; surgery was performed under local anesthesia at an outpatient center, which provided van transportation to and from the client's home. Mrs. Quick arranged to have a friend stay with her for a few days after surgery, and a parish helper from her church provided assistance with heavy household chores during the convalescent period. An examination in the eye clinic on the first postoperative day revealed immediate improvement in distance vision. Close vision was corrected with new reading glasses, prescribed 2 months postoperatively.

ASSESSMENT CRITERIA
Physical

Vision: visual acuity, visual fields, extraocular muscle function, external ocular structures, and ophthalmoscopic examinations, including measurements of dioptric power for lens to be implanted

Hearing: simple assessment of ability to hear spoken word

Primary sensory function: light touch, pain, vibration, and position

Mental status: level of consciousness, orientation, attention and concentration, memory, thought content and processes, mood and affect

Muscle strength, gait, and equilibrium

Coordination and fine motor function

Impact of vision changes on performance of activities of daily living

Dietary habits, presence of digestive disturbances

Patterns of elimination

Past and present health status

Usual medications, including over-the-counter preparations, and problems with adherence

Temperature, pulse, respiration, and blood pressure

Presence of any signs or symptoms of infection

Psychosocial

Elements of life-style: description of typical day, recreation/leisure profile, occupational profile, living environment profile

Family profile, resources/support systems used

Health maintenance behaviors

Knowledge of eye function and the nature of cataracts

Knowledge of planned surgical procedure, preoperative and postoperative care

Verbalization of fears about eye surgery

Signs or symptoms of anxiety

Spiritual

Personal belief/value system

Customary religious practices

Incorporation of spiritual resources into personal support system

Mrs. Quick demonstrated visual changes characteristic of senile cataracts. Surgery was recommended because her poor vision was seriously interfering with everyday activities.

Other physical findings were within normal limits for a 75-year-old woman. She demonstrated a high degree of functional ability and had no history of other serious illness.

Mrs. Quick is a retired widow with no close relatives; this may lead to feelings of loneliness. She has friends who have offered substantial support. In fact, her visual deterioration has made her increasingly dependent upon these friends for assistance with essential errands. The resulting decreased independence may have lowered her self-esteem. Leisure activities, both solitary and social, have been curtailed by declining vision.

Mrs. Quick lives alone and normally does all of her own housework. Postoperative activity restrictions mandate that she secure temporary help or defer doing certain tasks, especially those requiring bending, stooping, lifting, and straining, until the healing process is complete. Mrs. Quick has previously used appropriate community resources such as van transportation and the parish helper service to assist in meeting her needs.

Before surgery Mrs. Quick lacked accurate knowledge about eye function, cataracts, cataract surgery, and requirements for preoperative and postoperative care. She also had fears related to the procedure and recovery process based on stories she had heard.

Mrs. Quick's regular church attendance and participation in church activities suggest that religious observances are a vital part of her life. She expresses concern that she has been unable to attend church recently because of her inability to drive. In addition, poor eyesight might make it difficult for her to read the Bible and other religious literature.

Mrs. Quick views the church as part of her support system, as evidenced by her willingness to use the parish helper service. During the postoperative convalescent period she would probably appreciate visits from church members and from her customary spiritual advisor. Improved vision should make it possible for her to eventually resume her customary religious practices.

NURSING CARE PLAN: LENS EXTRACTION WITH IMPLANT

Nursing diagnoses	Expected client outcomes	Nursing strategies
Knowledge deficit regarding cataracts, cataract surgery, and preoperative and postoperative care; related to lack of previous experience	Upon completion of teaching sessions, client and significant other will demonstrate accurate knowledge of cataracts, cataract surgery, and preoperative and postoperative care	Provide teaching materials before surgery, to be used at the client's own pace at home Use materials with large print, or have someone read printed instructions to client Give verbal instructions clearly, concisely, slowly, in a low-pitched tone of voice Do teaching in a quiet environment Do teaching in small increments Use teaching materials at a level consistent with client's ability Whenever possible, instruct a second person who can provide essential care in the event that the client forgets or is unable to follow instructions
Fear related to knowledge deficit and inherent dread of possible blindness	Client's level of apprehension will be reduced before surgery	Ask client to verbalize specific concerns Do teaching to correct knowledge deficits Communicate true facts of a positive nature—for example, "Cataract surgery has a 95% success rate"; avoid using cliches such as "Everything will be fine" Provide opportunity for contact with someone who has had successful cataract surgery

Continued.

NURSING CARE PLAN: LENS EXTRACTION WITH IMPLANT—cont'd

Nursing diagnoses	Expected client outcomes	Nursing strategies
Potential for injury (eye injury or other personal injury) related to alterations in vision, fatigue, and knowledge deficit regarding postoperative eye care	Client will remain free of injury throughout the postoperative period	Advise client to rest upon returning home the day of surgery and, if possible, to have another person stay in the home for 1-2 days postoperatively when the eye is most vulnerable to the effects of trauma Instruct client to ambulate slowly and carefully and to exercise special caution when ambulating with operated-on eye covered, getting up at night, going up or down stairs, going outdoors, or driving a car When the surgical eye patch is removed on the first postoperative day, teach client to wear glasses for protection during the day and an eye shield at night Teach client not to rub or scratch the operated-on eye at any time Instruct client to place pillows at the operated-on side at bedtime to prevent rolling onto operated eye while asleep Teach client not to perform activities that increase intraocular pressure until the physician gives permission: heavy lifting (more than 5 pounds); straining; stooping; vigorous exercise; sexual relations; violent sneezing, nose blowing, or coughing; retching or vomiting; straining to pass feces; if cold symptoms, nausea, or constipation develop, the client should contact the physician about treatment for symptomatic relief Instruct client that severe pain or bleeding or marked loss of vision in the operated-on eye should be reported immediately to the physician
Potential for infection related to postoperative status, decreased immune response, and knowledge deficit regarding basic aseptic precautions	Client will remain free of infection throughout the postoperative period	Before surgery, instruct client to wash face thoroughly with antibacterial solution prescribed by physician to decrease bacterial flora of skin Instruct client in administration of antimicrobial drugs (eye drops and oral medication) to be taken before and after surgery; emphasize the importance of taking all of the prescribed medication Upon discharge from the recovery room, instruct client to keep the eye patch in place until the doctor removes it the following day Instruct client to wash hands thoroughly before doing eye care and to keep all equipment meticulously clean When the eye patch is removed on the first postoperative day, instruct client to wash area around operated-on eye gently with a clean cloth and warm water several times daily to remove crusts from eyelashes and maintain cleanliness of surrounding skin Teach client how to instill eye drops into the lower conjunctival sac without touching the cornea Instruct client to report severe pain, fever, increased redness and swelling, purulent drainage, or marked decrease in vision promptly to the physician

NURSING CARE PLAN: LENS EXTRACTION WITH IMPLANT—cont'd

Nursing diagnoses	Expected client outcomes	Nursing strategies
Alteration in comfort: postoperative pain related to surgical tissue trauma	Client will maintain a satisfactory comfort level throughout the postoperative period	Advise client to have a nonnarcotic analgesic (aspirin, acetaminophen, or ibuprofen) available at home on the day of surgery and to use it as directed; if the physician does not specify a particular medication, suggest that client use whatever she normally takes to relieve headache Suggest quiet diversional activities (watching television, reading, visiting with friends) to distract attention from discomfort Recommend having sunglasses available to decrease photophobia
Impaired home maintenance management; related to postoperative activity restrictions	Client will follow instructions regarding limitations on strenuous activity while maintaining a safe home environment	Counsel client to plan for surgery by scheduling the procedure at a convenient time, arranging the home so that frequently used items are within easy reach, preparing meals in advance, and securing temporary household help if necessary Explore community resources for help with cleaning and grocery shopping Emphasize the importance of following physician's instructions even if some household chores must be deferred For clients who have no help at home, advise home health nurse follow-up to assess adequacy of home maintenance and assist in solving problems

EVALUATION

1. After completing planned instruction, client and significant other demonstrate accurate recall of material covered in teaching sessions.
2. Prior to surgery the client verbalizes feeling less apprehensive about the surgery.
3. When reporting for postoperative check-ups, the client shows no sign of injury.
4. When reporting for check-ups, the client is free of infection.
5. Throughout the convalescent period the client verbalizes reasonable freedom from pain.
6. When reporting for check-ups, the client states that she is following postoperative orders and is able to maintain her own household adequately.

NURSING ALERTS

1. For clients who reside in long-term-care facilities such as nursing homes, care must be coordinated with staff in those facilities.
2. Clients with impaired mental status require very close supervision to prevent postoperative injury.
3. Clients who have lens extraction without an intraocular lens implant will have very poor vision in the operated-on eye until accommodation is restored with glasses or contact lenses. Cataract glasses do not restore normal vision—there is considerable distortion of the optical image. These clients require extensive guidance in learning to perform daily activities safely.

4. Many elderly persons become fatigued by the activities associated with outpatient surgery, and fatigue increases the risk for injury. A high anxiety level is also a risk factor for injury.
5. The client must exercise caution to avoid traumatizing the eye that was operated on, bumping the head, falling down, or performing activities that increase intraocular pressure (straining, bending, lifting, stooping, rapid head movements).
6. Trauma or increased intraocular pressure may result in complications such as hemorrhage or lens displacement.
7. Elderly persons have increased risk for infection because of the decrease in immunological defense mechanisms associated with the aging process.

Bibliography

Breitung JC: Caring for older adults, Philadelphia, 1987, WB Saunders Co.

Carpenito LJ: Nursing diagnosis: application to clinical practice, Philadelphia, 1987, JB Lippincott Co.

Carver JA: Cataract care made plain, American Journal of Nursing 87(5):626, 1987.

Eliopoulos C: Gerontological nursing, ed 2, Philadelphia, 1987, JB Lippincott Co.

Gioiella EC and Bevil CW: Nursing care of the aging client, Norwalk, Conn, 1985, Appleton-Century-Crofts.

Gittinger JW: Ophthalmology: a clinical introduction, Boston, 1984, Little, Brown & Co.

Gordon M: Manual of nursing diagnosis, 1988-1989, St Louis, 1989, The CV Mosby Co.

Lent-Wunderlich E and Ott MJ: Helping your patient through eye surgery, RN 49(6):43, 1986.

McFarland GK and McFarlane EA: Nursing diagnosis and intervention: planning for patient care, St Louis, 1989, The CV Mosby Co.

McKoy K: Cataracts and intraocular lenses: from cloudy to clear, Nursing Clinics of North America 16(3):405, 1981.

Sagaties MJ: Preparing patients for cataract surgery, Nursing 17(6):324, 1987.

Yurick AG, et al: The aged person and the nursing process, ed 3, Norwalk, Conn, 1989, Appleton & Lange.

Brain Tumor

Tally N. Bell

KNOWLEDGE BASE

1. The early warning signs of a brain tumor can be mistakenly attributed to age-related mental changes or other disease processes, which the elderly can ignore since gradual health deterioration is accepted by many elders as normal. This attitude, or fear of cancer, can result in significant treatment time being lost.

2. Brain tumors in the elderly are more likely to be malignant than benign. Aging of the immune system and homeostatic mechanisms puts the elder at an increased risk of developing malignant lesions.

3. Even though a tumor is benign, disability and death may occur because of the pressure exerted on brain tissue.

4. The possibility exists that there is an increased incidence of autoimmune reactions associated with aging, which could potentiate the cancerous process. Compromised immune function decreases an elder's resistance to bodily insults.

5. A grand mal seizure is a sign that something is awry in the nervous system and that further investigation is warranted. It is often the first indicator of a cerebral tumor.

6. The symptoms of a brain tumor result from both local and general effects of the tumor. Infiltration, invasion, destruction of brain tissue, and pressure leading to nerve and circulatory damage, edema, increased intracranial pressure (ICP), and shifting of brain mass may result.

7. A lesion in the left side of the brain results in abnormalities of the right side of the body. Symptoms may include changes in personality or judgment, abnormal sensations (paresthesias), visual abnormalities (diplopia or decreased acuity), report of unusual odors, headache, hearing loss, inappropriate behavior, incontinence, seizures, and aphasia.

8. Irregular pupil shape can be within normal limits for an elderly client, thus adding an important consideration to evaluation of the pupils during the neurological examination. Cataracts and lens implants are also concerns.

9. Reaction time lengthens in later years. This is important to consider in assessing a client's response to verbal commands, as well as for other neurological assessments.

10. A brain tumor increases intracranial pressure by increasing the bulk of brain tissue. The tumor may develop rapidly or slowly, diffusely or locally; thus the ability of the brain to compensate varies; the onset and progression of symptoms are indicators of the brain's inability to compensate.

11. Changes in level of consciousness are the earliest and most sensitive indicators of increasing intracranial pressure and are the single most important clinical observation in any neurological client. Brain herniation or direct destruction of tissue results with increased intracranial pressure.

12. Neurologically compromised clients can have impaired protective reflexes, which puts them at risk of aspiration. Side-lying positions help protect the airway of the client who has an impaired gag/cough reflex. It is important to consider the client's potential for increased ICP when determining what positions are the most appropriate.

13. A number of body positions can cause intracranial pressure to increase. Proper positioning to minimize adverse effects for the client at risk of increased intracranial pressure in-

cludes the following: preventing pressure on the jugular veins to facilitate proper drainage of blood from the brain; maintaining head elevation to facilitate venous drainage from the brain; preventing the client from actively turning himself or herself, which can cause a Valsalva maneuver; and preventing hip flexion, which increases intraabdominal pressure, leading to increased intrathoracic and intracranial pressure.

14. An increased P_{CO_2} is the most potent cerebrovascular vasodilator and will cause increased intracranial pressure by increasing the cerebral blood volume. Arterial blood gas determinations are a helpful diagnostic tool. A client with an ineffective respiratory pattern and/or inadequate airway clearance can require intubation and mechanical hyperventilation to treat or prevent increased intracranial pressure. Hypoxia, although not as potent a cerebrovascular dilator as hypercarbia, will also cause an increase in intracranial pressure. Coughing is important to clear the airway but will increase ICP in the process.

15. Stress, painful procedures, and prolonged nursing care can cause dangerous increases in ICP in a client who is at risk.

16. Straining and constipation can cause the client to perform a Valsalva maneuver and increase the intracranial pressure.

17. An excess of fluids can cause cerebral edema and increase the intracranial pressure. The client should not receive 5% dextrose in water, since free water fluids can cause an increase in ICP. Insensible fluid losses from diaphoresis, hyperventilation, or other causes should be considered when the fluid restriction is determined.

18. Hyperthermia increases cerebral metabolism and is known to increase ICP. It is also seen in the very late stages of increased ICP.

19. Steroids are known to be effective in the treatment of brain tumors. Antacids/gastric acid inhibitors are administered concurrently because steroids cause gastric irritation and because of the stress ulceration that can occur.

20. Diuretics decrease the fluid volume in the brain and effect a decrease in the ICP. Diuretic therapy can cause electrolyte imbalances, as well as disturbances in other body systems. A urine drainage catheter is indicated to ensure accurate output recordings.

21. Seizure activity causes an increase in metabolic waste products within the brain, increasing ICP. Anticonvulsants can be given prophylactically to prevent further seizure activity, but must reach therapeutic levels to be effective.

22. The neurological status must be evaluated carefully before range-of-motion exercises are performed, particularly to the lower extremities, since they can cause increases in ICP.

23. Codeine is generally considered safe to administer to a client with neurological impairment, although narcotics and other central nervous system depressants can mask important central nervous system signs. Age-related changes decrease the sensitivity to pain and change the way in which the central nervous system receives the sensory input of pain and interprets it.

24. A compromised neurological status can cause an elder to be unaware that he or she is neglecting self-care activities.

25. Immobility in the elderly can cause permanent functional loss, impaired skin integrity, and increased risk of urinary and respiratory infection.

26. Disorientation and confusion in the neurologically compromised client increases his or her risk of injury.

27. Restraining an elderly client for safety can increase confusion and contribute to increases in intracranial pressure and alterations in thought processes.

28. Unnecessary stimuli can contribute to altered thought processes through sensory overload and increased confusion, as well as potentially increase the ICP.

29. A fast, hurried approach can cause a confused client to feel threatened. A nurse should approach from the side on which the client's visual field is not distorted and speak in a clear and calm voice.

30. If the neurological deficits do not resolve, it is important that significant others understand the disease process and how to assist the client.

31. If short-term memory has declined, long-term memory will probably remain intact. An elderly client is capable of acquisition and retention of new information, but teaching him or her about a disease process and/or new skills can require a longer period of time and special techniques to ensure successful mastery of the information. This age-related change is compounded in the neurologically compromised elder.

32. The elderly need to retain the right to accept or refuse treatment and to choose treatment that will allow them to maintain their desired quality of life.

CASE STUDY

Mr. Dotson, a 76-year-old engineer, was admitted to the hospital 3 days ago following a grand mal seizure that occurred while he was visiting neighbors with his wife. The subsequent workup revealed a mass in the left frontoparietal lobe, which was biopsied and found to be a grade III astrocytoma.

The client reports that for the past 3 months he has been having frontal headaches that often were accompanied by nausea and were unrelieved by over-the-counter analgesics. He has noted progressive weakness and decreased sensation on his right side. He states that he has been "afraid" to seek medical attention. His wife states that he "hasn't seemed the same person lately and has been drowsy a lot." She says that his speech has been slower and that sometimes "he has trouble finding the right words to say." Since admission he has remained alert with occasional disorientation and has experienced no further seizure activity. His speech continues to be slow.

The Dotson's physician explains that the astrocytoma affects the connective tissue of the brain and that its fingerlike projections infiltrate into normal tissues. Since the tumor is not well encapsulated, surgical excision does not remove the complete tumor. Treatment options are fully explained to Mr. and Mrs. Dotson, and they jointly opt for radiation therapy only. Mr. Dotson asks to return home as quickly as possible.

ASSESSMENT CRITERIA
Physical

History
  Onset and progression of symptoms
  Medication history
  Past and present medical problems
Neurological examination
  Baseline vital signs
  Signs and symptoms of increasing intracranial pressure
  Changes in level of consciousness
  Lethargy, drowsiness, agitation
  Alert or comatose
  Responsive to stimuli
  Current affect and behavior (e.g., tone of voice, facial expression, demeanor)
  Mental/intellectual function
    Insight
    Cerebration rate
    Orientation to time, place, person
    Memory: immediate, recent, remote
    Concentration
    Judgment/reasoning
    Hallucinations
    Abstraction

Protective reflexes (gag, cough, corneal)
Deep tendon reflexes
Pathological reflexes (e.g., Babinski)
Onset, frequency, duration of headache, nausea, or vomiting
Clinical presentation of seizure activity; frequency, pattern, and duration
Postictal deficits
Signs and symptoms of tentorial (uncal) herniation
  Ipsilateral fixed, dilated pupil
  Contralateral hemiparesis or hemiparalysis
  Increased systolic blood pressure with widening pulse pressure
  Bradycardia/bradypnea
  Changes in respiratory pattern/character
Motor dysfunction
  Hemiparesis (contralateral or ipsilateral)
  Gait
  Balance/coordination
  Self-care abilities
  Ambulation/mobility
Bowel and bladder continence
Sensory-perceptual alterations
  Vision
    Changes in extraocular movement
    Visual field deficits
    Pupillary changes; size, shape, reactivity
    Papilledema
  Smell
    Obnoxious odors
    Loss of smell
Communication pattern; verbal and nonverbal
  Aphasia
  Dysphasia
  Inflections
Laboratory and diagnostic test results
  CT scan
  Brain imaging (MRI, CT)
  Skull x-ray films
  Blood and urine analysis
Review of other body systems

Psychosocial

Alterations in sleep/wake patterns
Judgment
Understanding of diagnosis
Personality/behavior changes
Meaning of diagnosis, prognosis
Coping strategies (adaptive or maladaptive)
Motivation for recovery
Support systems (family, friends, community groups)
Evidence of response to loss

Spiritual

Religious practices and beliefs
Faith affiliation
Ability to participate in usual religious practices
Source of strength and hope

Mr. Dotson's history and baseline assessment reveal a number of abnormal neurological signs and symptoms and many implications for developing the nursing care plan. A grand mal seizure is a sign that something is awry in the nervous system and that further investigation is warranted. It is often the first indicator of a cerebral tumor. Mr. Dotson reports a history of frontal headaches with nausea, as well as progressive weakness and decreased sensation on his right side. A lesion in the left side of the brain, in this case the left frontoparietal lobe, is consistent with clinical abnormalities of the right side of the body. His reported speech difficulties also can occur with frontoparietal brain tumors.

Mr. and Mrs. Dotson have no children. Both have brothers and sisters who live out of state. Only one sister is healthy and active. Mr. and Mrs. Dotson have been encouraged to call her.

 ## NURSING CARE PLAN: BRAIN TUMOR

Nursing diagnoses	Expected client outcomes	Nursing strategies
Anxiety related to unknown procedure and increased awareness of death, hospitalization, and cancer diagnosis	Client and wife will demonstrate mild to moderate signs of anxiety	Observe for verbal and/or nonverbal signs of anxiety Assess client and wife's understanding of the cancer diagnosis and their readiness to learn
	Client and wife will verbalize understanding of procedures and disease process	Provide information on treatments, procedures, radiation therapy, and potential side effects Allow opportunities for client and wife to ask questions or raise concerns regarding the disease process and hospitalization; answer questions honestly; offer realistic hope
	Client and wife will demonstrate appropriate grieving and coping behaviors	Provide opportunities for client to discuss death and dying, if he so chooses; allow client and wife time to grieve Encourage open communication between client and significant other regarding their concerns Provide active listening Accept client and wife's coping behaviors; assist them in identifying other strategies, such as imagery, music therapy, relaxation Determine if spiritual leader is to be notified; if so, call and document
Altered cerebral tissue perfusion; related to increased intracranial pressure secondary to the tumor	Client will maintain optimal neurological functioning	Monitor and report any subtle or obvious changes in level of consciousness, such as restlessness, irritability, lethargy, confusion, and agitation Perform frequent respiratory assessments, especially noting respiratory pattern, rate, and character; report signs of inadequate respiration or airway clearance immediately Perform neurological assessment, including all vital signs, on admission and on an ongoing basis; the frequency of the examination should be increased if any abnormal findings are present or if any deteriorating changes in the client's neurological status are detected; report any significant changes immediately Monitor and document additional neurological signs indicating increased ICP (see Assessment Criteria); report any signs immediately Monitor and document headache, nausea and/or vomiting Maintain head and neck in neutral position Elevate the head of the bed 30 degrees continuously

Continued.

NURSING CARE PLAN: BRAIN TUMOR—cont'd

Nursing diagnoses	Expected client outcomes	Nursing strategies
		Assist client to turn every 2 hours or as neurological condition warrants; teach client to assume position to prevent hip flexion
		Plan rest periods between nursing care activities
		Institute a bowel care program per standard protocol or physician order
		Decrease environmental stimuli
		Restrict fluids, as ordered
		Administer diuretics as ordered; monitor for effects and side effects
		Maintain accurate intake and output recordings
		Regulate temperature of environment to promote normothermia; report significant elevations of temperature immediately; obtain order for cooling blanket or antipyretics, as needed
		Administer steroids and antacids/gastric acid inhibitors as ordered
		Evaluate other potential causes for restlessness and agitation (i.e., pain, decreased respiratory rate, confusion)
	Client will maintain patent airway and normal P_{O_2} and P_{CO_2}	Perform ongoing respiratory assessments, including assessment of cough reflex and auscultation of breath sounds
		If client is unable to clear airway, suction no more than 15 seconds, as needed, or per standard protocol; preoxygenate with 100% oxygen before, during, and after suctioning, or per protocol policy
		Monitor arterial blood gas values and other laboratory and x-ray data
		Monitor sputum for signs of infection; report to physician as indicated
		Administer oxygen therapy, as ordered
	Client will not be injured if seizure activity occurs	Monitor closely for signs of seizure activity and report immediately; carefully document seizure activity that occurs
		Remain with client
		If client is not in bed, lower to floor; remove close objects to prevent injury
		Loosen tight clothing, especially around the neck
		If teeth are not clenched, use padded tongue blade to protect tongue and mouth
		Administer anticonvulsants, as ordered; monitor for effects, side effects, and blood levels
Pain: headache; related to increased intracranial pressure and direct pressure on brain tissue	Client will indicate verbally and/or nonverbally relief of pain	Assess vital signs
		Assess for verbal or nonverbal indicators of pain
	Client and wife will be able to explain the drug and nondrug treatments for pain	Assess severity, duration, site, and quality of pain
		Administer analgesics, as ordered; note effects and side effects
		Explore nonpharmacological methods to treat the client's pain, such as cool cloth to forehead, therapeutic touch, visual imagery, distraction, or an ice pack to head
		Carefully assess and monitor client's emotional status in relation to his pain
		Teach client and wife medication regimen
Impaired physical mobility related to compromised neurological status	Client will maintain an optimal level of mobility	Assess ability to transfer and ambulate safely
		Position weak extremities functionally to prevent deformities
		Request consultation with physical therapist to develop an exercise program, including range of motion, based on client's neurodeficits and physician orders and prognosis; involve wife in program

NURSING CARE PLAN: BRAIN TUMOR—cont'd

Nursing diagnoses	Expected client outcomes	Nursing strategies
		Assess lower extremities every day for signs of tenderness, redness, warmth, increase in size, and/or presence of Homans' sign
		Apply antiembolism hose or sequential compression devices, as ordered
		Obtain consultation with occupational therapist to evaluate need for assistive devices
		Assist client with ambulation and transfers, as ordered
		Encourage use of remaining areas of functioning
		Perform ongoing assessments to detect additional problems caused by immobility, such as pressure sores and depression
		Instruct client and wife about importance of frequent position changes in bed or chair
Potential for self-care deficits related to right-sided weakness and disorientation secondary to brain tumor	Client will demonstrate ability to perform activities of daily living (ADLs) within physical and mental ability	Help client to identify self-care deficits
		Assist client in ADL routine only to the extent needed, so that functioning is maximized and independence promoted
		Ensure proper mouth care, per standard protocol, and observe for the development of mucositis
		Provide frequent rest periods, if needed, during ADLs
		Involve wife in providing client's ADLs, as her comfort level and the client's comfort level permit
		Assist wife to develop a plan for ADLs when client returns home, based on home assessment
Potential for injury related to altered neurological status, disorientation, and potential seizure activity	Client will not experience preventable injuries	Assess deficits that increase risk for injury; develop compensation and prevention strategies
		If client has a potential for choking, ensure staff presence during meals and provide suction equipment
		Instruct client and wife to use unaffected side or thermometer to test temperature of bath water, foods, and drinking liquids
		Institute safety measures such as bed in low position, side rails up, no smoking while alone, and call light within reach
		Avoid use of arm, leg, hand, and/or chest restraints; use only if all other solutions fail
		Ensure that glasses, hearing aids, and/or prosthetic devices are worn
		Reorient client to environment as needed
		Ensure that seizure precautions are maintained
		Avoid any substances such as hot coffee or a heating pad that may result in a burn
Altered nutrition: less than body requirements; related to radiation therapy, loss of appetite, headache, and nausea	Client will have adequate nutrient intake Client will have adequate fluid intake within ordered restrictions	Assess current nutritional status
		Request consultation from a dietician to establish a dietary plan
		Assess client's ability to feed self and swallow
		Assess food preferences and intolerance to specific foods
		Monitor intake and output
		Establish schedule for weighing client
		Establish schedule for antiemetics and pain medication in relation to food and fluid intake
		Consider small, frequent feedings and supplemental high-nutrient feedings
		Assess need for additional nutritional support, such as total parenteral nutrition
		Alert staff to potential for choking; develop additional strategies if this occurs (see care plan for impaired swallowing, p. 87)
		Provide preferred fluids
		Provide oral care before feedings and at bedtime
		Teach wife nutritional care for home care
		Teach wife Heimlich maneuver for home care

Continued.

NURSING CARE PLAN: BRAIN TUMOR—cont'd

Nursing diagnoses	Expected client outcomes	Nursing strategies
Altered thought processes; related to brain tissue destruction or pressure secondary to brain tumor	Client will compensate for deficits in orientation and short-term memory	Assess mental status on a weekly basis Place clock and calendar within client's line of vision Help client to utilize visual and verbal clues to maintain orientation Instruct staff members to introduce themselves and orient client during care Use client's name when speaking to him Monitor response to noise and activity levels in the environment, and modify the environment accordingly Use calm, slow approach Encourage wife to talk with client about familiar people and events
Potential for infection related to radiation and hospitalization	Client will report symptoms of infection	Monitor complete blood count and other laboratory studies Perform multisystem assessments to detect signs and symptoms of infection, reporting promptly any detected Follow universal blood and body secretion precautions, including good hand-washing and aseptic practices Teach client and wife proper hand-washing technique Assist client and wife in identifying significant symptoms and encourage them to report
Potential for impaired skin integrity related to radiation therapy	Client's skin integrity will be maintained	Visually inspect area of head and surrounding areas where the radiation is received to note hair loss and the status of skin Carefully wash the scalp, ear, and neck with warm water and mild soap; avoid temperature extremes; pat dry and apply mild lotion for dryness; make sure not to wash off portal marks Teach client and wife to avoid ointments containing zinc during treatments Provide stockinette cap or other protective head cover Protect irradiated area from tape, sunlight, and trauma
Body image disturbance related to neurological deficits and hair loss	Client will verbalize feelings about body image change	Provide opportunities for client to discuss feelings regarding changes in his body Instruct staff to maintain eye contact during interactions Offer suggestions for ways client can deal with the alopecia associated with radiation and with neurological changes Inquire about wish to have chaplain or other support person or group to visit; provide opportunities to interact with others Provide assistance with bathing and grooming to the extent needed
Impaired verbal communication related to tissue damage secondary to astrocytoma	Client will maintain effective communication	Request consultation from speech therapist for evaluation and recommendations to staff Evaluate client's need for alternate communication systems (e.g., picture cards and word boards) Assist client with nonverbal ways to communicate; allow client adequate time to respond Instruct and encourage wife in use of communication-enhancing strategies See care plan on impaired communication, p. 19

NURSING CARE PLAN: BRAIN TUMOR—cont'd

Nursing diagnoses	Expected client outcomes	Nursing strategies
Potential for altered health maintenance; related to lack of knowledge about treatment implications and return to the home setting	Client and wife will participate in the treatment/discharge plan Client will express feelings and expectations about treatment Client will explain plans for home care	Assess client and wife's feelings and level of anxiety about post-hospital care Assess knowledge of disease, treatment plan, and prognosis Involve client and wife in treatment and discharge plans Allow client control in decision making as appropriate and as condition permits Support client and wife's decisions Emphasize the importance of completing the course of radiation therapy Explain that some side effects of the radiation therapy can have delayed onset Teach client (if capable) and wife all aspects of care and treatment requirements Help client and wife to identify post-discharge community support resources such as church-based programs, home health agencies, and hospice programs Obtain social services consultation to assist in identifying services, equipment, and resources for home care

EVALUATION

1. The client maintains optimal neurological functioning.
2. The client maintains a patent airway, and P_{CO_2} and P_{O_2} remain within normal limits.
3. The client remains free of preventable injury.
4. Client and wife verbalize an understanding of care-giving procedures and information regarding the disease process.
5. Client and wife demonstrate involvement in the treatment and discharge plan.
6. Client and wife demonstrate verbal and/or nonverbal behavior to indicate mild to moderate anxiety.
7. The client's verbal and/or nonverbal behavior indicates control of pain.
8. The client maintains an optimal level of mobility.
9. The client maintains skin integrity as evidenced by the absence of skin breakdown over the irradiated area.
10. The client expresses his feelings about changes in body image.
11. The client maintains an effective means of communication.
12. The client has an adequate nutrient and fluid intake.
13. The client compensates for deficits in orientation and short-term memory.
14. The client reports symptoms of infection.
15. The client demonstrates the ability to perform activities of daily living within his physical and mental abilities.

NURSING ALERTS

1. Consult a significant other to obtain or validate the history if the client's mental condition makes him an unreliable source of information.
2. Be cautious not to misinterpret the significance of tremors as a finding in the neurological examination; determine whether the elder had the tremors before this episode.
3. Diuretic therapy decreases the fluid volume in the brain, which allows more space for the brain tumor to increase in size. Monitor closely for neurological changes if diuretics are utilized.
4. Monitor continuously for signs of increasing intracranial pressure. Elevated intracranial pressure requires immediate and intensive nursing and medical management.
5. Restlessness and agitation can be due to factors other than neurological deterioration—for example, pain, the need for a change of position or for elimination, or altered thought processes.
6. White blood cell counts can be falsely elevated in the client receiving steroids.
7. It is important to weigh the benefits of a nursing intervention against the risk of increasing intracranial pressure in a client with compromised neurological status.

Bibliography

Carpenito L: Nursing diagnosis: application to clinical practice, ed 3, Philadelphia, 1989, JB Lippincott Co.

Eliopoulos C: A guide to the nursing of the aged, Baltimore, 1987, Williams & Wilkins.

Hodges K: Meningioma, astrocytoma, and germinoma: case presentations of three intracranial tumors, Journal of Neuroscience Nursing 21(2):113, 1989.

Johanson BC et al: Standards for critical care, ed 3, St Louis, 1988, The CV Mosby Co.

Long BC and Phipps WJ, editors: Medical-surgical nursing: a nursing process approach, ed 2, St Louis, 1989, The CV Mosby Co.

Matteson V and McConnell E: Gerontological nursing: concepts and practice, Philadelphia, 1988, WB Saunders Co.

McIntire S and Cioppa A: Cancer nursing: a developmental approach, New York, 1984, John Wiley & Sons.

McNally J, Stair J, and Somerville E, editors: Guidelines for cancer nursing practice, Orlando, 1985, Grune & Stratton, Inc.

Rudy E: Advanced neurological and neurosurgical nursing, St Louis, 1984, The CV Mosby Co.

Vogt G, Miller M, and Esluer M: Mosby's manual of neurological care, St Louis, 1985, The CV Mosby Co.

Ziegfeld C, editor: Core curriculum for oncology nursing, Philadelphia, 1987, WB Saunders Co.

Chronic Subdural Hematoma

Tally N. Bell

KNOWLEDGE BASE

1. Chronic subdural hematomas occur with an increased incidence in the elderly.
2. The diagnosis of a chronic subdural hematoma in elders can be delayed as the result of several factors:
   a. Many clients do not lose consciousness at the time of the trauma.
   b. Signs and symptoms may be misinterpreted as age-related changes.
   c. The trauma may have been considered minor and because the symptoms may be delayed, the event is forgotten.
3. Early recognition and accurate diagnosis, followed by prompt evacuation of the hematoma, are critical in preventing permanent brain damage.
4. The typical signs of increasing intracranial pressure resulting from a hematoma are as follows:
   a. Decline in the level of consciousness
   b. Diminished motor response to verbal commands
   c. Diminished response to painful stimuli
   d. Slowed pupillary reactions
   e. Changes in vital signs
5. Although all of the signs are important, a deterioration in the level of consciousness is the most crucial indicator of increasing intracranial pressure. Thus assessment of level of consciousness (LOC) is the single most important clinical observation in any neurological client. Brain herniation may occur with increased intracranial pressure (ICP).

6. The mortality rate in elders with subdural hematoma is high because of the complications arising from other chronic disease conditions, their lack of reserve in all organs and tissues, and the decreased efficiency of all the systems in responding to the trauma.
7. An increased PCO_2 is the most potent cerebrovascular vasodilator and will cause intracranial pressure to increase by increasing the cerebral blood volume. A client with an ineffective respiratory pattern and/or inadequate airway clearance can require intubation and mechanical hyperventilation to treat or prevent increased intracranial pressure. Hypoxia, although not as potent a cerebrovascular dilator as hypercarbia, will also cause an increase in intracranial pressure. Arterial blood gas determinations are a helpful tool.
8. A number of body positions can cause intracranial pressure to increase. It is important to properly position the client to minimize adverse effects. Proper positioning for the client who is at risk of increased intracranial pressure includes the following:
   a. Preventing pressure on the jugular veins to facilitate proper drainage of blood from the brain
   b. Maintaining head elevation to facilitate venous drainage from the brain
   c. Preventing the client from actively turning himself or herself, which can cause a Valsalva maneuver

d. Preventing hip flexion, which increases intraabdominal pressure, which in turn increases the intrathoracic pressure and results in an increase in intracranial pressure

9. Neurologically compromised clients can have impaired protective reflexes, which puts them at risk of aspiration. Side-lying positions can help protect the airway of the client who has an impaired gag/cough reflex. It is important to consider the client's potential for increased ICP when determining what positions are the most appropriate.

10. If the gag/cough reflexes are absent, a nasogastric (NG) tube will facilitate gastric emptying and minimize the risk of aspiration. However, insertion of the NG tube can increase ICP.

11. Straining and constipation can cause the client to perform a Valsalva maneuver and increase the intracranial pressure.

12. An excess of fluids can cause cerebral edema and increase the ICP. The client should not receive 5% dextrose in water, since free water fluids can cause an increase in ICP. Insensible fluid losses from diaphoresis, hyperventilation, or other causes should be considered when the fluid restriction is determined.

13. Diuretics will decrease the fluid volume in the brain and effect a decrease in ICP. Diuretic therapy can cause electrolyte imbalances, as well as disturbances in other body systems. A urine drainage catheter is indicated to ensure accurate output recordings.

14. Hyperthermia increases cerebral metabolism and is known to increase ICP. It is also seen in the very late stages of increased ICP.

15. The use of steroids to help stabilize the cell wall membrane and support the stress response remains a controversial therapy. Antacids/gastric acid inhibitors are administered concurrently because steroids cause gastric irritation and because of the stress ulceration that can occur.

16. Coughing is important to clear the airway but will increase ICP in the process.

17. Suctioning clears the airway but causes hypercarbia and hypoxia during the process. Preoxygenation helps decrease the risk of hypoxia.

18. It is important to weigh the benefits of a nursing intervention against the risk of increasing intracranial pressure in a client with a compromised neurological status. Pacing nursing interventions and giving rest periods are important to prevent increased intracranial pressure.

19. The presence of a chronic subdural hematoma places the client at risk for developing seizure activity. Seizure activity causes an increase in metabolic waste products within the brain, causing an increase in ICP. Anticonvulsants can be given prophylactically to prevent seizure activity, but must reach therapeutic levels to be effective. If central nervous system depressants are utilized, they will mask the neurological signs that indicate increasing ICP.

20. The neurological status must be evaluated carefully before range-of-motion exercises are performed, particularly to the lower extremities, since they can cause increases in ICP.

21. The cerebral atrophy associated with aging allows an increase in space to occur as the brain separates from the dura mater. Because of this increased spatial compensation and the slow development of a chronic subdural hematoma, there may not be any signs or symptoms of increased intracranial pressure until the intracranial contents are compromised. A major goal of nursing management is to implement ongoing neurological assessments to detect increases in intracranial pressure so it can be prevented or treated immediately.

22. Neurological diseases are a frequent cause of disability in the elderly. Differentiating neurological disease from age-related changes often requires careful assessment and diagnostic tests, such as CT brain scans, electroencephalograms, and magnetic resonance imaging.

23. Irregular pupil shape can be within normal limits for the elderly client, thus requiring baseline data to make any inferences. Cataracts may be present, making pupil checks difficult.

24. The cerebral blood vessels and the meninges are less elastic in the elderly, resulting in an increased risk of damage to these areas when head trauma occurs.

25. Whether there is a reduction in cerebral blood flow as a normal age-related change is controversial. Cerebral blood flow plays an important role in the compensatory reactions of the intracranial contents that occur as intracranial pressure increases.

26. Slower synaptic transmission in elders is due to decreased neurotransmitter production. As a result, reaction time lengthens in later years. This is important to consider in assessing a client's response to verbal commands, as well as other reaction times.

27. Disorientation and confusion in the neurologically compromised client increase his or her risk of injury.

28. Restraining an elderly client can increase confusion and contribute to increases in ICP and alterations in thought processes.

29. Unnecessary stimuli can contribute to altered thought processed through sensory overload and increased confusion, as well as potentially increase ICP. A fast, hurried approach can cause a confused client to feel threatened.

30. If the neurological deficits do not resolve, it is important that significant others understand the disease process and how to assist the client.

31. Codeine is generally considered safe to administer to a client with a chronic subdural hematoma. However, narcotics can mask important central nervous system signs. Age-related changes cause a decreased sensitivity to pain and a change in the way in which the central nervous system receives the sensory input of pain and interprets it.

32. If short-term memory has declined, long-term memory usually remains intact in the elderly. Capabilities for acquisition and retention of new information are not lost with aging, but teaching the client about his or her disease process and/or new skills can require a longer period of time and special techniques to ensure successful mastery of the information. This age-related change is compounded in the neurologically compromised elder.

CASE STUDY

Mr. Thomas, 72 years old, is admitted to the hospital this morning. His daughter, with whom he lives, states that her father has had frequent headaches for the past week and upon waking this morning was confused and agitated. His neurological examination shows a well-nourished male who is somewhat lethargic and disoriented to time and place. His pupils are equal, with the left pupil reacting slower than the right pupil. Left extremity strength is less than right extremity strength. No sensory deficits are noted. His past history includes a fall 4 weeks ago; he hit the right side of his head on a chair as he fell. He was seen by his physician after this fall and was monitored at home, with no apparent changes in level of consciousness during the immediate postinjury phase. His daughter reports that during the past week he has seemed "slower mentally and has been very forgetful," progressing to his confusional state this morning. A CT scan shows a chronic subdural hematoma in the right temporoparietal region. Mr. Thomas is scheduled for evacuation of the subdural hematoma in the morning.

ASSESSMENT CRITERIA

General

Baseline vital signs
History (may need family/significant other to assist)
   Onset, progression, and duration of symptoms
   Description of head trauma, past and present
   Past and present medical problems, including neurological system
   Medication history
   Alterations in sleep/wake patterns
   Past episodes of trauma

Physical

Neurological examination: watch for increasing intracranial pressure
   Changes in level of consciousness (e.g., lethargic, drowsy, agitated, obtunded, comatose)
   Personality or behavior changes
   Impairment in mental/intellectual functioning (e.g., loss of insight, slow cerebration, confusion, defects in judgment or reasoning, hallucinations, difficulty with abstraction)
   Motor dysfunction, particularly contralateral hemiparesis or hemiparalysis
   Sensory-perceptual alterations
   Cranial nerve dysfunction
   Pupillary changes: note irregularities in size, shape, and/or reactivity
   Disorientation to time, place, person, or self
   Gait, balance, or coordination disturbances
   Changes in extraocular movements
   Visual-field defects
   Changes in speech pattern
   Presence of papilledema
Evaluate for presence of:
   Protective reflexes: gag, cough, and corneal
   Deep tendon reflexes
   Pathological reflexes (e.g., Babinski)
   Abnormal muscle movement
Evaluate for:
   Headache
   Nausea or vomiting
   Seizure activity
   Bleeding or loss of cerebrospinal fluid from the ears or nose
Evaluate for signs of tentorial (uncal) herniation:
   Ipsilateral fixed, dilated pupil
   Contralateral hemiparesis or hemiparalysis
   Increased systolic blood pressure with widening pulse pressure
   Bradycardia
   Bradypnea
   Changes in respiratory pattern
Immediate, recent, and remote memory loss
Bowel and/or bladder dysfunction
Signs of external head trauma (i.e., lacerations, ecchymoses, or swelling)
Laboratory and diagnostic test results, including arterial blood gas values, CT scan, skull x-ray films
Communication pattern, verbal and nonverbal
Review of other body systems
Presence of self-care deficits

Psychosocial

Self-esteem
Coping strategies, adaptive or maladaptive
Support systems
Risk factors in life-style (e.g., smoking, alcohol consumption)

Spiritual

Religious practices and beliefs
Source of strength and hope

Mr. Thomas' assessment demonstrates a number of clinical signs and symptoms that are consistent with a diagnosis of chronic subdural hematoma. The neurological examination shows several abnormal findings, including lethargy, disorientation to time and place, and a recent event of confusion and agitation. The history, supplied by Mr. Thomas' daughter, reveals a traumatic fall, 4 weeks before his hospital admission, in which the client sustained a blow to the right side of his head. His left pupil currently shows diminished reactivity, and his left extremity strength is weaker than the right. Both of these findings are consistent with a lesion in the right side of the brain.

A chronic subdural hematoma characteristically develops slowly, which accounts for the 4-week interval between Mr. Thomas' fall and the diagnosis. During that time, however, he had begun to demonstrate decreased mentation, forgetfulness, and confusion. The abnormal neurological findings can be attributed to increasing intracranial pressure as the chronic subdural hematoma begins to expand past the client's ability to compensate. The presence of these abnormal neurological findings and the client's risk of increasing intracranial pressure have many implications for development of the nursing care plan.

 NURSING CARE PLAN: CHRONIC SUBDURAL HEMATOMA

Nursing diagnoses	Expected client outcomes	Nursing strategies

Altered cerebral tissue perfusion; related to presence of a chronic subdural hematoma	Client will maintain optimal neurological functioning, preoperatively and postoperatively	Monitor and report any subtle or obvious changes in level of consciousness, such as restlessness, irritability, lethargy, confusion, and agitation
		Perform frequent respiratory assessments, especially noting respiratory pattern and rate; report signs of inadequate respiration or airway clearance immediately
		Perform neurological assessment, including all vital signs, on admission and on an ongoing basis; the frequency of the examination should be increased if any abnormal findings are present or if any deteriorating changes in the client's neurological status are detected; report any changes immediately
		Monitor and document additional neurological signs indicating increased ICP; report immediately:
		  Dilated, fixed, or sluggish pupils (usually ipsilateral)
		  Motor paresis or paralysis (usually contralateral)
		  Elevated systolic blood pressure and widening pulse pressure
		  Bradypnea and alterations in respiratory pattern
		  Additional signs as listed under Assessment Criteria
		Monitor and document headache, nausea and/or vomiting
		Maintain head and neck in neutral position
		Elevate the head of the bed 30 degrees continuously
		Passively turn and position the client every 2 hours or as neurological condition warrants
		Plan rest periods between nursing care activities
		Position to prevent hip flexion
		Institute a bowel care program per protocol
		Decrease environmental stimuli
		Restrict fluids, as ordered
		Administer diuretics, such as mannitol and furosemide, as ordered; monitor for effects and side effects
		Maintain accurate intake and output record

Continued.

NURSING CARE PLAN: CHRONIC SUBDURAL HEMATOMA—cont'd

Nursing diagnoses	Expected client outcomes	Nursing strategies
Altered cerebral tissue perfusion; related to presence of a chronic subdural hematoma—cont'd	Client will maintain optimal neurological functioning, preoperatively and postoperatively—cont'd	Keep temperature of environment so that it promotes normothermia Report significant elevations of temperature immediately; obtain order for cooling blanket or antipyretics, as needed Administer steroids and antacids/gastric acid inhibitors, as ordered Evaluate other potential causes for restlessness and agitation Perform ongoing assessments of all body systems
	Client will maintain patent airway	Perform ongoing respiratory assessments, including assessment of cough reflex and auscultation of breath sounds Suction no more than 15 seconds, as needed, or per hospital policy Oxygenate with 100% oxygen before, during, and after suctioning, or per hospital policy Monitor arterial blood gas values and other laboratory and x-ray data Monitor sputum for signs of infection and report to physician as indicated Administer oxygen therapy, as ordered
	Client will not be injured if seizure activity occurs	Monitor closely for signs of seizure activity and report immediately; carefully document seizure activity that occurs Institute seizure precautions per hospital protocol Administer anticonvulsants, as ordered Monitor for effects, side effects, and blood levels
Mobility, impaired physical; related to altered neurological status	Client will maintain an optimal level of mobility	Position weak extremities functionally to prevent deformities Perform passive range-of-motion exercises every 8 hours, as neurological condition permits Assess lower extremities every day for signs of tenderness, redness, warmness, increase in size, and/or presence of Homans' sign Encourage deep breathing every 2 hours Apply antiembolism hose or sequential compression devices, as ordered Assess breath sounds every 8 hours and as necessary Obtain physical and occupational therapy consultations, as appropriate, for evaluation and to obtain assistive devices, if required Assist client with ambulation and transfers, as activity is ordered Perform ongoing assessments to detect additional problems caused by immobility, such as pressure ulcers and depression
Injury, potential for; related to altered neurological status and altered thought processes	Client will not experience preventable injuries	Assess risk factors; plan compensation Institute safety measures, such as bed in low position, side rails up, no smoking while alone, and call light within reach Avoid use of arm, leg, hand, and/or chest restraints unless all other measures fail Ensure that glasses, hearing aids, prosthetic devices are worn Monitor for signs of sensory-perceptual alterations Reorient to environment, as needed
	Client will maintain mentation at the highest level possible	Place clock and calendar within client's line of vision Encourage client to utilize visual and verbal clues Use client's name when speaking to him Monitor sleep/wake patterns Monitor noise and activity levels in environment Use calm, slow approach

NURSING CARE PLAN: CHRONIC SUBDURAL HEMATOMA—cont'd

Nursing diagnoses	Expected client outcomes	Nursing strategies
Potential for aspiration related to compromised neurological status	Client will have decreased potential for aspiration	Assess for presence of gag and cough reflexes Monitor arterial blood gas values and chest x-ray films and lung sounds Position on side, if appropriate Provide mechanical soft diet, if gag reflex intact and as ordered Obtain order for NG tube and gastric suctioning, if needed
Fear related to lack of knowledge, neurological deficit, and potential changes in quality of life	Client and significant other's verbal and nonverbal behavior will demonstrate positive coping	Assess level of anxiety Encourage client and/or significant other to verbalize their fears, concerns, and questions Listen actively to expressions of feelings Discuss positive coping strategies Allow present coping behaviors Provide information in small, clear steps, and give client adequate time to process information; speak with slow, distinct speech Answer questions about client's physical condition honestly Prepare client and significant other through preoperative teaching what to expect postoperatively, such as hair being shaved, increased monitoring and assessments, postoperative routines, possible drainage from burr holes, and dressing changes
	Client and significant other will demonstrate understanding of hospital procedures, diagnostic testing, and routines	Offer explanation of all procedures and tests before they occur Provide opportunities for client and significant other to ask questions Maintain calm and slow pace when giving care Allow significant others to spend time with client Reinforce the gains the client makes Involve chaplaincy and social services, as appropriate
Body image disturbance related to neurological deficits and temporary loss of hair (postoperatively)	Client will verbalize feelings about body image	Assess client's perception of self Provide client and significant other with opportunities to ask questions regarding neurological deficits Provide assistance with grooming and dressing only to the extent needed After surgery, assist client with alternates to deal with hair loss, such as a stocking cap Encourage decision making
Pain; headaches	Client's verbal and nonverbal behavior will indicate relief of pain	Assess for verbal and nonverbal indicators of pain Administer analgesics, as ordered; note effects and side effects Assess severity, duration, site, and quality of pain Explore nonpharmacologic methods to treat the client's pain, such as a cool cloth to the forehead, therapeutic touch, visual imagery, distraction, or an ice pack to the head Decrease environmental stimuli
Total self-care deficits; related to compromised neurological status and confusion	Client will participate in activities of daily (ADLs) living to the extent possible	Help client to identify self-care deficits Request consultation with occupational therapist for retraining for ADLs Assist client in ADL routine only to the extent that is needed Ensure proper mouth care, per hospital protocol, and observe for the development of mucositis Provide frequent rest periods, if needed, during ADLs Assist with bathing, mouth care, personal hygiene, dressing and feeding, as necessary Involve significant others in providing for client's ADLs, as their comfort level and the client's comfort level permit

Continued.

NURSING CARE PLAN: CHRONIC SUBDURAL HEMATOMA—cont'd

Nursing diagnoses	Expected client outcomes	Nursing strategies
Infection, potential for; related to burr holes (postoperatively)	Client's surgical site will remain free of infection	Observe burr hole sites for signs of redness, swelling, drainage, leakage, and/or exudate Perform dressing changes, as ordered Monitor temperature every 4 hours Monitor laboratory work for elevated white blood cell count Obtain cultures of burr hole drainage if infection suspected, per hospital protocol Maintain aseptic techniques, and utilize universal blood and body secretion protocols during dressing changes
Potential for altered health maintenance; related to unmet needs after dismissal from acute care	Client and significant other will participate in treatment discharge plan	Assess knowledge of treatment/discharge plan and readiness to learn Involve significant others in treatment/discharge plan, particularly if client's neurological status remains compromised
	Client and family will be able to identify community resources	Help client and significant other to identify community support programs, such as support groups, home health agencies, church-based programs; obtain social services consultation to assist in identifying discharge options, such as returning to home, rehabilitation facility, or skilled nursing facility

EVALUATION

1. The client maintains optimal neurological functioning.
2. The client remains free of injury if seizure activity occurs.
3. The client achieves an optimal level of mobility and compensates for neurological motor deficits.
4. The client experiences no preventable injury.
5. The client maintains a level of orientation relative to his condition.
6. Client and significant other verbalize an understanding of hospital procedures, diagnostic testing, and routines.
7. Client and significant other describe or demonstrate required post-hospital care and safety measures.
8. Client and significant other demonstrate verbal and nonverbal behavior of increased confidence related to health management.
9. The client verbalizes feelings about his body image.
10. The client describes a method of pain management.
11. The client demonstrates an ability to perform activities of daily living within his physical and mental ability.
12. The client remains free of infection, as evidenced by a normal temperature and no redness, swelling, or exudate at the surgical site.

NURSING ALERTS

1. Consult a significant other to obtain or validate the history if the client's mental condition makes him an unreliable source of information.
2. Be cautious not to misinterpret tremors as part of the aging process. Establish a baseline for the client.
3. Diuretic therapy decreases the fluid volume in the brain, which allows more space for the hematoma to increase in size. Monitor closely for neurological changes.
4. Monitor continuously for signs of increasing intracranial pressure. Elevated intracranial pressure requires immediate and intensive nursing and medical management.
5. Restlessness and agitation can be due to reasons other than neurological deterioration. The need for a change of position, the need for elimination, or altered thought processes are other potential causes.
6. White blood cell counts may be falsely elevated in a client receiving steroids.

Bibliography

Adelstein W: Head injury perils, Geriatric Nursing 10:285, Nov/Dec 1989.

Burgraf V and Stanley M: Nursing the elderly: a care plan approach, Philadelphia, 1989, JB Lippincott Co.

Carpenito L: Nursing diagnosis: application to clinical practice, ed 3, Philadelphia, 1987, JB Lippincott Co.

Eliopoulos C: A guide to the nursing of the aged, Baltimore, 1987, Williams & Wilkins.

Hickey J: The clinical practice of neurological and neurosurgical nursing, ed 2, Philadelphia, 1986, JB Lippincott Co.

Johanson BC et al: Standards for critical care, ed 3, St Louis, 1988, The CV Mosby Co.

Matteson V and McConnell E: Gerontological nursing: concepts and practice, Philadelphia, 1988, WB Saunders Co.

Rudy E: Advanced neurological and neurosurgical nursing, St Louis, 1984, The CV Mosby Co.

Taylor C and Cress S: Nursing diagnosis cards, Springhouse, Pa, 1987, Springhouse Corp.

Vogt G, Miller M, and Esluer M: Mosby's manual of neurological care, St Louis, 1985, The CV Mosby Co.

Meningitis: Lumbar Puncture

Margherita P. Nahrup

KNOWLEDGE BASE

1. Pneumococcal meningitis is the most common type of meningitis in adults over the age of 40.

2. Pneumococcal meningitis is one form of bacterial meningitis. Bacterial meningitis may be defined as a pyrogenic infection that involves the pia-arachnoid layers of the meninges, the subarachnoid space, and the cerebrospinal fluid. The inflammation spreads quickly via the exudate by means of the cerebrospinal fluid. Hydrocephalus may be caused by accumulation of exudate upon the choroid plexus. This causes the arachnoid villi to be plugged, causing an obstruction in the ventricles. The prognosis in meningitis depends on how extensive the infection is and on the speed of effective treatment.

3. The following complications commonly occur if the infection is widespread and goes untreated: Fibrosis and tissue formation occur in the arachnoid layer of the brain. Adhesions and effusions of the subarachnoid space can develop, causing a disruption in the normal cerebrospinal fluid drainage system, which may result in hydrocephalus and subsequent increased intracranial pressure.

4. During the seventh and eighth decades of life, changes in the cerebrum become more pronounced. It is known that structural changes occur within the meninges and in cerebral blood flow. These factors, combined with hypertension, could potentiate a decrease in neurological compensatory mechanisms (the Monro-Kellie hypothesis), which could further impair vascular response to the presence of the exudate, resulting in increased intracranial pressure. The accumulating exudate, coupled with a decrease in compensatory mechanisms, would contribute to the presence of disorientation in the client's clinical picture.

5. Two neurological signs are indicative of meningeal irritation: (a) Kernig's sign, the inability to extend the legs completely without extreme pain, and (b) Brudzinski's sign, flexion of the hip and knee when the neck is flexed.

6. When a client presents with signs of meningeal irritation (i.e., stiff neck), Brudzinki's sign, and Kernig's sign, further neurological tests are usually done to rule out specific illnesses. These tests include a CT scan, which shows the density of brain tissue; an angiogram, which gives a picture of the circulation of the brain; a nuclear magnetic resonance imaging (NMR) scan, which provides an image of brain tissue without the use of radiation; and a spinal tap, which is used to examine the cerebrospinal fluid, which circulates in the spinal column and around the brain. The cerebrospinal fluid is tested for color, consistency, and number and type of cells present.

7. Fear of paralysis from a spinal tap is common among clients. However, there is no risk of this because the needle is inserted below the level of the cord, into the lumbar interspace of L4-L5 or into L5-S1. Clients need to be instructed that they may feel a sharp pain shooting down one leg as a result of a nerve root being brushed or irritated, and they should be reassured that this pain is harmless.

8. The client's blood pressure must be monitored closely because of the risk associated with high blood pressure and the greater probability of subsequent increased intracranial pressure, which might contraindicate a spinal tap procedure. The spinal tap might be contraindicated because of the risk of brainstem herniation, which could occur through the procedure site as a result of increased intracranial pressure. This same risk of herniation may still exist after the procedure;

therefore the client is monitored closely after the procedure for changes in blood pressure or for signs of increased intracranial pressure.

9. Early signs of increased intracranial pressure include the following: restlessness; disorientation; lethargy; headache; contralateral hemiparesis; ipsilateral pupil dilated; visual blurring or diplopia; elevated systolic blood pressure and widening pulse pressure; slowed respiration and altered pattern.

10. If the client is very anxious about a spinal tap, a mild tranquilizer may be prescribed and the nurse or assistant will help the client maintain the proper position for the procedure. The client is either on one side with both knees and head flexed or positioned on the edge of the bed with feet supported and leaning over the bedside table. The client should be instructed to lie still during the procedure.

11. During the procedure the physician will inject a local anesthetic with small needle. The spinal needle will then be inserted into the subarachnoid space. A small prick and a burning sensation may be felt at this point, followed by a pressure sensation as the needle enters the subarachnoid space. Once the needle is within the subarachnoid space, the physician withdraws three to five tubes of cerebrospinal fluid for analysis. The opening pressure of the cerebrospinal fluid is also measured while the needle is still in the subarachnoid space. When the physician is finished, he or she withdraws the needle and applies an adhesive bandage.

12. After the spinal tap, the physician may order the client to lie flat for up to 24 hours. Vital signs and neurological checks will be performed frequently for the first few hours following the procedure.

13. The most common complication of a spinal tap is severe headache, which is experienced more acutely in the upright position. This headache can be minimized by having the client remain flat, drink fluids, and take acetaminophen.

14. Other complications include nausea, malaise, and irritation or a hematoma at the procedure site. Pain in a leg or a buttock can occur as a result of local nerve root irritation by the needle. Some clients experience vomiting. The most severe complication is brain herniation resulting from sudden pressure changes within the cranium. If this occurs, it is generally during the procedure; however, it can occur later.

CASE STUDY

Mr. Maxwell, 73 years old, has had hypertension for 10 years and arthritis for 18 years. He recently returned from a trip to the Cayman Islands with his wife of 35 years. He had a severe ear infection while on their trip. A local island physician had prescribed an antibiotic. Mr. Maxwell complained of flu-like symptoms upon their return flight and attributed them to the ear infection and fatigue from the trip. His symptoms of nausea, vomiting, chills, and fever have escalated since Mr. and Mrs. Maxwell's return. The evening before admission Mr. Maxwell was complaining of a stiff neck. The next morning, upon admission to the hospital, his wife reported that he was confused when he woke up; frightened, she brought him to the hospital.

Upon admission he was alert but slightly disoriented to time. His blood pressure was 160/88, and his neurological assessment showed positive Kernig's and Brudzinski's signs. A lumbar puncture (spinal tap) was ordered to rule out the diagnosis of pneumococcal meningitis.

ASSESSMENT CRITERIA
Physical

Neurological
  Mental status changes
  Cranial nerve assessment
  Motor and sensory function
  Kernig's sign
  Brudzinski's sign
  Signs of meningeal irritation
  Discomfort/pain
  Activity that exacerbates or relieves discomfort or pain
  Tremors/seizure activity
Musculoskeletal
  Muscle tone and strength
  Coordination, gait
  Presence of bone degeneration
  Calcification of the spinal column
  Changes in the spinous process
Vital signs
Onset and duration of symptoms
Presence of vomiting
Demographic data (age, height, weight)
Medications
Current treatments
Visual and auditory abilities
Diet
Activity patterns
Past medical conditions
History of infections

Psychosocial

Coping mechanisms
Anxiety level

Support systems
Risk factors (smoking, drinking, etc.)
Recent travel
Understanding of processes and cause

Spiritual

Religious beliefs or practices

Mr. Maxwell's recent trip to the Cayman Islands and the ear infection he had during the trip may be viewed as predisposing factors to his acquiring meningitis. The flu-like symptoms he continued to experience, his fatigue, and his stiff neck were also indicative of meningeal involvement.

The confusion with which Mr. Maxwell awoke can be attributed to an increase in exudate pooling at the base of the brain, causing inflammation and blockage of cerebrospinal fluid flow.

Because of Mr. Maxwell's history of hypertension, close monitoring for the presence of increased intracranial pressure would be warranted. His age would assist in narrowing down the type of organism causing the bacterial meningitis, since pneumococcal meningitis usually occurs in the very young and those over the age of 40. Therefore, because of this factor and the other presenting symptoms, the spinal tap was ordered to rule out pneumococcal meningitis.

Mr. Maxwell's wife seems to be a good source of support for him.

The presence of Kernig's and Brudzinski's signs indicates meningeal irritation. And Mr. Maxwell's stiff neck was an early sign of meningeal irritation, which was caused by a spasm of the extensor muscles in the neck; forceful flexion causes pain.

In the presence of meningitis, Kernig's sign is present, which results in pain and spasm of the hamstring muscles when an attempt is made to extend the knee. This discomfort is caused by inflammation of the meninges and spinal roots. The presence of Brudzinski's sign is caused by exudate around the spinal roots in the lumbar region.

NURSING CARE PLAN: MENINGITIS—LUMBAR PUNCTURE

Nursing diagnoses	Expected client outcomes	Nursing strategies
Fear or anxiety related to the spinal tap procedure	Client will express feelings regarding spinal tap procedure	Assess client knowledge base Encourage verbalization of fears or anxiety
	Client will verbalize the steps and rationale for performing a spinal tap procedure	Teach relaxation and imagery techniques Review steps of procedure with client; instruct client in maintaining the proper position during the tap Discuss reasons for performing a spinal tap
	Client will verbalize an understanding of the risk factors involved in a spinal tap procedure	Review what client can expect during and after the procedure Discuss headache as the most common risk factor and its treatment Discuss other possible complications, such as nausea, vomiting, pain in a leg or buttock, fever Reassure client that he will be monitored closely and kept comfortable after the procedure
Potential for injury related to disorientation and possible seizure activity	Client will be free from preventable injuries	Schedule neurological assessments Assess orientation and understanding of restricted movement Be attentive to premonitory signs of an impending seizure, such as tremors, increased disorientation, or restlessness Use a calm, slow voice to give reassurance during spinal tap procedure and during care; orient frequently Schedule monitoring and care at frequent intervals Request wife to be present or provide staff at mealtime if potential for seizure is high Keep side rails up and bed in low position Provide adequate but dimmed lighting in room and bathroom Keep noise to a minimum; avoid startling the client

Continued.

NURSING CARE PLAN: MENINGITIS—LUMBAR PUNCTURE—cont'd

Nursing diagnoses	Expected client outcomes	Nursing strategies
Potential for altered tissue perfusion; related to increased intracranial pressure secondary to meningitis	Client will experience prompt treatment for increased intracranial pressure	Assess signs of increased intracranial pressure and report any changes (see Knowledge Base)
	Client will verbalize understanding of rationale for testing and treatments	Maintain bed at 30 degrees of elevation Instruct client to keep head in good alignment Provide rest periods during care Discuss with client's wife the importance of keeping him calm and avoiding agitation
Potential for altered nutrition and hydration; related to nausea, vomiting, and increased needs secondary to the infectious process	Client will consume adequate nutrients and fluids	Assess current nutritional and hydration status Request consultation from a dietitian to plan nutritional intake Instruct client to drink fluids in small amounts frequently Explain the purpose of the intravenous fluids Request an antiemetic, and plan for food and fluid intake 30 minutes after administering Provide supplemental feedings within the dietary plan

EVALUATION

1. The client is able to verbalize fears and concerns regarding the spinal tap procedure.
2. The client feels comfortable asking caregivers for information regarding areas of concern.
3. The client is able to verbalize the reasons for performing a spinal tap.
4. The client is able to give an explanation of how the procedure will be done.
5. The client is able to describe what will be expected of him during and after the procedure.
6. Client and wife are able to verbalize the risks involved in a spinal tap procedure.
7. The client remains free from preventable injuries.
8. The client has adequate nutrient and fluid intake.

NURSING ALERTS

1. Monitor the client's blood pressure closely before and after the spinal tap procedure.
2. If the client remains too confused, be sure his wife or a significant other is informed of the procedure's risks as well as the client.
3. Be sure that the client has not taken any anticoagulant medications, especially aspirin products, recently; they may cause prolonged bleeding or clotting time, particularly at the procedure site. Check the prothrombin time and the partial thromboplastin time.

4. Obtain a neurological baseline assessment before the procedure to be able to monitor neurological changes accurately.
5. Obtain a signed permit for the procedure, since it is considered invasive.
6. Be attentive to the client's intracranial pressure during diagnostic procedures.

Bibliography

Adams RD and Victor M: Principles of neurology, ed 3, New York, 1985, McGraw-Hill Book Co.

Bass B and Vandervoort M: Post-lumbar puncture headache, Canadian Nurse 4(84):15, 1988.

Eliopoulos C: Gerontological nursing, ed 2, Philadelphia; 1987, JB Lippincott Co.

Fisher J: What you need to know about neurological testing, RN 1(50):47, 1987.

Hickey J: Neurological and neurosurgical nursing, ed 2, Philadelphia; 1986, JB Lippincott Co.

Long BC and Phipps WJ, editors: Medical surgical nursing: a nursing process approach, ed 2, St. Louis, 1989, The CV Mosby Co.

Sternbach GL: Lumbar puncture, Topics in Emergency Medicine 10(1):1, 1988.

Yurick AG et al: The aged person and the nursing process. Norwalk, Conn, 1989, Appleton & Lange.

GENITOURINARY SYSTEM

Hyperplasia of the Prostate

Roberta Purvis Bartee

KNOWLEDGE BASE

1. The muscle tone of genitourinary structures decreases with age.
2. Aging reduces bladder size and capacity.
3. The pressure and speed of the urinary stream diminish with age, as a result of a reduction in the elasticity of the bladder.
4. A reduced sensitivity to the voiding urge is associated with the aging process.
5. The prostate is located at the base of the bladder, circumferential to the proximal urethra.
6. Cellular proliferation of smooth muscle and connective and glandular tissue characterizes hyperplasia of the prostate.
7. Hormonal changes in men over 50 may stimulate hyperplasia.
8. Hyperplasia of the prostate occurs most frequently among whites, then among blacks, and least frequently among Orientals.
9. The incidence of hyperplasia does not correlate with the incidence of cancer, and hyperplasia does not necessarily progress to urinary obstruction.
10. Pain with hyperplasia is unusual.
11. Symptoms of hyperplasia are more related to location than to size of the enlargement. Hyperplasia of the median and lateral lobes of the prostate tends to be more symptomatic than that of the posterior lobe.
12. Urinary flow may become compromised gradually or abruptly by hyperplasia.
13. Symptoms of hyperplasia reflect compromised bladder evacuation, obstructed urinary flow, bladder neck compromise, and irritable bladder.
14. The collection of symptoms associated with hyperplasia of the prostate is called prostatism and may include the following:
    a. Hesitancy, frequency, urgency, dysuria, nocturia
    b. Incomplete bladder emptying, acute retention
    c. Stream interruption
    d. Straining to initiate and maintain flow
    e. Lack of stream force
    f. Reduction in stream caliber
    g. Dribbling after voiding
    h. Urinary incontinence
15. Progressive urethral compression by hyperplastic tissues may be compensated for by bladder hypertrophy.
16. Ruptured bladder vessels or irritated bladder mucosa cause hematuria.
17. Gross hematuria among elderly men most frequently is attributed to hyperplasia of the prostate.
18. Client teaching prior to diagnostic tests increases comfort, the ability to participate, and the accuracy of the results. Assessments and safety precautions prevent injury from falls caused by orthostatic hypotension, which may occur at the end of the examination while the client changes from the lithotomy position. The following diagnostic categories are associated with hyperplasia of the prostate:
    a. Urine studies (urinalysis, specific gravity, chemistries), hematology (complete blood count, white blood cell count with differential, coagulation studies) and blood chemistries (glucose, protein, electrolytes, pH, blood urea nitrogen, creatinine, alkaline phosphatase) determine the client's health status and the probability of hyperplasia-induced abnormalities.
    b. Cystoscopic examination with urethral scope insertion provides access to visualize, evaluate, irrigate, biopsy, and photograph genitourinary (GU) structures. Preparation includes hydration and medication.

c. Radiological tests of the kidneys and GU tract detect possible damage caused by hyperplasia. Preparation for various tests may include nothing-by-mouth status, bowel cleansing, and investigation for iodine or shellfish allergy.

d. Urodynamic studies evaluate pressure, flow rate, and bladder and sphincter muscle competency. Pretest voiding is not necessary, because micturation is evaluated during the studies. The bladder may be catheterized to determine filling and evacuation capabilities.

19. Fluid intake and warm sitz baths may relieve urethral discomfort experienced after invasive diagnostic testing.

20. The following contribute to urinary retention: delay in voiding; chilling; medication (tranquilizers, decongestants, antidepressants, anticholinergics); infection.

21. Alcohol and caffeine may cause bladder irritability and rapid filling.

22. Large amounts of fluid ingested at a time lead to overdistension of the bladder.

23. Incomplete urine evacuation is an underlying cause of overflow incontinence and may cause infection, increased pressures within the genitourinary tract, and compromised renal integrity.

24. Calculi formation and urinary tract infection are promoted by stasis and an alkaline urine.

25. Acid-ash foods and cranberry, plum, and cherry juice acidify the urine.

26. In elders, sepsis develops rapidly and may be asymptomatic until the end stages of sepsis.

27. Elders are vulnerable to untoward reactions to antibiotics because of reduced renal and hepatic efficiency and disrupted normal flora caused by decreased intestinal motility.

28. Client teaching and principles of treatment for hyperplasia of the prostate center around maintaining or restoring urinary flow, preventing or treating urinary tract infection, and preserving hydration status.

CASE STUDY

Sixty-eight-year-old Mr. Albert had experienced occasional urine dribbling and nocturia in the past. He had attributed these symptoms to aging. Despite the limitation dribbling had placed on social activities, he and Mrs. Albert decided to visit their grandsons.

Limiting fluid intake before the trip and during the visit reduced Mr. Albert's nocturia and prevented dribbling. He had no problems on the long flight home.

The next day Mr. Albert experienced increasing dysuria and was alarmed to see bloody urine. Worrying about failing health and wondering how serious the bleeding was, he prayed en route to the clinic in the retirement center where he lived.

During the assessment he shared his fears. His history revealed occasional hesitancy and a diminished urine flow force. Mr. Albert denied sensations of inadequate bladder emptying or urgency. He reported no other health problems and was not taking medication. A urine specimen was obtained. The physical examination showed a marginally enlarged prostate. He was referred to a urologist that afternoon. A catherterized specimen revealed a 75-ml postvoid residual of cloudy urine, so laboratory, cystoscopic, and urodynamic studies were arranged. Diagnostic results showed normal renal function and prostatic hyperplasia.

Conservative, nonsurgical management was chosen, and future evaluations of his status were planned. The clinic nurse and urologist continued to plan Mr. Albert's care.

ASSESSMENT CRITERIA
Physical

General health
Medical-surgical experience
Nutritional status
Use of prescribed and over-the-counter medications
Relation of hydration status to health problem
Level of activity
Quality of sleep
Changes in level of comfort
Nocturia
Dysuria
Urinary elimination patterns
Presence of hesitancy or dribbling and force of stream
Other symptoms of infection (e.g., chills and fever)
Presence of distended bladder
Urethral discharge
Hyperplasia (palpated by digital rectal examination)
Integrity of renal function and genitourinary tract as shown by urine studies

Psychosocial

Role in family and community
Social activities
Use of leisure time
Communication skills
Anxiety management
Significance of health problem
Access to health care

Spiritual

Practice of religious activities
Relationship of spiritual belief to health

Mr. Albert's age, urinary hesitancy with diminished flow, dribbling, and nocturia are consistent with prostatism (symptoms of hyperplasia of the prostate). Hyperplasia may create urinary obstruction sufficient to cause urinary retention or infection or to damage bladder and kidney tissue. Mr. Albert's dysuria and hematuria may be caused by infection or tissue damage.

Fluid limitation, Mr. Albert's effort to control the symptoms, impairs hydration and compromises renal function, promoting urinary tract infection.

The fears Mr. Albert expresses need to be explored. Lack of information or misinformation may be the source of many fears. Enabling Mr. Albert to express his fears provides opportunities to assess his range of fears, offer information, and make appropriate referrals.

Mr. Albert readily made use of the convenient health care offered in the retirement community. We are left to wonder if his wife accompanied him or even knew about his prob-

lem. She could be a valuable resource and support person for Mr. Albert. She may need clarification of misconceptions and fears about her husband's health problem.

At the clinic, urinalysis and culture and sensitivity testing provided information about Mr. Albert's hydration status, urinary pH, and the presence or likelihood of an infection. The 75-ml postvoid residual quantified Mr. Albert's retention. Blood studies and cystoscopic and urodynamic studies provided information about Mr. Albert's health status, revealing function and degree of compromise of bladder and kidney tissue. Test results in the diagnostic process helped to rule out bladder or prostatic carcinoma.

Nonsurgical management hopefully will alleviate Mr. Albert's symptoms. The symptoms may persist or escalate, requiring surgery. Mr. Albert needs to understand that the clinical course of hyperplasia of the prostate may not be predictable. Regular assessments will be necessary to evaluate his progress.

NURSING CARE PLAN: HYPERPLASIA OF THE PROSTATE

Nursing diagnoses	Expected client outcomes	Nursing strategies
Knowledge deficit related to unfamiliar situation secondary to prostatic hyperplasia and normal aging of the genitourinary tract	Client will explain how hyperplasia causes symptoms	Allow client to express feelings
	Client will describe relationship of prostate to bladder and urethra	Assess client's knowledge of structure and function of GU tract and prostate gland
		Briefly describe how structure and function of the GU tract are affected by hyperplasia; encourage questions
		Instruct client to drink at least 2000 ml of non-caffeinated beverages per day
	Client will state reasons for avoiding bladder distension and dehydration	Instruct to void at regular intervals; avoid over-distension
		Teach importance of reporting changes in voiding patterns or comfort to health care provider
	Client will compare symptoms of hyperplasia with normal aging of the GU tract	Provide information about age-related genitourinary changes
		Document outcome of client teaching
Anxiety related to changes in urinary function, fear of the unknown regarding diagnostic tests, and threat to privacy	Client will report reduced anxiety	Incorporate spouse, support persons in care so client can be realistically assured
	Client will identify areas of anxiety and methods of coping	Help to identify areas of anxiety and describe prior techniques of management
		Provide client with other stress-reduction techniques, such as relaxation, imagery, music therapy
		Support client's use of prayer as a coping strategy
	Client will ask questions about health status and diagnostic processes	Encourage client to ask questions
		Provide privacy
	Client will describe diagnostic preparation, purposes, and expectations	Teach preparation, purpose, and expectations for planned diagnostic tests
		Use terms about structures and function that the client is familiar with
		Document outcome of client teaching

Continued.

NURSING CARE PLAN: HYPERPLASIA OF THE PROSTATE—cont'd

Nursing diagnoses	Expected client outcomes	Nursing strategies
Fluid volume deficit related to inadequate fluid intake	Client will have moist mucous membranes	Assess amount of fluid intake; investigate causes of insufficient intake (mobility, access, knowledge) Teach signs of inadequate fluid intake and that thirst may not be a reliable sign
	Client will describe the relationship of hydration to renal function	Teach relationship of hydration to renal function
	Client will describe plans for 2000-ml fluid intake to be ingested throughout the day	Plan fluid intake of 2000 ml to be ingested throughout the day Instruct client to consume fluids 2 hours before bedtime
	Client will ingest 2000 ml of fluid daily	Instruct client to avoid consuming large amounts of fluid at one time Assess cardiovascular and renal tolerance of fluids Assess hydration status from laboratory data (specific gravity) and accurate intake record
Potential for infection related to urine stasis and diagnostic instrumentation	Client will report any symptoms of infection promptly	Assess integrity of healing reserve and immune system: blood nutrition, hydration, GU status Assess threats to immunity: invasive procedures, urinary retention, compromise to immunity or healing

	Client will relate how an acid urine will decrease the risk of infection	Monitor vital signs
		Practice scrupulous hand washing
		Teach the client cleansing of penis and foreskin
		Promote bladder emptying
		Monitor urine pH, maintaining an acid urine
		Encourage daily fluid intake of 2000 ml
		Frequently assess for infection after urine retention episodes and invasive maneuvers: changes in mentation or vital signs or clarity, odor, or color of urine
		Relate vital signs to client baseline values
		Assess for warm (vasogenic) and cold (hypovolemic) shock:
		  Urinary output: diminished in cold shock; normal in early warm shock
		  Skin: pale in cold shock; dry, flushed in warm shock
		Investigate reports of pain
		Obtain midstream specimen for urinalysis, culture and sensitivity
		Use strict asepsis if bladder catheterization is ordered; select nontraumatizing catheter type and size; do not force catheter if obstruction is encountered; gently rotate catheter in place during deep breath by client
		Teach client to report signs of infection to health care provider

	Client will name medications and state administration times and side effects	Administer antibiotics as ordered Explain purpose, dosage schedule, importance of taking all prescribed medication to maintain satisfactory blood titers Teach side effects, importance of reporting them to physician Document outcome of client teaching

NURSING CARE PLAN: HYPERPLASIA OF THE PROSTATE—cont'd

Nursing diagnoses	Expected client outcomes	Nursing strategies
Sleep pattern disturbance related to occasional nocturia	Client will report increase in restful sleep	Assess perceptions about sleep pattern change with client and spouse Assess time of awakenings, encourage client to identify a pattern Investigate cause of awakenings Limit daytime naps
	Client will establish sleep routines	Establish regular bedtime routines, and consider scheduling a regular wake-up time during the night for voiding

	Client will list activities that induce or support uninterrupted sleep	Teach evening and bedtime measures to induce and maintain sleep:
		    Assessment for bladder distension
		    Avoidance of fluids during the 2 hours before bedtime
		    Avoidance of caffeine and alcohol in the evening
		Document outcome of client teaching

Altered urinary elimination patterns; related to decreased bladder tone, obstructed passage, incomplete emptying	Client will report feeling of postvoid evacuation	Assess perception, sensation of the need to void Assess times and situations of urine loss Assess bladder for retention (150 ml of urine distorts percussion; 500 ml creates visible distension) Assess for flank, bladder, or scrotal pain Review usual voiding pattern
	Client will record time and amount of each voiding	Teach client to record and report voiding time and amounts Assess intake and output, urine specific gravity Assess blood urea nitrogen and serum creatinine
	Client will report plan for spacing fluid throughout the day	Teach client to space fluid intake throughout the day

	Client will list strategies to prevent retention	Teach methods to reduce retention and enhance voiding:
		    Avoid caffeine and alcohol
		    Respond immediately to voiding urge
		    Use relaxation techniques prior to voiding
		    Palpate bladder for fullness before and after voiding
		    Stand to void; bend at waist to expel more urine
		    Stimulate voiding (hands in water, running water)
		    Credé's maneuver (if not contraindicated): massage lower abdomen toward midline and toward pubis with fingertips to manually express residual urine
		    Provide private, safe, and convenient toileting facilities
		    Teach client that postvoid dribbling may be related to inadequate emptying
		    With physician's order, aseptically catheterize client to slowly decompress bladder and measure postvoid residual; select least traumatizing catheter size and type

	Client will report increased comfort after sitz baths	Provide warm sitz baths to relieve congestion Prostatic massage (if ordered) temporarily relieves congestion Document outcome of client teaching

Continued.

NURSING CARE PLAN: HYPERPLASIA OF THE PROSTATE—cont'd

Nursing diagnoses	Expected client outcomes	Nursing strategies
Body image disturbance related to change in health status	Client will view self more positively, as evidenced by verbal reports	Assist the client in identifying impact of present health problem
	Client will list troublesome aspects of health status	Help client to identify and express feelings regarding change in health status
		Provide information to help and encourage client to identify and understand available options for management/resolution
	Client will state some self-care strategies for handling troublesome aspects of hyperplasia	Offer self-care strategies for troublesome aspects of hyperplasia
		Identify health resources
		Document outcome of client teaching
Impaired social interaction; related to occasional unpredictable dribbling	Client will report decreased incidents of dribbling	Assess degree and times of dribbling
		Suggest protective products and strategies for managing social events (padding, toilet access, ease of departure)
		Instruct client to void at scheduled intervals and completely empty the bladder
		Assess amount and time of intake and output
		Teach methods of skin protection to keep the area clean and dry
		Assess support systems
	Client will develop and maintain social contact and interchange	Encourage social contact and interchange to prevent isolation (telephone, mail)
		Suggest home entertaining
		Document outcome of client teaching

EVALUATION

1. The client lists the manifestations of prostatic hyperplasia.
2. The client describes the relationship of the prostate to the bladder and the urethra.
3. The client explains the importance of preventing bladder distention.
4. The client identifies areas of anxiety and methods of coping.
5. The client asks questions regarding his health status and diagnostic processes.
6. The client briefly describes preparation, purpose, and expectations prior to invasive tests.
7. The client explains the relationship of hydration to renal function.
8. The client's laboratory data show a normal range of hydration.
9. The client spaces 2000 ml of fluid intake throughout the day.
10. The client names his prescribed drugs and states dosage times and side effects.
11. Client and spouse describe the client's pattern of sleep changes and remedial strategies to address them.
12. The client explains the relationship of caffeine, alcohol, bedtime fluids to nocturia.
13. The client records voiding times consistently.
14. The client expresses his feelings regarding body image.
15. The client lists positive characteristics of his present health status.
16. The client relates options for management and resolution of the present situation.
17. The client utilizes self-care strategies for managing troublesome aspects of hyperplasia.
18. The client voids on schedule and empties the bladder.
19. The client identifies protective strategies and actions that make possible increased social interaction.

NURSING ALERTS

1. Anticipate a possible narrowed urethra (silent hyperplasia) when catheterizing an elderly man.
2. Prostatic symptoms may be exacerbated by medications that reduce the response to the voiding urge (sedatives, hypnotics, strong analgesics, tricyclic antidepressants, phenothiazines) or cause parasympathetic inhibition of bladder contractions and sphincter relaxation (over-the-counter nasal decongestants and cold preparations, anticholinergics, antihistamines, antihypertensives, antiparkinson drugs, bronchodilators).

3. Rectal stimulation inherent in prostatic palpation or massage may induce bradycardia.
4. Prostates inflamed by infectious agents may cause sepsis if they are massaged or palpated.
5. Prevent contamination of urine specimens by palpating the prostate after the specimen is collected.
6. Cranberry juice may cause calculi formation in poorly hydrated elders.
7. Exercises of starting and stopping urine flow to increase the strength of the pelvic floor are contraindicated in clients with a history of urinary retention.
8. A 1-degree temperature elevation in the elderly is significant as a sign of infection.

Bibliography

Brundage DJ: Age related changes in the genitourinary system. In Mattheson MA and McConnell ES: Gerontological nursing: concepts and practice, Philadelphia, 1988, WB Saunders Co, pp 279-289.

Carter MA: Nursing role in management: male reproductive problems. In Lewis SM and Collier IC: Medical-surgical nursing: assessment and management of clinical problems, ed 2, New York, 1987, McGraw-Hill Book Co, pp 1425-1440.

Ebersole P and Hess P: Toward healthy aging: human needs and nursing response, ed 3, St Louis, 1985, The CV Mosby Co.

Ebert NJ: Elimination in the aged. In Yurick AG et al: The aged person and the nursing process, ed 3, Norwalk, Conn, 1989, Appleton & Lange, pp 582-600.

Folk-Lighty ME and Lewis SM: Nursing role in management: urological problems. In Lewis SM and Collier IC: Medical-surgical nursing: assessment and management of clinical problems, ed 2, New York, 1987, McGraw-Hill Book Co, pp 1153-1187.

Gioiella EC and Bevil CW: Nursing care of the aging client: promoting healthy adaptation, Norwalk, Conn, 1985, Appleton-Century-Crofts.

Grayhack JT and Kozlowski JM: Benign prostatic hyperplasia. In Gillenwater JT et al: Adult and pediatric urology, vol 2, Chicago, 1987, Year Book Medical Publishers, pp 1062-1125.

Johnson DE, Swanson DA and von Eschenbach AC: Tumors of the genitourinary tract. In Tanagho EA and McAninch JW: Smith's general urology, ed 12, Norwalk, Conn, 1988, Appleton & Lange, pp 330-434.

Kim MJ, McFarland GK and McLane AM: Pocket guide to nursing diagnoses, ed 3, St Louis, 1989, The CV Mosby Co.

Lerner J and Khan Z: Mosby's manual of urologic nursing, St Louis, 1982, The CV Mosby Co.

McAninch JW: Symptoms of disorders of the genitourinary tract. In Tanagho EA and McAninch JW: Smith's general urology, ed 12, Norwalk, Conn, 1988, Appleton & Lange, pp 29-37.

McConnell EA and Zimmerman MF: Care of patients with urologic problems, Philadelphia, 1983, JB Lippincott Co.

Olshansky EF: Nursing assessment: reproductive system. In Lewis SM and Collier IC: Medical-surgical nursing: assessment and management of clinical problems, ed 2, New York, 1987, McGraw-Hill Book Co, pp 1325-1347.

Smeltzer SCO: Assessment of renal and urinary function. In Brunner LS and Suddarth DS: Textbook of medical-surgical nursing, ed 6, Philadelphia, 1988, JB Lippincott Co, pp 992-1008.

Specht J: Genitourinary problems. In Carnevali DL and Patrick M: Nursing management for the elderly, Philadelphia, 1986, JB Lippincott Co, pp 447-466.

Tanagho EA: Anatomy of the genitourinary tract. In Tanagho EA and McAninch JW: Smith's general urology, ed 12, Norwalk, Conn, 1988, Appleton & Lange, pp 1-15.

Tanagho EA: Urodynamic studies. In Tanagho EA and McAninch JW: Smith's general urology, ed 12, Norwalk, Conn, 1988, Appleton & Lange, pp 452-472.

Transurethral Resection of the Prostate

Roberta Purvis Bartee

KNOWLEDGE BASE

1. The prostate is located at the base of the bladder, circumferential to the proximal urethra.
2. If cellular proliferation of the periurethral glands becomes adenomas, the condition is known as hyperplasia of the prostate. It is thought that hormonal imbalance is the trigger for the cellular proliferation. The adenomas increase in size and number, compressing the true prostate toward the fibrous capsule. The prostatic urethra and outlet of the bladder may be obstructed by the increased mass of tissue.
3. Urinary flow from the bladder may be gradually or abruptly compromised by hyperplasia as the urethra is narrowed. Obstruction results in increased pressure within the bladder, ureters, and kidneys, causing structural and functional damage to each of those tissues.
4. Prostatic hyperplasia may remain stable in some men and not require surgery. Even with surgery, hyperplasia may recur.
5. Urinary retention, chronic urinary tract infections, gross hematuria with clots, or renal symptoms are indications for transurethral resection of the urethra (TURP).
6. Preoperative anxieties include embarrassment from lack of privacy, fear of impotence, and fear of change in sexual functioning.
7. Vasectomies are done in conjunction with the TURP to prevent epididymitis.
8. The leading causes of postprostatectomy death are myocardial infarction and cardiopulmonary failure.
9. Large amounts of irrigant (800 to 1000 ml) are absorbed into the venous sinusoids during surgery and may cause water intoxication (TUR syndrome). Cerebral and pulmonary edema result. Fluid shifts are seen more frequently in clients with hyponatremia, hypoproteinemia, and reduced serum osmolality. Cerebral edema can also occur. Disorientation and agitation are early signs. Encephalophathy, caused by metabolized glycine (ammonia) from the operative irrigant, is seen especially among men with compromised hepatic function, obstructive uropathy, urinary tract infection, or skeletal muscle atrophy. Visual disturbance of short duration occurs from the direct effect of glycine or occipital cortical edema.
10. Other complications of TURP are hemorrhage, infection, and bladder perforation.
11. Blood loss increases proportionately with gland size. Postoperatively, bladder distension increases bleeding by opening up the operative site of the prostatic fossa.
12. Bladder spasms are a response to the trauma on bladder mucosa. The irrigant and catheter contribute to the bladder spasms, which give the sensation of needing to urinate and are a cramping pain. Increased spasms indicate a distended bladder as a result of an obstructed catheter or a clot occluding the bladder outlet. Bladder spasms increase bleeding.
13. Maintaining a patent catheter and administering belladonna and opium suppositories relieve bladder spasms. Teaching the client about the spasms preoperatively will help the client recognize early symptoms and receive prompt intervention. After surgery, the client is reminded not to strain and to try to avoid urinating around the catheter.
14. Persistent bladder spasms or failure of the catheter to drain requires immediate attention. There is a possibility of hemorrhage with clot retention, displacement of the catheter, or perforation of the bladder during surgery.
15. Following a TURP, a large (no. 24 Fr) three-way Foley catheter with a 30-ml balloon is usually inserted into the bladder. The catheter is used for both bladder irrigation and drainage. The large catheter lumen is needed to evacuate clots formed as a result of bleeding in the prostatic fossa.
16. The purpose of constant irrigation is to keep the bladder free from clots that would block the drainage of urine. Faster rates of irrigation are needed when urine is bloody, because dilute urine prevents clot formation.

17. Bleeding can be expected to diminish within 24 hours. After the urine clears, the urinary catheter is removed. Early catheter removal reduces the incidence of stricture formation.
18. After catheter removal, fluid intake relieves dysuria and frequency and clears any new bleeding and tissue fragments.
19. Clients at risk for requiring recatheterization tend to have had preoperative total urinary retention, gross hematuria, or surgical specimens greater than 30 g.
20. After catheter removal, serial voidings are collected, saved, allowed to settle, and visually inspected for sedimentation and color. The expectation is for the specimens to become progressively more clear.
21. Client teaching is a critical factor in the recovery process. Following are areas to be included:
    a. About 2 weeks after surgery as healing occurs, desiccated tissue sloughs out. There is a potential for bleeding to occur. The client is instructed that clot formation would obstruct urine flow, so he should notify his physician if the urine is thick with blood or he cannot urinate.
    b. Sexual activity is delayed until after healing occurs, because orgasm causes the prostate to contract, which would potentiate bleeding.
    c. Epithelialization of the prostatic fossa may take 6 to 12 weeks.
    d. Physiological impotence is associated less frequently with TURP than with other surgical approaches.
    e. Retrograde ejaculation can be expected. Semen flows into the bladder because of the surgical injury to the bladder sphincter. Evidence of regrograde ejaculation is cloudy urine and lack of urethral ejaculate. The client should be told that there is a decreased probability of fertility but that the procedure does not affect orgasm or erection.
    f. Limitations in physical activity, lifting, and riding in a car will be clarified by the physician.
    g. Urinary continence should improve with time. Kegel exercises are helpful in strengthening the perineal muscles.

CASE STUDY

Recurrent episodes of urinary tract infections and retention gradually responded less vigorously to treatment over the years, becoming intolerable for Mr. Benjamin. A transurethral resection of the prostate was scheduled. At 75 Mr. Benjamin was well nourished and healthy except for findings indicating long-standing prostatic hyperplasia. Preoperative preparations were completed prior to hospitalization. Mr. Benjamin seemed anxious on admission.

Under regional anesthesia, surgery extended beyond an hour before 25 g of hyperplastic tissue was removed. Mr. Benjamin was short of breath at the end of the procedure and reported a dimming of the operating room lights.

Postoperatively his skin was warm and dry. Vital signs were within normal range. The catheter drained bloody urine, a few clots, and some tissue plugs. Analgesia, bladder irrigation, and intravenous fluid were ordered.

He was seen by the resident after becoming disoriented and confused and attempting to remove the catheter. Catheter traction was discontinued, and laboratory specimens were drawn. During the night, the catheter drainage began to lighten as numerous clots and plugs were evacuated. The next morning he was oriented and reported clear vision. Later that week, the catheter was removed, and he was discharged 5 days postoperatively.

ASSESSMENT CRITERIA
Physical
Preoperative
Knowledge of operative course and expectations
Vital signs
Concurrent health problems
General health, multisystem status
Nutritional status
Height and weight: usual, current, ideal
Results from blood chemistry, complete blood count, coagulation, urinalysis
Level of activity
Mobility
  Gait
  Coordination
  Balance
  Flexibility
Urinary elimination
  Voiding pattern
  Urine color, clarity
  Dysuria, frequency, urgency
  Bladder distensions, residual
Bowel elimination
  Stool amount, frequency, consistency
  Presence of blood
  Constipation
  Diarrhea

Cardiopulmonary
  Heart sounds
  Peripheral pulses
  Edema
  Lung sounds
  Cough
  Smoking history
Pain
  Location
  Characteristics
  Duration
  Exacerbating and relieving factors

Postoperative

Vital signs
Mentation
Reassessment of systems
Urethral catheter integrity: flow, character, amount
  of urine
Catheter effluent: arterial versus venous drainage
Bladder distension, spasms
Hydration status
TUR syndrome: visual disturbance, fluid overload,
  mentation changes
Laboratory data: chemistries, osmolality, urine
  culture
Comfort
Sepsis
Peripheral vascular integrity
Post–catheter removal assessments: voiding status,
  quality and quantity of urine

Psychosocial

Convalescence expectation and knowledge of home
  care
Support systems
Roles, intimacy, sexual activity
Health care resources; insurance
Anxiety level
Meaning of surgery

Spiritual

Impact on spirituality and religious practices
Perception of inner strength to deal with the surgery
  and recovery
Ability to identify source of strength and hope
Support from beliefs during illness experience
Desire for visit from a religious representative during
  hospitalization

Mr. Benjamin's symptoms of recurrent urinary tract infection and urine retention became intolerable and refractory to treatment, making him a candidate for prostatic surgery. The surgical approach selected, transurethral resection, was based on his health status and the size and location of hyperplasia. Mr. Benja-

---

min's health and nutritional status will enhance healing and somewhat reduce operative risk.

Evidence of long-standing hyperplasia needs to be quantified for the effect it may have on his postoperative course, immune status, and renal integrity. The history of retention suggests an enlarged bladder and loss of tone, which may complicate the period after catheter removal. His history of recurrent episodes of urinary tract infection may increase the risk for sepsis.

Surgery lasted longer than an hour, and 25 g of tissue was removed. Surgeries of long duration and with removal of large amounts of tissue increase the risk for systemic absorption of operative irrigant, which can cause the TUR syndrome. Mr. Benjamin's shortness of breath may be related to anxiety, fluid overload, or a cardiopulmonary event; more assessment data are needed. His experience of the lights dimming is an effect of TUR syndrome on vision.

Postoperatively, Mr. Benjamin was stable and began drinking fluids before becoming disoriented and confused. He may have been having bladder spasms caused by bladder irritability, or distension caused by a nonpatent catheter. He may have been in fluid overload from operative irrigant absorption, or from intravenous fluids. The stress response to surgery causes fluid retention, which contributes to fluid overload.

Mr. Benjamin's change in mentation (disoriented, confused) may have reflected fluid overload or a hemodynamic, cerebral, or cardiac event. Change in mentation may be the only symptom of sepsis in elders who are unable to mount a significant white blood cell or febrile response to infectious agents. Laboratory tests were performed to provide information about hematological and electrolyte status and the client's immune response. Blood cultures were done to identify any infectious agents; the results were negative.

Mr. Benjamin's catheter drainage continued to lighten as clots and tissue plugs were evacuated. The next morning he was oriented and regained visual acuity. Resolution of both problems may be attributed to the short duration of the TUR syndrome.

Mr. Benjamin continued to have an uneventful recovery. After his catheter was removed, he established a satisfactory voiding pattern of clearing urine without retention or bladder spasm and was discharged.

NURSING CARE PLAN: TRANSURETHRAL RESECTION OF THE PROSTATE

Nursing diagnoses	Expected client outcomes	Nursing strategies
Anxiety related to hospitalization, the operative course, and fear of impotence	Client will experience mild to moderate anxiety	Assess level of knowledge about hospitalization, surgery, and TUR
	Client will discuss the surgical event and postoperative course	Prepare client for surgery by providing and clarifying information:
		Assessments during perioperative time
		Catheter: purpose, irrigation, character of flow
		Comfort: sensations of bladder spasms, remedies
		Mobility and nutrition
		Hydration: requirements, relation to operative course
		Intravenous fluids
	Client will identify coping mechanisms	Assess client's coping methods and assist with use
	Client will express concerns to the nurse	Provide for privacy, opportunities to discuss concerns
		Incorporate support system in teaching (with the client's permission).
	Client will list resources available for present health problem	Provide access to post-hospital resources as appropriate: social services, church groups, Meals on Wheels
		Provide home care information: activity, voiding, comfort, preservation of surgical site integrity, and reportable phenomena
	Client will discuss home care	Document outcome of client teaching
Potential for fluid volume excess related to absorption of bladder irrigation solution	Client will experience prompt intervention in response to TUR syndrome	Evaluate intake and output
		Assess for other factors that may be the cause of symptoms
		Administer diuretics as ordered; monitor response
		Document outcome of client teaching
Altered urinary elimination: retention; related to surgical debris and insufficient bladder evacuation	Client will not experience urinary retention	Observe for bladder distension and amount of catheter output and characteristics frequently, on scheduled basis and as necessitated by ongoing assessments
	Client will state the function of the urinary catheter	Maintain patency of catheter by irrigating and monitoring for clots
		Encourage fluid intake to 3000 ml/day
		Explain purpose of the catheter (hemostasis, drainage)
		Maintain unkinked gravity flow line below bladder
		Assess meatus for bleeding or drainage; cleanse meatus around the catheter, and teach client importance for tissue integrity and infection control
		Record urinary output, distinguishing from irrigant
		Maintain continuous or intermittent irrigation (as ordered) to three-way catheter, facilitating removal of surgical debris (clots, tissue plugs, mucus)
	Client's urine color will progressively clear from shades of red to yellow	Monitor urine color; adjust irrigant rate, frequency to prevent clot formation, obstruction
		Empty bladder prior to catheter removal for accurate subsequent assessments of voiding pattern

NURSING CARE PLAN: TRANSURETHRAL RESECTION OF THE PROSTATE—cont'd

Nursing diagnoses	Expected client outcomes	Nursing strategies
	Client will void within 6 hours of catheter removal	Record times and amounts of voids to identify patterns; expect first void within 6 hours of catheter removal 150-250 ml of urine should be voided every 3-4 hours Should Foley bag fail to deflate: roll, compress filling ports; if unsuccessful, notify surgeon Assess need for recatheterization; if so, notify surgeon

	Client will discuss home-care procedures for bladder hydration and management and list reportable symptoms	Instruct for home care:
		  Identify factors affecting bladder function: medications, caffeine, alcohol, chilling
		  Avoid forced or delayed voidings; bladder capacity may increase during next 2 postoperative months
		  Cleanse tract daily with 2000 ml of oral fluid
		  Teach use, purpose, side effects of medicines
		  Notify physician of retention, voiding changes
		  Instruct client to return to physician for evaluation of progress and recurrence
		Document outcome of client teaching

Fluid volume deficit related to hemorrhage secondary to surgical disruption of vessels	Client will experience prompt treatment for signs of volume depletion
	
	Client catheter system will remain functionally in place
		Monitor vital signs and mentation
		Assess complete blood count and coagulation studies
		Prevent catheter displacement
		Calculate fluid intake and urinary output
		Maintain irrigation (continuous or intermittent) of bladder as ordered
		Observe urine flow for amount, clarity
		Differentiate venous (darker, less viscous) from arterial (bright, numerous clots) bleeding
		Avoid trauma to surgical site:
		  No rectal manipulation (tubes, enemas, thermometers)
		  No straining at stool; prevent constipation with juices, fiber, hydration
		  Minimize prolonged periods of sitting

	Client and significant other will discuss points of home care	Instruct for home care:
		  Hydration: 2000 ml daily to flush tract
		  Hematuria: intermittent for 4-6 weeks during fossa healing, or initiated by colon contractions of bowel movements; rare after 21 days
		  Voiding: note and report changes in pattern, difficulty in voiding, retention
		  Protect surgical site: no enemas, rectal temperatures, straining at stool or voiding
		  Avoid increased intraabdominal pressure caused by prolonged sitting or lifting more than 20 pounds
		  Instruct to resume sexual activity after surgeon verifies prostatic fossa healing
		Document outcome of client teaching

NURSING CARE PLAN: TRANSURETHRAL RESECTION OF THE PROSTATE—cont'd

Nursing diagnoses	Expected client outcomes	Nursing strategies
Potential for infection related to surgically disrupted tissue integrity (prostatic fossa), invasive procedures (surgery, catheterization, irrigations), and compromised ability of immune system to mount a response (aging process)	Client will present no manifestation of local or systemic infection	Assess client's immune integrity and risks for infection: blood and urine studies, nutritional status, concurrent health problems, genitourinary history (retention, infection) Evaluate vital signs according to client's established baseline values Assess mentation for early sign of sepsis

	Client's drainage will remain closed, functional, and sterile	Assess for meatal drainage
		Assess for pain; note location, characteristics, exacerbating and relieving factors
		Maintain closed-system drainage for urinary catheter
		Offer cranberry, plum, or cherry juice to maintain acid urine
		Maintain scrupulous catheter system care:
		  Frequent handwashing, continuous urine assessments
		  Teach client rationale for aseptic practices
		  Cleanse meatus with soap and water every 4 hours; teach client importance of cleansing during home care
		  Maintain gravity flow by keeping tubing and container below bladder
		  Prevent drainage system contact with floor

	Client will explain home care and reportable symptoms of infection	Instruct client for home care:
		  Reportable symptoms: fever, pain, foul urine odor
		  Cloudy urine resolves with healing
		  Medication protocol: antibiotics, antiseptics as ordered
		  Hand washing, aseptic practices
		Document outcome of client teaching

Pain related to surgical trauma, bladder spasms, and urinary retention	Client will express increased comfort	Assess level of comfort: identify and investigate source of discomfort and characteristics Assess verbal and nonverbal behaviors and vital signs indicating discomfort
	Client will report decreased back pain	Relieve back pains (from operative lithotomy position) with massage and application of warmth Relieve postspinal headache with bed rest and analgesia Assess and intervene to promote urinary flow Assess location of catheter Irrigate catheter (as ordered) to promote flow and remove debris Assess and intervene for bladder spasms Teach client symptoms of bladder spasms: presence of severe lower abdominal discomfort; severe urge to void or defecate
	Client will report relief of bladder spasms	Assess patency of catheter Medicate for bladder spasms, noting relief effect Use noninvasive methods of pain control: relaxation, deep breathing, imaging Hydrate with at least 2000 ml daily
	Client will explain home care measures to promote comfort	Provide sitz baths to relieve voiding discomfort Instruct for home care: methods to prevent or relieve bladder spasms and dysuria; report pain to physician Document outcome of client teaching

Continued.

NURSING CARE PLAN: TRANSURETHRAL RESECTION OF THE PROSTATE—cont'd

Nursing diagnoses	Expected client outcomes	Nursing strategies

Urge incontinence: related to irritable bladder after surgery, catheter removal, and diminished capacity resulting from catheterization	Client will report improved urinary continence
	Client will void at first urge
	
	Client will perform exercises to improve muscle tone
	
	Client will space fluid intake of 2000 ml throughout the day
	Client will list agents that cause diuresis
	
	Client will not require protective devices to remain dry
		Assess voiding habits, incontinence, dribbling, and degree of retention
		Instruct client to prevent bladder overfilling: void frequently and at first urge
		Inform that sitz baths provide comfort for urgency and dysuria
		Offer encouragement that dribbling may resolve
		Provide exercises to help improve muscle tone:
		  Press together, then relax muscles of buttocks 10-20 times per hour
		  Stop urine stream in midvoid; then continue
		Instruct client not to limit fluid intake
		Space fluid intake of 2000 ml throughout the day
		Avoid diuretic effect of alcohol, caffeine
		Note and report dysuria, frequent small voided amounts, changes in urine characteristics
		Avoid straining to micturate
		Encourage client to discuss any problems with surgeon on postoperative visit
		Document outcome of client teaching.

Potential altered tissue perfusion; related to venous stasis secondary to TURP	Client will have fewer risk factors for altered tissue perfusion Client will experience prompt intervention for calf pain or ischemic change Client will gradually increase activities Client will drink adequate fluids	Evaluate presence of risk factors: history of deep vein thrombosis (DVT), peripheral vascular disease, diabetes, immobility, obesity, age, large prostate resection, sustained lithotomy operative position, length of surgery, hydration status Assess tissue perfusion of extremities; note calf tenderness. Encourage leg and foot movement Administer low-dose heparin as ordered; monitor platelet count during therapy Advance activity as ordered, tolerated Encourage fluid intake to prevent dehydration, which induces thrombus formation Assess for pulmonary embolus: dyspnea, substernal pain, weakness, tachycardia Document outcome of client teaching
Potential for altered sexuality patterns; related to retrograde ejaculation and fear of impotence	Client will verbalize feelings about threat to sexuality Client will describe expected effects of TURP on sexuality	Preoperatively assess client information and concerns regarding impact of prostate surgery on sexual activity Assess client's level of comfort in discussing fears Establish comfortable and private environment Give client an opportunity to discuss fears about sexuality Describe expected effects of TURP on sexuality, including retrograde ejaculation Inform client that physiological impotence occurs less frequently after TURP than after other surgical approaches Instruct client that sexual activity may be resumed after fossa healing, with advice of the surgeon Document outcome of client teaching

EVALUATION

1. The client uses past successful coping mechanisms during hospitalization.
2. The client verbalizes concerns to the nurse.
3. The client lists possible resources to assist with current health situations.
4. The client is able to discuss the surgical event and the postoperative course.
5. The client experiences prompt intervention if cardiopulmonary, cerebral, or renal compromise occurs.
6. Client and significant other understand the purpose of the urinary catheter.
7. The client recalls home care instructions for bladder management, hydration, comfort, and reportable phenomena.
8. The client's catheter system remains in place and patent.
9. The client's surgical site is not traumatized.
10. The client experiences relief from bladder spasms.
11. The client drinks 2000 ml of fluid throughout the day.
12. The client voids frequently, at scheduled intervals.
13. The client consistently performs sphincter-strengthening exercises.
14. The client lists agents causing diuresis.
15. The client progressively increases levels of activity.
16. The client's extremities remain adequately perfused, without pain, edema, or redness.
17. The client describes the expected effects of TURP on sexuality and discusses his feelings about them.

NURSING ALERTS

1. Investigate changes in postoperative mentation: TUR syndrome? Neurological, cardiovascular, or renal event? Ammonia intoxication? Early sepsis? Bladder spasms? Bladder distension?
2. Normal temperature for elders may be less than 98.6° F. Baseline data are important for future interpretations.
3. Indiscriminate bladder palpation or percussion may traumatize the surgical site.
4. Supervise sitz baths; monitor for heat-induced orthostatic hypotension.
5. Avoid rectal manipulations (temperatures, enemas, tubes), which may traumatize the prostatic surgical site.
6. Methantheline bromide (Banthine) for bladder spasm is contraindicated in clients with glaucoma, bronchial asthma, or cardiopulmonary disease.

Bibliography

Ashby D: Hyponatremia after transurethral resection of the prostate, Journal of Post Anesthesia Nursing 3:121, 1988.

Brundage DJ: Age related changes in the genitourinary system. In Matteson MA and McConnell ES: Gerontological nursing: concepts and practice, Philadelphia, 1988, WB Saunders Co. pp 279-289.

Brunner LS and Suddarth DS: Management of the male patient with disorders related to the reproductive system. In Brunner LS and Suddarth DS: Textbook of medical-surgical nursing, ed 6, Philadelphia, 1988, JB Lippincott Co, pp 1152-1170.

Carter MA: Nursing role in management: male reproductive problems. In Lewis SM and Collier IC: Medical-surgical nursing: assessment and management of clinical problems, ed 2, New York, 1987, McGraw-Hill Book Co, pp 1425-1440.

Creel DJ, Wang JM, and Wong KC: Transient blindness associated with transurethral resection of the prostate, Archives of Opthalmology 105:1537, 1987.

Feldstein MS and Benson NA: Early catheter removal and reduced length of hospital stay following transurethral prostatectomy: a retrospective analysis of 100 consecutive patients, Journal of Urology 140:532, 1988.

Folk-Lighty ME and Lewis SM: Nursing role in management: renal and urological problems. In Lewis SM and Collier IC: Medical-surgical nursing: assessment and management of clinical problems, ed 2, New York, 1987, McGraw-Hill Book Co, pp 1153-1187.

Grayhack JT and Kowlowski JM: Benign prostatic hyperplasia. In Gillenwater, JY et al: Adult and pediatric urology, vol 2, Chicago, 1987, Year Book Medical Publishers, pp 1062-1125.

Greene LF: Transurethral prostate resection: technique. In Greene LF and Segura JW, editors: Transurethral surgery, Philadelphia, 1979, WB Saunders Co, pp 108-164.

Johnson DE, Swanson DA, and von Eschenbach AC: Tumors of the genitourinary tract. In Tanagho EA and McAninch JW: Smith's general urology, ed 12, Norwalk, Conn, 1988, Appleton & Lange, pp 330-434.

Kim MJ, McFarland GK, and McLane AM: Pocket guide to nursing diagnoses, ed 3, St Louis, 1989, The CV Mosby Co.

Lerner J and Khan Z: 1982, Mosby's manual of urologic nursing, St Louis, 1982, The CV Mosby Co.

Lewis SM: Nursing assessment: urinary sytem. In Lewis SM and Collier IC: Medical-surgical nursing: assessment and management of clinical problems, ed 2, New York, 1987, McGraw-Hill Book Co, pp 1135-1152.

McConnell EA and Zimmerman MF: Care of patients with urological problems, Philadelphia, 1983, JB Lippincott Co.

Olshansky EF: Nursing assessment: reproductive system. In Lewis SM and Collier IC: Medical-surgical nursing: assessment and management of clinical problems, ed 2, New York, 1987, McGraw-Hill Book Co, pp 1325-1347.

Smeltzer SCO: Assessment of renal and urinary function. In Brunner LS and Suddarth, DS: Textbook of medical-surgical nursing, ed 6, Philadelphia, 1988, JB Lippincott Co, pp 992-1008.

Smeltzer SCO: Management of patients with renal and urinary dysfunction. In Brunner LS and Suddarth DS: Textbook of medical-surgical nursing, ed 6, Philadelphia, 1988, JB Lippincott Co, pp 1009-1032.

Tanagho EA: Urodynamic studies. In Tanagho EA and McAninch JW: Smith's general urology, ed 12, Norwalk, Conn, 1988, Appleton & Lange, pp 452-472.

Urinary Incontinence

Joan D. Nelson

KNOWLEDGE BASE

1. Urinary incontinence is the involuntary loss of urine from the lower urinary tract.
2. Two to four million elderly people living in the community have at least some degree of urinary incontinence, and nearly 50% of the institutionalized elderly are incontinent.
3. Incontinence is second only to cognitive dysfunction as the cause of admission to nursing homes.
4. The following are some of the high-risk factors for urinary incontinence: being female, acute illness, urinary tract infection, prostatic hyperplasia in men, constipation and stool impaction, neurological impairment, new environment, impaired mobility and/or dexterity, impaired cognition, and depression.
5. Urinary tract infections are one of the most common health problems among the elderly. The elderly person may be asymptomatic or have nonspecific symptoms such as fever and/or vomiting. There is a 96% chance of bacteriuria after an indwelling catheter connected to straight drainage has been present for 4 days.
6. Effects of aging on the urinary system include the following:
   a. Decreased bladder capacity
   b. Increased voiding frequency and volume of residual urine
   c. Varying urge to void; urge may not occur until bladder is filled to capacity
   d. Detrusor hyperreflexia
   e. Sphincter weakness
7. Nursing diagnoses related to incontinence include the following:
   a. *Stress* incontinence is the loss of urine that occurs with increased intraabdominal pressure caused by weakening of pelvic floor and levator ani muscles; the condition can be treated with Kegel exercises and medications.
   b. *Urge* incontinence is involuntary urination occurring soon after a strong urgency to void. (Treatments are discussed in this care plan.)
   c. *Reflex* incontinence is involuntary loss of urine caused by completion of the spinal cord reflex arc in the absence of higher neural control. Treatments relate to stimulating the reflex arc in order to stimulate bladder emptying.
   d. *Functional* incontinence is an inability to reach the toilet in time because of environmental barriers, cognitive dysfunction, or physical limitations (treatment is discussed in care plan).
   e. *Total* incontinence is the continuous or unpredictable loss of urine, which is often diagnosed after treatment has failed; the condition is usually controlled with some type of catheter or protective garments.
   f. Urinary *retention* results from high urethral pressure, which inhibits voiding until high abdominal pressure causes urine to be involuntarily lost, or high urethral pressure can inhibit complete emptying of bladder (also known as overflow incontinence). This problem is treated according to which of the various causes is present.
8. Medications may play a major role in creating urinary incontinence (see the Nursing Alerts section).
9. In order for an elderly client to have urinary control, the following criteria must exist:
   a. Integrity of the genitourinary system
   b. Cognitive ability to cooperate with teaching
   c. Mobility
   d. Motivation to desire control
10. Urodynamic testing may not be appropriate for the aging client, since many continent elderly people demonstrate diagnostic abnormalities. These tests are expensive and uncomfortable, increase the danger of infection, and probably will not change the mode of treatment.
11. Elderly people who experience urinary incontinence suffer from guilt and loss of self-esteem, self-confidence, and self-worth and undergo physical and psychosocial decline as well as social disengagement. Common responses to incontinence are a depressive reaction, insecurity, and apathy.
12. Factors that often affect urine control in aging women include atrophic vaginitis, urethritis, urethral prolapse, pelvic floor relaxation, cystocele or rectocele, uterine prolapse, estrogen depletion, and chronic urinary tract infection (especially in institutionalized women).
13. Factors that may affect urine control in aging men include chronic urinary tract infection and enlarged prostate gland.

14. Medications are available to treat specific types of incontinence, but unwanted side effects may outweigh the benefits.
15. Irregularity of bowels, especialy constipation or fecal impaction, may cause urinary incontinence because of abdominal fullness and pressure.
16. Frequent urination to avoid "accidents" may contribute to urgency in the elderly, since the bladder is rarely allowed to be fully expanded.
17. The diminished vision, mobility, and energy that accompany aging necessitate increased time to reach the toilet, which, in turn, necessitates the ability to delay urination.
18. Kegel exercises, which are used to improve pelvic floor muscles, are as follows:
    a. Place a finger inside your rectum or vagina; try to squeeze around finger. This will identify the muscle to exercise, which is the same muscle that holds back gas or a bowel movement.
    b. *Never* use abdominal, buttock, or leg muscles; place a hand on your abdomen to feel if you are contracting an abdominal muscle.
    c. Strength will build slowly; there will be no instant results.
    d. Squeeze the muscle you identified, and hold for a count of 10.
    e. Relax the muscle for a count of 10. (This is equally important.)
    f. Do this 15 times three times a day, working up to 25 exercises at one time.
    g. You should notice improvement in approximately 2 weeks.
    h. These exercises cannot harm you in any way.
19. Bladder training programs
    a. *Bladder retraining* restores the normal voiding pattern and continence. Remove the indwelling catheter, and treat any urinary tract infection. Initiate a toileting schedule, progressively lengthening or shortening the toileting interval (e.g., upon awakening; every 2 hours during day and evening; before going to bed; every 4 hours at night). The client's voiding and continence pattern must be monitored as:
       (1) Frequency, timing, and amount of continent voids
       (2) Frequency, timing, and amount of incontinent episodes
       (3) Fluid intake
       (4) Postvoid volumes
       Instruct the client on techniques to trigger voiding if there is difficulty, such as running water, stroking the inner thigh, or suprapubic tapping. (The client must be mentally and physically capable and motivated.) If the client is voiding frequently (every 2 hours or less), perform a postvoid residual determination to ensure complete emptying of the bladder. If frequency and enuresis continue in the absence of infection, rule out other reversible causes such as medications, hyperglycemia, congestive heart failure, bladder instability, and fear of incontinence.
    b. *Scheduled toileting* to avoid incontinence episodes begins with establishing a fixed schedule, usually every 2 hours while awake. This method is beneficial for moderate or even severe mental or physical dysfunction, but the staff must be motivated.
    c. *Habit training* to avoid incontinence uses a flexible toileting schedule based on pattern of incontinence. Reinforcement techniques are used with this program, which is beneficial for clients with moderate to severe mental or physical dysfunction if the staff is motivated.
20. Cooperation among nurse's aides, nurses, and physicians is the key to success in working with incontinent clients.
21. Medications used for stress incontinence include the alpha adrenergics:
    a. Phenylpropanolamine, 50 mg one to two times a day
    b. Ephedrine, 25 to 50 mg one to four times a day
    c. Ornade, 25-mg capsule one to two times a day
22. Medications used for urge incontinence are the following:
    a. Propantheline, 15 to 30 mg two to four times a day
    b. Urised, 1 to 2 tablets one to four times a day
    c. Oxybutynin chloride, 5 mg two to three times a day

CASE STUDY

Eighty-year-old Mrs. Moore, a nursing home resident, was discharged 5 days ago from an acute care hospital where she was diagnosed and treated for an acute episode of diverticulosis. During her hospital stay Mrs. Moore became disoriented to time and place and incontinent of urine. Her restricted mobility because of arthritis, combined with her disoriented state, led to multiple unsuccessful attempts to find the bathroom and several "near fails." An indwelling Foley catheter was inserted, and a Posey jacket was ordered to keep Mrs. Moore from getting out of bed without assistance. The catheter and Posey jacket were removed the day of discharge, and Mrs. Moore was returned to her room at the nursing home.

Mrs. Moore is no longer disoriented but is continuing to have incontinence problems and states, "By the time I realize I have to go, it's too late to get there." Mrs. Still, the charge nurse, observes that Mrs. Moore is spending more time alone in her room and less time with her friends and activities.

Further assessment shows that her limited mobility improves after she is out of bed in the morning and that she needs assistance only with early-morning dressing and toileting. Her problem, since returning from the hospital is: "I have to urinate every 1 to 2 hours, and when I get the urge to go I have to go right away; if I get too far away from the toilet, I just can't move fast enough to get there. I guess this happens to all us old and useless people." Mrs. Moore is also refusing fluids, except coffee with meals and juice in the morning, in an attempt to control voiding.

ASSESSMENT CRITERIA
Physical

Toileting patterns
  Frequency
  Schedule
  Nocturia
  Sensation for need to void
  Ability to empty
Incontinence pattern
  Amount
  Onset
  Duration
  Frequency
  Aggravating and alleviating factors
  Dribbling
  Urgency
  Pain/burning
History of renal dysfunction
  Urinary tract infections
  Obstructions
  Blood urea nitrogen, creatinine
Urine characteristics
  Color
  Odor
  Appearance
  pH
  Specific gravity
  Glucose
  Proteins
  Ketones
  Red blood cells, white blood cells
  Bacteria
Intake and output

Medical-surgical history
  Congestive heart failure
  Neuropathies
  Cerebrovascular
  Diabetes
Medication history and current prescription and over-the-counter drugs
Mobility
  Gait
  Coordination
  Speed
  Flexibility of joints
  Activity/exercise patterns
  Weakness
Self-care abilities
  Remove and replace clothing
  Need for assistive devices
  Speed of ambulation to toilet
  Barriers, side rails, distance to toilet
  Visual or auditory deficits
  Activity tolerance
Nutrition and hydration
  Current weight, usual and ideal weight
  Nutrient intake: adequacy and patterns
  Hydration: amount, type, pattern
Bowel elimination
  Patterns
  Consistency; constipation, impactions
  Ease of elimination
  Laxative use
  Incontinence
Abdomen
  Bladder distension
  Tenderness
  Masses
  Softness
  Muscle tone
Genitalia
  Uterine prolapse
  Cystocele, rectocele
  Pelvic floor strength

Psychosocial

Self-described life-style
Health perceptions
Health maintenance behaviors
Knowledge of problem and treatment
Support system
Coping patterns
Risk factors (e.g., smoking, drinking)
Motivation to be continent
Present emotional status
  Level of anxiety
  Depression
  Feelings about recent hospitalization
Cognitive functioning
  Long-term and short-term memory
  Orientation
  Judgment

Spiritual

Ability and desire to participate in religious practices
Feelings of isolation, hopelessness, lack of control

Mrs. Moore's incontinence is an involuntary urination pattern occurring promptly after an urgent signal to void, which is characteristic of urge incontinence. Also, Mrs. Moore is physically incapable of reaching the toilet quickly because of her restricted mobility related to osteoarthritis and rheumatoid arthritis.

Symptoms such as a mild cystocele, a history of "difficult childbirth," slightly diminished sphincter muscle tone, and somewhat relaxed abdominal and pelvic floor muscles are suggestive of stress incontinence.

There are no signs of urinary retention, as noted by the voiding pattern of 50 to 100 ml of urine expelled about every 2 hours. The postvoid urinary residual measures at 75 ml, which is within normal limits for a client of this age, and the bladder is not palpable.

Urinalysis results are nonsignificant; urine is negative for white blood cells, red blood cells, protein, glucose, ketones, and bacteria. Although Mrs. Moore does not have any symptoms of urinary tract infection, there is a potential for infection because of the recent use of a retention catheter and the diminishing immune function typical of aging.

The intake of fluids has diminished to less than 1000 ml daily, and urinary output is estimated at 800 ml daily (difficult to measure because of "accidents").

Mrs. Moore is alert and oriented to time, place, and person, and short-term and long-term memory are intact. Her affect is "sad" and apathetic, yet she also appears tense. She is "disgusted" with her inability to control her bladder and her inability to function more quickly and effectively. She spends most of her day in her room, near the bathroom, and has become very inactive and immobile. Activities of daily living are performed awkwardly and slowly because of arthritic deformities of both hands, but she requires assistance only with early-morning dressing and bathing.

NURSING CARE PLAN: URINARY INCONTINENCE

Nursing diagnoses	Expected client outcomes	Nursing strategies

Fluid volume deficit related to inadequate fluid intake	Client will drink 2000 ml of appropriate fluid in each 24-hour period	Assess client's preference in liquids and provide those liquids
		Explain the reason to drink adequate amount of fluid
		Increase client's hydration level by:
		  Encouraging fluid intake of 1200 ml 7:00 AM to 3:00 PM, 600 ml 3:00 PM to 7:00 PM, 200 ml 7:00 PM to 7:00 AM, and limiting fluids after 7:00 PM to avoid urgency at night or enuresis
		  Keeping accurate intake and output records, noting volume of each voiding and incontinence pattern
		  Discouraging the use of caffeinated beverages and artificial sweeteners, which cause bladder irritation
		Instruct client to avoid large fluid intake just before a meal
		Involve client in planning for fluid intake

Alteration in urinary elimination; related to suspected stress incontinence	Client will demonstrate an absence of, or decreased episodes of, incontinence	Assess incontinence patterns and concomitant events
		Increase bladder capacity as follows:
		  Determine time lapsed between urge to void and actual voiding; personnel must respond promptly to client's request for assistance in toileting
		  Once client is placed on toilet, encourage her to "hold off" urinating as long as possible
		  Give positive reinforcement for client's efforts
		  Discourage frequent voiding as result of habit or anxiety and not need

Continued.

NURSING CARE PLAN: URINARY INCONTINENCE—cont'd

Nursing diagnoses	Expected client outcomes	Nursing strategies
	Client will state techniques that increase bladder control	Instruct client in techniques that strengthen sphincter and muscle control relating to urination by: Teaching Kegel exercises Starting and stopping stream while voiding Instructing client to schedule voiding or setting a voiding schedule with client that involves drinking a measured amount of fluid and voiding at specific times; this requires a commitment of both staff and client for consistency
	Client will state how she can alter some factors contributing to incontinence	Teach healthy nutritional habits by: Encouraging daily intake of fiber, fresh fruits and vegetables, and fluids to ensure regular bowel elimination and avoid abdominal pressure on bladder Avoiding use of laxatives and enemas that develop dependency Advising that caffeinated beverages and grapefruit juice act as diuretics as well as bladder irritants Encouraging client to respond promptly to urge to defecate
Alteration in urinary elimination: functional incontinence; related to decreased dexterity of upper extremities	Client will state factors contributing to functional incontinence	Discuss with client the incontinent episodes, reenact with her exactly what occurs, and discuss possible solutions: "What goes through your mind when you first realize you have to urinate?" "How easy is it to remove clothing in order to urinate?" Encourage client to schedule toileting upon arising in morning; after meals, before bedtime, before becoming involved in a lengthy activity, and before and after exercise Resolve environmental barriers by: Providing call light Having bedpan or commode within reach at night Installing grab bars around toilet Using raised toilet seat Leaving bathroom door ajar if it is difficult to turn knob Using night-light in bedroom and bathroom Discuss appropriate clothing, use of Velcro instead of zippers and buttons, loops at waist of underpants to hook fingers through and remove pants easily and quickly
	Client will demonstrate exercises that improve mobility, dexterity, and urine-controlling muscle	Discuss with client types of activities she prefers—walking, dancing, swimming, aerobics, knitting, sewing, painting—and arrange a routine that will maintain walking muscle strength, and hand and finger dexterity: Kegel exercises for pelvic floor muscles three times a day for 10 minutes each time; should see improvement within 2 weeks if done consistently Water exercise classes or measuring out a mile walk within nursing home halls (a chalkboard or bulletin board at end of mile to mark off achievement is positive reinforcement) Regularly scheduled group exercise classes Manual-dexterity activities (sewing, knitting, etc.) Positive reinforcement for exercising efforts and signs of motivation toward continence is essential

NURSING CARE PLAN: URINARY INCONTINENCE—cont'd

Nursing diagnoses	Expected client outcomes	Nursing strategies
		Avoid encouragement of incontinence or negative reinforcement by routine use of pads, diapers, or other depersonalizing procedures, since they trap urine and enhance bacterial growth; avoid placing client on toilet following incontinence episode, unless overflow incontinence has been identified; if incontinence occurs, assist with clean-up as quickly as possible and with minimal conversation; this should not be a socializing event
Potential for infection: urinary; related to altered immune response (age-related) and recent catheter insertion	Client will experience prompt detection of urinary tract infection	Instruct client to report any "feverish" feelings, chills, lower abdominal discomfort, urgency in voiding, dysuria, lower back or flank pain, changes in color, odor or amount of urine, return or increase of incontinence
		Instruct client to report any symptoms of infection, the most common in the elderly being "not feeling well," loss of appetite, odorous urine, lack of clear urine, and increased disorientation
		Request order for urinalysis
		Note white blood cell count and bacterial level
	Client will demonstrate habits that decrease the potential for urinary tract infection	Stress importance of maintaining optimal fluid intake to prevent urinary tract infections, urinary stasis, dehydration, and concentrated urine
		Teach client importance of changing clothes and cleansing perineum promptly if incontinent
		Review use of cranberry juice to maintain acidity of urine and prevent infection; avoid caffeinated beverages and artificial sweeteners
		Reinforce hygiene measures such as: Washing hands after each toileting Cleansing perineal area from front to back when bathing or after toileting Showering instead of bathing, to prevent bacteria from entering urethra Completely emptying bladder, which is achieved most effectively by upright or forward-bent position during voiding
Disturbance in self-concept and self-esteem; related to urinary incontinence and recent hospitalization	Client will identify personal strengths	Assess cognition, motivation to be continent, and willingness to participate in care plan through communication and mental status testing
		Encourage verbalization of anger, frustration, helplessness; explore previously used coping techniques when problems arise; convey to client that incontinence can be controlled, and discuss mutual goals to give client sense of control; explore and stress positive personality characteristics
		Encourage client to discuss recent hospitalization and to air feelings about use of jacket and indwelling catheter
	Client will attain continence by following nursing care plan and mutually determined goals	Encourage use of clothes that are easily and quickly removed
		Anticipate continence and demonstrate positive attitude
		Encourage return to social activities
		Assist with grooming
		Suggest limited use of sanitary pads for social outings

EVALUATION

1. Urinary incontinence is eliminated or diminished.
2. The client maintains fluid intake at 2000 ml daily.
3. The client exercises consistently and correctly.
4. The client is participating in nursing home activities and maintaining social contacts.
5. The client reports symptoms of urinary tract infection promptly for timely intervention.
6. The client makes positive statements about herself and her ability to care for herself.

NURSING ALERTS

1. Muscle relaxants, sedatives, narcotics, and hypnotics relax urine-controlling muscles and reduce awareness of the need to void.
2. Diuretics increase urine volume, frequency, and urgency.
3. Antidepressants, alcohol, tranquilizers, and antipsychotic drugs reduce the motivation toward continence.
4. Anticholinergics may produce urinary retention.
5. Antihypertensives and calcium channel blockers relax smooth muscles, which may induce urinary incontinence.

Bibliography

Burgio LD, Jones LT, and Engel BT: Studying incontinence in an urban nursing home, Journal of Gerontological Nursing, 14(4):40, 1988.

Carnevali DL and Patrick M: Nursing management for the elderly, Philadelphia, 1986, JB Lippincott Co.

Carpenito LJ: Nursing diagnosis: application to clinical practice, Philadelphia, 1987, JB Lippincott Co.

Cormack D: Geriatric nursing: a conceptual approach, Oxford, England, 1985, Blackwell Scientific Publications.

Gordon M: Manual of nursing diagnosis, 1988-1989, St Louis, 1989, The CV Mosby Co.

Greengold BA and Ouslander JG: Bladder retraining, Journal of Gerontological Nursing, 12(6):31, 1986.

Kim MJ, McFarland GK, and McLane AM: Pocket guide to nursing diagnoses, ed 3, St Louis, 1989, The CV Mosby Co.

Lederer JR, et al: Care planning pocket guide: a nursing diagnosis approach, Menlo Park, Calif, 1988, Addison-Wesley Publishing Co.

Smith D: Continence restoration in homebound, Nursing Clinics of North America 1:207, March 23, 1988.

Taylor K and Henderson J: Effects of biofeedback and urinary stress incontinence in older women, Journal of Gerontological Nursing 12(9):25, 1986.

Turnink PM: Alteration in urinary elimination, Journal of Gerontological Nursing 14(4):25, 1988.

Wells TJ: The rehabilitation management of urinary incontinence, Topics in Geriatric Rehabilitation, vol 3, no. 2, January 1988.

Whitman S and Kursh ED: Curbing incontinence, Journal of Gerontological Nursing 13(4):35, 1987.

Yu LC: Incontinence stress index: measuring psychological impact, Journal of Gerontological Nursing 13(7):18, 1987.

Yu LC et al: Measuring stress associated with incontinence: the ISQ-P tool, Journal of Gerontological Nursing 15(2):9, 1989.

ENDOCRINE, NUTRITIONAL, AND METABOLIC DISEASES

Diabetes Mellitus

Christine Clarkin

KNOWLEDGE BASE

1. There is a greater incidence of diabetes and of glucose intolerance in the population over 65 than in the population as a whole. It is estimated that 15% to 20% of persons over 65 have diabetes.
2. There appears to be decreased production of insulin in advanced age, and less efficient peripheral utilization of insulin.
3. The percentage of body fat normally increases with aging, and this increased adiposity can increase insulin resistance.
4. Changes in diet to more convenient, easy-to-chew, high-fat foods are often preferred by older people. Many do not like to sit down and eat alone; consequently they eat one large meal daily and snack continuously throughout the day.
5. As physical activity decreases with aging, metabolic rates decline and the rate of energy expenditure decreases, as does sensitivity to insulin.
6. The abnormal formation of collagen in persons with diabetes suggests that they are aging at an accelerated rate.
7. Capillary membrane thickening, believed to be responsible for many of the complications of diabetes, is a normal part of the aging process, but it occurs at a more rapid pace in a person with diabetes.
8. The premature atherosclerosis of diabetes is another finding that suggests diabetes causes accelerated aging.
9. Most older people will not present with diabetic ketoacidosis. Many will present with mild symptoms of increased urination, thirst, or increased hunger, associated with an infection such as vaginitis, a furuncle, or a urinary tract or respiratory infection.
10. Most older people will have type II diabetes, which is characterized by insulin resistance, with or without insulin deficiency.
11. Type II diabetes may be present for years before it is recognized. A 2-hour glucose tolerance test is the best vehicle for diagnosing diabetes.
12. In the early stages of type II diabetes the fasting blood glucose level may be within normal limits, while the 2-hour level is elevated. Urine tests do not serve as useful screening tools because the renal threshold tends to increase with age, meaning that the urine will not show glucose until the blood level is very high.
13. Type II diabetes may be managed by a calorie-restricted diet, exercise, and weight loss. If these measures fail to control the blood glucose level, oral hypoglycemic drugs may be used.
14. Sulfonylurea compounds are the class of drugs used in the United States at this time as an adjunct to dietary control. Their dosages, duration of action, and half-lives vary considerably. These drugs are believed to stimulate insulin release by the pancreas temporarily, then increase peripheral utilization of insulin, and decrease hepatic glucose production.
15. Most of the oral hypoglycemic agents must be taken in coordination with food intake, preferably half an hour before meals.
16. If oral hypoglycemic agents do not succeed in lowering the blood glucose to safe levels, the individual may be placed on insulin therapy.

17. Complicated medication and diet plans may be difficult for an elder with memory impairment to manage.
18. Declining financial resources may make it difficult for an elderly person to obtain their medications and appropriate test materials.
19. Decreasing vision resulting from aging and the development of cataracts, one of the consequences of hyperglycemia, may cause a person to make errors in insulin administration, self-monitoring, inspecting the body for sores, and protecting himself or herself from environmental hazards.
20. To be successful in maintaining themselves at home, most older diabetics require an effective network of family, friends, and health care providers.

CASE STUDY

Lila Freeze, a plump 74-year-old, is admitted to the hospital with nausea and vomiting, hyperglycemia, and cellulitis of the left foot. She looks flushed, and her skin and buccal membranes are dry, with moderate tenting of the skin on her forearms. She is weak but able to respond appropriately to assessment questions about her orientation to time and place. Her breathing is not labored, at 26 breaths/min. Her abdomen is soft and protruding, with bowel sounds heard in all four quadrants. She complains of mild tenderness over her low abdomen and states that she has had urinary frequency and urgency for the past week. She has some pretibial edema on both legs, with more pronounced swelling on her left foot from the ankle down. A ¾-inch crack is noted in the heel of her left foot, with no drainage noted. There are numerous fissures on the heel of the right foot, but no redness or drainage. She says the leg has not caused her any pain at all. The nails of both feet are thick and opaque, and the nail beds of her fingers are pale. She has had diabetes for 20 years; for the last 7 years she has been insulin treated. She has not taken her insulin for 3 days. She does own a home glucose meter but has not used it "for weeks." She is taking chlorothiazide (Diuril), 500 mg daily, for her hypertension. Her temperature is 102.6° F, her pulse is full and bounding at 92 beats/min, and her blood pressure is 160/92. Admission laboratory test results are as follows: glucose, 312 mg/dl; sodium, 133 mEq/L; potassium,

3.7 mEq/L; chloride, 97 mEq/L; carbon dioxide, 24 mEq/L; blood urea nitrogen (BUN), 20 mg/dl; creatinine, 1 mg/dl. Her urine shows a trace of protein, hemoglobin, glucose, and ketones, more than 50 WBC's, and 4.32 RBC's. Her hemoglobin is 12.1 g/dl; hematocrit, 36; and white blood cell (WBC) count, 12,800/mm³. Admitting orders include 2000 ml of normal saline given intravenously at 125 ml/hr; vital signs every 4 hours for 2 days; intravenous antibiotics (gentamicin and cefazoxole); bed rest; glucose monitoring before each meal and bed time snack; Diuril (500 mg daily); and an insulin infusion of 50 units of Regular Humulin in 250 ml of normal saline, to infuse to 5 units/25 ml/hr.

Mrs. Freeze tells you that she supports herself and her daughter on her social security income. She has been eating one meal each day at the local senior citizen meal site and snacking for the other two meals. Unable to drive, she has missed eating with her friends and her weekly bridge games. She is a smoker but does not use alcohol.

ASSESSMENT CRITERIA
Physical
Neurological
   Mental alertness, memory, ability to make simple computations
   Response to touch, pain
   Vision changes, blurring, difficulty with accommodation; "floaters or dark threads in line of sight"
Integument
   Dry skin and buccal membranes
   Poor skin turgor
   Soft, dull eyes
   Pretibial edema, pale nail beds
   Hard lumpy areas (lypohypertrophy) resulting from overuse of an area for injections
   Any interruptions in skin integrity
Vital signs
Cardiovascular/respiratory
   Heart sounds
   Shortness of breath
   Presence of cough and sputum production
   Presence of respiratory infection
Gastrointestinal
   Appearance of mouth, teeth, gums, tongue
   Presence of bowel sounds
   Diarrhea, constipation, nausea, vomiting
   Time and content of last meal

Genitourinary
    Frequency, quantity, appearance of urine
    Vaginal itching, symptoms of yeast infection in
      the female
    Impotence in the male
Musculoskeletal
    Muscle tone and strength
    Deformities
    Typical activity pattern, including exercise type
      and amount

Psychosocial

Self-described life-style, health perceptions
Health maintenance behaviors, knowledge of disease
    and treatments
Ability to plan and prepare meals
Presence or absence of adequate support systems
Presence of risk factors (e.g., drinking, smoking)

Spiritual

Inability to participate in or attend religious activities
Feelings of social isolation

Mrs. Freeze's lack of pain in the reddened left foot may indicate loss of sensory function related to diabetic neuropathy.

The dry skin and buccal membranes and poor skin turgor are evidence of fluid deficit. Pretibial edema and pale nail beds are indications of decreased peripheral tissue perfusion. Mrs. Freeze also has skin interruption on the heels of both feet, with the fissure on the left foot running through several skin layers, accompanied by redness and swelling.

Mrs. Freeze's increased pulse rate, blood pressure, and temperature confirm the nursing diagnosis of hyperthermia. Her respiratory rate is elevated at 26 breaths/min, but she does not exhibit the deep, rapid respiratory movements characteristic of Kussmaul respiration.

Because of Mrs. Freeze's age and her hypertension, she is evaluated for evidence of heart failure, with respiratory effort and any rales in her chest being noted. She shows no problem in this area.

The presence of bowel sounds indicates that peristalsis is present. Mrs. Freeze's nausea and vomiting are indications of fluid deficit. Her habits of eating only one meal per day and snacking the rest of the day may result in consumption of nutritionally inadequate foods and a high calorie intake.

Mrs. Freeze's history of urinary frequency is a further indication of fluid deficit. It may be a consequence of hyperglycemia or a urinary tract infection.

The obvious deformities in the feet may have occurred with aging or as a result of long-standing diabetes. Asking her about the number of hours spent watching television may provide information indicating a sedentary life style.

Mrs. Freeze's failure to use the glucose meter may be a result of lack of knowledge, or it may be the result of her having inadequate funds to purchase strips for her meter. This situation may be regarded as evidence to support the nursing diagnoses of altered health maintenance. Mrs. Freeze's eating habits may be due to lack of knowledge about the importance of diet to diabetes control or may be due to her lack of needed resources for food preparation. The fact that Mrs. Freeze is on a fixed income and supporting her daughter may indicate that she will need financial support on her return home.

Mrs. Freeze feels isolated from her friends and community as a result of her foot problem and consequent immobility.

NURSING CARE PLAN: DIABETES MELLITUS

Nursing diagnoses	Expected client outcomes	Nursing strategies
Hyperthermia	Client will have normal body temperature	Monitor blood pressure, pulse, and respiration every 4 hours Administer antipyrretics for temperature elevation Keep room cool
Impaired skin integrity	Client will have skin intact with resolution of erythema Client will utilize methods for reducing swelling Client will visually inspect feet and will use appropriate footwear	Assess wound and surrounding skin every 4 hours Avoid prolonged soaking of feet Apply lotion to dry skin twice a day Instruct client not to walk barefooted at any time Instruct client to keep feet and legs level with body to reduce swelling Encourage client to stay off her feet until they heal, avoiding walking, running, etc., as much as possible Teach client and her daughter to check client's feet for sores, cracks, etc., and to check footwear for cracks or rough areas that may injure her feet
Altered health maintenance related to sick day management of diabetes: Lack of glucose monitoring Omission of insulin dose for two days	Client and daughter will state sick day rules and will describe the appropriate actions to take when client is ill and unable to eat Client will be able to use the glucose meter correctly and will state that she will call physician if blood glucose results are >300 or urine ketone check is positive	Assess client and daughter's present knowledge of sick day management and what they want to know Determine if client and daughter need information or assistance in applying information Utilize written charts and audiovisual materials when instructing client and daughter Teach client and daughter the rules of sick day management; explain the importance of following through with client's treatment even if she is ill and unable to eat Have client demonstrate testing her own blood and urine; instruct client to contact physician if blood glucose results are >300 or urine ketone check is positive Allow client and daughter to practice applying sick day rules Provide client with a copy of discharge guidelines covering medications, treatments, and dietary instructions
Altered health maintenance related to diabetes complications	Client's health maintenance measures will be restored: Sustains no further injury to feet Monitors blood glucose and urine as instructed Takes her insulin as directed Gets adequate nutrition Monitors hypertension with daily blood pressure checks Takes Diuril as directed for hypertension	Evaluate client's willingness and ability to inspect her feet daily; evaluate availability of suitable footwear Evaluate and support as client monitors blood glucose and urine ketones as instructed Advise client never to omit insulin without calling physician Evaluate ability of client's daughter to assist in food preparation and obtain food Instruct client and daughter in procedure for checking blood pressure and recording results; evaluate systems used for remembering blood pressure medicine

NURSING CARE PLAN: DIABETES MELLITUS—cont'd

Nursing diagnoses	Expected client outcomes	Nursing strategies
	Establishes adequate support systems	Explore additional available resources for client, such as home health nurses Provide client with guidelines for health maintenance: when to call physician for emergencies; visiting primary physician every 3 months, ophthalmologist and dentist yearly
Social isolation related to foot problems inability to drive and to participate in communal meals and bridge games with friends	Client will experience relief from feelings of isolation and will take steps to reestablish contact with her bridge and lunch companions	Encourage client to express feelings and concerns Encourage client to maintain phone contact with her friends Explore with client the possibility of having her friends join her in her home for a meal or bridge game, with her friends bringing food with them Explore client's spiritual concerns (e.g., her contacts, if any, with a church group in her area)

EVALUATION

1. The client has adequate tissue perfusion, as evidenced by the following: blood pressure, pulse, and respiration within client's normal ranges; skin warm, dry, and usual color; usual mental status being maintained; decreased signs of redness and swelling of the feet.
2. The client discusses a plan to reduce her smoking.
3. Client and daughter demonstrate the checking of blood pressure and state the importance of taking blood pressure medication as directed.
4. The client establishes adequate hydration, as evidenced by the following: no further vomiting; urine output greater than 30 ml/hr; fluid intake greater than output; improved skin turgor; stable weight; moist tongue and buccal membranes; BUN, creatinine, sodium, chloride, and potassium within normal limits; blood glucose less than 180 mg/dl.
5. The client's body temperature has returned to normal.
6. The client's skin is intact; her wound exhibits decreased swelling and redness and no drainage.
7. The client keeps her feet and legs elevated to reduce swelling.
8. Client and daughter demonstrate proper care for the wound.
9. The client uses appropriate footwear.
10. Client and daughter are able to state the rules of sick day management and state that they will obtain the needed supplies for use at home.
11. The client demonstrates correct testing of her blood and urine and states that she will call her physician if her blood glucose results are greater than 300 or if a urine ketone check is positive.
12. The client describes a plan to continue health maintenance measures after discharge, including caring for feet and using appropriate footwear, monitoring blood glucose and urine ketones as instructed, taking her insulin as instructed, making plans for meal management, and contacting available resources for assistance.
13. The client expresses relief of feelings of isolation. She reestablishes contact with her friends by telephoning them and considers options for meeting with friends while she is confined to her home. She explores available community resources, with the intent of easing her isolation.

NURSING ALERTS

1. The complications of diabetes may tip a client over to incontinence at the same time that further alterations in vision or neuropathic changes may place him or her at increased risk for falls.
2. The impact of other diseases—for example, arthritis—on diabetes may range from difficulty with preparing food to problems with drawing up insulin or operating a portable glucose meter.
3. Although home monitoring of blood glucose levels has been a tremendous help to many people with diabetes, it is not universally appropriate for elders with diabetes. Elderly clients need careful evaluation and assistance to determine which, if any, of the home blood glucose meters are appropriate for their use. Monitoring supplies are costly, ranging from 50 to 75 cents per test, 2 dollars per day for some individuals. Fixed incomes and limited financial reserves may make home blood glucose monitoring impractical for many older diabetics.

4. Chlorothiazide (Diuril) is an effective antihypertensive agent, often used as a first choice in treating hypertension in diabetics. Thiazide diuretics may cause increased insulin resistance and consequent increases in blood glucose levels. Expect increased blood glucose levels if dosages of thiazide diuretics are increased, and decreasing blood glucose levels as dosages are tapered.

5. A regular exercise program, consistent with each client's physical ability, is an essential factor in controlling blood glucose levels and in preventing obesity, improving cardiovascular status, and helping prevent depression. Coexisting medical problems, such as heart disease, arthritis, and peripheral vascular disease, must be considered when an exercise program is recommended to the elderly diabetic. Clients with open lesions on their feet are usually advised against any exercises that depend on weight bearing.

6. Dietary restrictions that are established with patience, and in a manner that considers the individual's life-style and resources, will be more likely to meet with success. Approaches that emphasize the negative concept of "cheating" will arouse guilt and defensiveness in clients and will rarely accomplish desired behavior changes.

7. Hyperosmolar nonketotic syndrome (HNKS) can be a serious threat to older diabetic clients. Age-related changes in the kidney, a higher thirst threshold, and decreased body water predispose older clients to this syndrome. Clients who cannot complain of thirst, those who are unable to obtain needed fluids, and those who are oversedated are particularly prone to this crisis. Frequent physician contact and periodic glucose and metabolic evaluation should help prevent HNKS.

Bibliography

Baker DE: New drug evaluation: nicarpidine, Practical Diabetology 2(3):13, 1989.

Carpenito LJ: Nursing diagnosis: application to clinical practice, Philadelphia, 1983, JB Lippincott Co.

Davidson, MB: Conclusions: aging—relation to diabetes and carbohydrate metabolism, Diabetes Spectrum 2(3):191, 1989.

Holvey M: Psychosocial aspects in the care of elderly diabetic patients, American Journal of Medicine, 80 (Suppl 5A) 1:54, May 16, 1986.

Kim MJ, McFarland GK, and McLane AM: Pocket guide to nursing diagnoses, ed 3, St Louis, 1989, The CV Mosby Co.

Laufer IJ: Diabetes in the elderly, Practical Diabetology, May-June 1985, p 7.

Lipson LG: Diabetes mellitus in the elderly: special problems, special approaches, New York, 1985, Pfizer, Inc, and Medica, Inc.

Levin RF et al: Diagnostic content validity of nursing diagnoses, Image: Journal of Nursing Scholarship 21(1):40, 1989.

Matz R: Diabetes mellitus in the elderly, Hospital Practice 21(3):195, 1986.

Puderbaugh U et al: Nursing care planning guides: a nursing diagnoses approach, Philadelphia, 1986, WB Saunders Co.

Yura H and Walsh MB: The nursing process, ed 5, Norwalk, Conn, 1988, Appleton & Lange.

Appendix

A

Alphabetical List of NANDA-Accepted Diagnoses

Activity intolerance
Activity intolerance, potential
Adjustment, impaired
Airway clearance, ineffective
Anxiety
Aspiration, potential for
Body image disturbance
Body temperature, altered, potential
Breastfeeding, effective
Breastfeeding, ineffective
Breathing pattern, ineffective
Cardiac output, decreased
Communication, impaired verbal
Constipation
Constipation, colonic
Constipation, perceived
Coping, defensive
Coping, family: potential for growth
Coping, ineffective family: compromised
Coping, ineffective family: disabling
Coping, ineffective individual
Decisional conflict (specify)
Denial, ineffective
Diarrhea
Disuse syndrome, potential for
Diversional activity deficit
Dysreflexia
Family processes, altered
Fatigue
Fear
Fluid volume deficit (1)
Fluid volume deficit (2)
Fluid volume deficit, potential
Fluid volume excess
Gas exchange, impaired

Grieving, anticipatory
Grieving, dysfunctional
Growth and development, altered
Health maintenance, altered
Health seeking behaviors (specify)
Home maintenance management, impaired
Hopelessness
Hyperthermia
Hypothermia
Incontinence, bowel
Incontinence, functional
Incontinence, reflex
Incontinence, stress
Incontinence, total
Incontinence, urge
Infection, potential for
Injury, potential for
Knowledge deficit (specify)
Mobility, impaired physical
Noncompliance (specify)
Nutrition, altered: less than body requirements
Nutrition, altered: more than body requirements
Nutrition, altered: potential for more than body
  requirements
Oral mucous membrane, altered
Pain
Pain, chronic
Parental role conflict
Parenting, altered
Parenting, altered, potential
Personal identity disturbance
Poisoning, potential for
Post-trauma response
Powerlessness
Protection, altered

From the Proceedings of the Eighth National Conference of the North American Nursing Diagnosis Association held in St. Louis, Missouri, March 13-16, 1988. Reflects revised taxonomy, Fall 1988.

Rape-trauma syndrome
Rape-trauma syndrome: compound reaction
Rape-trauma syndrome: silent reaction
Role performance, altered
Self care deficit, bathing/hygiene
Self care deficit, dressing/grooming
Self care deficit, feeding
Self care deficit, toileting
Self-esteem disturbance
Self-esteem, chronic low
Self-esteem, situational low
Sensory/perceptual alterations (specify) (visual,
  auditory, kinesthetic, gustatory, tactile, olfactory)
Sexual dysfunction
Sexuality patterns, altered
Skin integrity, impaired
Skin integrity, impaired, potential
Sleep pattern disturbance

Social interaction, impaired
Social isolation
Spiritual distress (distress of the human spirit)
Suffocation, potential for
Swallowing, impaired
Thermoregulation, ineffective
Thought processes, altered
Tissue integrity, impaired
Tissue perfusion, altered (specify type) (renal,
  cerebral; cardiopulmonary, gastrointestinal,
  peripheral)
Trauma, potential for
Unilateral neglect
Urinary elimination, altered patterns
Urinary retention
Violence, potential for: self-directed or directed at
  others

Appendix

B

Preventive Health History Form

1. Name _____ ( ) 2. Sex M _____ F _____ ( )
   Address _____
3. Date _____ / _____ / _____ ( )
       Month   Date   Year
4. Age _____ ( ) 5. Place of birth _____ ( )
6. Current doctor:
   Name _____ Phone # _____
   Address _____ ( )
7. Who to contact in case of emergency:
   Name _____ Phone # _____ ( )
   Relationship _____ ( )
   Address _____
8. Religion _____ ( )
9. Marital status _____ ( )
10. Whom do you live with? Check all that are appropriate:
    Friend _____ Spouse _____ Children _____ Other _____
             ( )   ( )   ( )   ( )
11. How many children do you have? _____ ( )
12. If you have any children, do they live nearby? Yes _____ No _____ ( )
                                                        (1)   (0)
13. Is your mother alive? Yes _____ No _____ ( )
                              (1)   (0)
14. If not, cause of death _____ ( )
15. Is your father alive? Yes _____ No _____ ( )
                              (1)   (0)
16. If not, cause of death _____ ( )
17. Do you have any brothers or sisters? Yes _____ No _____ ( )
                                              (1)   (0)
18. If yes, do they live nearby? Yes _____ No _____ ( )
                                      (1)   (0)
19. If they are no longer alive, please give the causes of their death:

    _____ ( )
20. Have you had any formal education beyond high school? Yes _____ No _____ ( )
21. Your occupation/profession is (was) _____ ( )
22. Are you retired? Yes _____ No _____ ( )
                          (1)   (0)
23. If not retired, are you working part-time? Yes _____ No _____ ( )
                                                    (1)   (0)
24. How do you usually get around? _____ ( )
25. Your last medical checkup was _____ / _____ ( )

From Kopf R, Salamon, MJ, and Charytan P: Journal of Gerontological Nursing 8:521, 1982.

26. Rate your general health:
Excellent _____ Good _____ Poor _____ ( )

27. List any illnesses that seem to run in your family.
_____
_____ ( )

28. Have you ever been hospitalized? Yes _____ No _____ ( )
If yes, how many times? _____ ( )
Give the dates and reasons for your hospitalization:
Date _____ / _____ ( )   Reason _____ ( )
     Month   Year
Date _____ / _____ ( )   Reason _____ ( )
     Month   Year
Date _____ / _____ ( )   Reason _____ ( )
     Month   Year

29. Have you ever had any operations (other than those listed above)?
Yes _____ No _____ ( )
   (1)   (0)
If yes, give the dates and types of operations:
Date _____ / _____ ( )   Type of operation _____ ( )
     Month   Year
Date _____ / _____ ( )   Type of operation _____ ( )
     Month   Year

30. Have you ever had any accidents or injuries (other than listed above)?
Yes _____ No _____ ( )
   (1)   (0)
If yes, give the dates and kind of accident or injury:
Date _____ / _____ ( )   Kind _____ ( )
     Month   Year
Date _____ / _____ ( )   Kind _____ ( )
     Month   Year

31. Do you have any of the following? If yes, check as many as apply.

Heart disease _____	Breathing problems _____	Bladder problems _____
Rheumatic fever _____	Osteoarthritis _____	Kidney problems _____
High blood pressure _____	Rheumatoid arthritis _____	Prostate problems _____
Stroke _____	Tuberculosis _____	Change of life
Leg cramps _____	Diabetes _____	symptoms _____
Bronchitis _____	Cancer _____	Nervousness _____
Angina _____	Thyroid _____	Headaches _____
Heart attack _____	Fever _____	Bleeding _____
Dizziness _____	Ulcers _____	Colitis _____
Asthma _____	Sinus problems _____	Falling _____
Seizures _____	Yellow eyes or skin _____	Other (explain) _____
Sadness _____	Anemia _____	
Gout _____	Diverticulitis _____	

32. Do you have any allergies? If yes, please check as many as apply.
Food _____ Drugs _____ Pollen _____ Other _____ ( )
    ( )   ( )   ( )   ( )

33. Are there any foods you can't eat? If yes, what are they?
_____ ( )

34. Do you have visual problems? Yes _____ No _____ ( )
                      (1)   (0)

35. Do you wear glasses? Yes _____ No _____ ( )
               (1)   (0)

36. Has there been any change in your vision recently? Yes _____ No _____ ( )
                                    (1)   (0)

37. When was your last examination? _____ / _____ ( )
                          Month   Year

38. Do you wear dentures? Yes _____ No _____ ( )
                 (1)   (0)

39. Do you have any problems with your teeth? Yes _____ No _____ ( )
                             (1)   (0)

40. Your last visit to the dentist was _____ / _____ ( )
                        Month   Year

41. How many glasses of wine, beer, or other alcohol do you drink a day? _____ ( )

42. Do you smoke? Yes _____ No _____ ( )
           (1)   (0)

43. How many cups of coffee do you drink a day? _____ ( )

44. How many cups of tea do you drink a day? _____ ( )

45. How many cups of cola do you drink a day? _____ ( )

46. Do you take any vitamins? Yes _____ No _____ ( )
                 (1)   (0)

47. If yes, what kind? _____ ( )

48. Do you exercise regularly? Yes _____ No _____ ( )
                 (1)   (0)

49. Has your weight changed recently? Yes _____ No _____ ( )
    ₍₁₎   ₍₀₎

50. Do you have any trouble sleeping? Yes _____ No _____ ( )
    ₍₁₎   ₍₀₎

51. Please list the foods that you eat on an average day, by meal.
    Breakfast _____   Lunch _____   Dinner _____
    _____   _____   _____
    _____   _____   _____

52. Do you take any of the following? If yes, check as many as apply.
    Sleeping pills _____   Blood pressure pills _____
    Nerve pills _____   Hormones _____
    Water pills _____   Heart pills _____
    Thyroid pills _____   Laxatives _____
    Aspirin/Tylenol _____   Cold/allergy pills _____
    Mylanta/Maalox _____   Sugar/diabetic pills _____
    Any other? Please list _____

53. Are the medications you take prescribed by your doctor?
    Yes _____ No _____ ( )
    ₍₁₎   ₍₀₎

54. What kind of home remedies do you use? _____
    _____
    _____

55. Please describe what you do on an average day using the times below:
    Awakening _____
    Morning _____
    Afternoon _____
    Evening _____

56. Do you feel that your present affection needs are satisfied?
    Yes _____ No _____ ( )
    ₍₁₎   ₍₀₎

57. If you wish to make any comment about the questionnaire, please use the remaining space.

Appendix
C

Normal Physical Assessment Findings in the Elderly

Cardiovascular changes

Cardiac output	Heart loses elasticity; therefore decreased heart contractility in response to increased demands
Arterial circulation	Decreased vessel compliance with increased peripheral resistance to blood flow resulting from general or localized arteriosclerosis
Arterial circulation	Decreased vessel compliance with increased peripheral resistance to blood flow resulting from general or localized arteriosclerosis
Venous circulation	Does not exhibit change with aging in the absence of disease
Blood pressure	Significant increase in the systolic, slight increase in the diastolic, increase in peripheral resistance and pulse pressure
Heart	Dislocation of the apex because of kyphoscoliosis; therefore diagnostic significance of location is lost
	Increased premature beats, rarely clinically important
Murmurs	Diastolic murmurs in over half the aged; the most common heard at the base of the heart because of sclerotic changes on the aortic valves
Peripheral pulses	Easily palpated because of increased arterial wall narrowing and loss of connective tissue: feeling of tortuous and rigid vessels
	Possibility that pedal pulses may be weaker as a result of arteriosclerotic changes; colder lower extremities, especially at night; possibility of cold feet and hands with mottled color
Heart rate	No changes with age at normal rest

Respiratory changes

Pulmonary blood flow and diffusion	Decreased blood flow to the pulmonary circulation; decreased diffusion
Anatomic structure	Increased anterior-posterior diameter
Respiratory accessory muscles	Degeneration and decreased strength: increased rigidity of chest wall
	Muscle atrophy of pharynx and larynx
Internal pulmonic structure	Decreased pulmonary elasticity creates senile emphysema
	Shorter breaths taken with decreased maximum breathing capacity, vital capacity, residual volume, and functional capacity
	Airway resistance increases: less ventilation at the bases of the lung and more at the apex

Data from Malasanos L et al: Health assessment, ed 3, St Louis, 1985, The CV Mosby Co; Blake D: Physiology and Aging Seminar for Nurses, Napa, Calif, May 1979; and Wardell S, editor: Acute interventions: nursing process throughout the life span, Reston Va, 1979, Reston Publishing Co.

Integumentary changes

Texture	Skin loses elasticity; wrinkles, folding, sagging, dryness
Color	Spotty pigmentation in areas exposed to sun; face paler, even in the absence of anemia
Temperature	Extremities cooler; decreased perspiration
Fat distribution	Less on extremities; more on trunk
Hair Color	Dull gray, white, yellow, or yellow-green
Hair distribution	Thins on scalp, axilla, pubic area, upper and lower extremities; decreased facial hair in men, women may develop chin and upper lip hair
Nails	Decreased growth rate

Genitourinary and reproductive changes

Renal blood flow	Because of decreased cardiac output, reduced filtration rate and renal efficiency; possibility of subsequent loss of protein from kidneys
Micturition	In men possibility of increased frequency as a result of prostatic enlargement
	In women decreased perineal muscle tone; therefore urgency and stress incontinence
	Increased nocturia for both men and women
	Possibility that polyuria may be diabetes related
	Decreased volume of urine may relate to decrease in intake but evaluation needed
Incontinence	Increased occurrence with age, specifically in those with dementia
Male reproduction	
Testosterone production	Decreases; phases of intercourse slower, lengthened refractory time
Frequency of intercourse	No changes in libido and sexual satisfaction; decreased frequency to one or two times weekly
Testes	Decreased size; decreased sperm count; diminished viscosity of seminal fluid
Female reproduction	
Estrogen	Decreased production with menopause
Breasts	Diminished breast tissue
Uterus	Decreased size; mucous secretions cease; possibility that uterine prolapse may occur as a result of muscle weakness
Vagina	Epithelial lining atrophies; narrow and shortened canal
Vaginal secretions	Become more alkaline as glycogen content increases and acidity declines

Gastrointestinal changes

Mastication	Impaired because of partial or total loss of teeth, malocclusive bite, and ill-fitting dentures
Swallowing and carbohydrate digestion	Swallowing more difficult as salivary secretions diminish
Esophagus	Decreased esophageal peristalis
	Increased incidence of hiatus hernia with accompanying gaseous distention
Digestive enzymes	Decreased production of hydrochloric acid, pepsin, and pancreatic enzymes
Fat absorption	Delayed, affecting the absorption rate of fat-soluble vitamins A, D, E, and K
Intestinal peristalsis	Reduced gastrointestinal motility
	Constipation because of decreased motility and roughage

Musculoskeletal changes

Muscle strength and function	Decrease with loss of muscle mass; bony prominences normal in aged, since muscle mass decreased
Bone structure	Normal demineralization, more porous
	Shortening of the trunk as a result of intevertebral space narrowing
Joints	Become less mobile; tightening and fixation occur
	Activity may maintain function longer
	Normal posture changes; some kyphosis
	Range of motion limited
Anatomic size and height	Total decrease in size as loss of body protein and body water occurs in proportion to decrease in basal metabolic rate
	Increased body fat; diminished in arms and legs, increased in trunk
	Decreased height from 2.5 to 10 cm from young adulthood

Nervous system changes

Response to stimuli	All voluntary or automatic reflexes slower
	Decreased ability to respond to multiple stimuli
Sleep patterns	Stage IV sleep reduced in comparison to younger adulthood; increased frequency of spontaneous awakening
	Stay in bed longer but get less sleep; insomnia a problem, which should be evaluated

Reflexes	Deep tendon reflexes responsive in the healthy aged
Ambulation	Kinesthetic sense less efficient; may demonstrate an extrapyramidal Parkinson-like gait
	Basal ganglions of the nervous system influenced by the vascular changes and decreased oxygen supply
Voice	Decreased range, duration, and intensity of voice; may become higher pitched and monotonous

Sensory changes

Vision	
Peripheral vision	Decreases
Lens accommodation	Decreases, requires corrective lenses
Ciliary body	Atrophy in accommodation of lens focus
Iris	Development of arcus senilis
Choroid	Atrophy around disk
Lens	May develop opacity, cataract formation; more light necessary to see
Color	Fades or disappears
Macula	Degenerates
Conjunctiva	Thins and looks yellow
Tearing	Decreases; increased irritation and infection
Pupil	May differ in size
Cornea	Presence of arcus senilis
Retina	Observable vascular changes
Stimuli threshold	Increased threshold for light touch and pain
	Ischemic paresthesias common in the extremities
Hearing	Less perceptible high-frequency tones, hence greatly impaired language understanding; promotes confusion and seems to create increased rigidity in thought processes
Gustatory	Decreased acuity as taste buds atrophy; may increase the amount of seasoning on food

Appendix

D

How Illness Changes with Age

Problem	Classic presentation in young patient	Presentation in elderly
Urinary tract infection	Dysuria, frequency, urgency, nocturia	Dysuria often *absent*, frequency, urgency, nocturia sometimes present. Incontinence, confusion, anorexia are other signs.
Myocardial infarction	Severe substernal chest pain, diaphoresis, nausea, shortness of breath	Sometimes no chest pain, or atypical pain location such as in jaw, neck, shoulder. Shortness of breath may be present. Other signs are tachypnea, arrhythmia, hypotension, restlessness, syncope.
Pneumonia (bacterial)	Cough productive of purulent sputum, chills and fever, pleuritic chest pain, elevated white blood count.	Cough may be productive, dry or absent; chills and fever and/or elevated white count also may be absent. Tachypnea, slight cyanosis, confusion, anorexia, nausea and vomiting, tachycardia may be present.
Congestive heart failure	Increased dyspnea (orthopnea, paroxysmal nocturnal dyspnea), fatigue, weight gain, pedal edema, night cough and nocturia, bibasilar rales	All of the manifestations of young adult and/or anorexia, restlessness, confusion, cyanosis, falls.
Hyperthyroidism	Heat intolerance, fast pace, exophthalmos, increased pulse, hyperreflexia, tremor.	Slowing down (apathetic hyperthyroidism), lethargy, weakness, depression, atrial fibrillation and congestive heart failure.
Depression	Sad mood and thoughts, withdrawal, crying, weight loss, constipation, insomnia.	Any of classic, plus memory and concentration problems, weight gain, increased sleep.

Appendix
E

Home Assessment Checklist

GENERAL HOUSEHOLD

1. Is there good lighting available, especially around stairwells?
2. Are there handrails (which can be easily grasped) on both sides of the staircases, designed to indicate when top and bottom steps have been reached?
3. Are top and bottom steps painted in easily seen colors? Are nonskid treads used?
4. Are the edges of rugs tacked down? (Suggest the use of wall-to-wall carpeting.)
5. Is a telephone present? Does the telephone have a dial that is easily readable? Are emergency numbers written in large print and kept near the telephone?
6. Are electrical cords, footstools, and other low-lying objects kept out of walkways?
7. Are electrical cords in good condition?
8. Is furniture arranged to allow for free movement in heavily traveled areas?
9. Is furniture sturdy enough to give support?
10. Is furniture designed to accommodate easy transfers on and off?
11. Is the temperature of the home within a comfortable range?
12. If fireplaces or other heating devices are present, do they have protective screens?
13. Are smoke detectors present (especially in the kitchen and bedroom)?
14. Are rapidly closing doors eliminated?
15. Are there alternative exits from the house?

From Tideiksaar R: New York, 1983, Ritter Department of Geriatrics and Adult Development, The Mount Sinai Medical Center.

16. Are basements and attics easy to get to, well lighted, and well ventilated?
17. Are slippers and shoes in good repair? Do they fit properly and have nonskid soles?

KITCHEN

18. Are there loose extension cords, small sliding rugs, slippery linoleum tiles present? (Suggest the use of rubber-backed, nonskid rugs and nonskid floor wax.)
19. Is the cooking stove gas or electric?
20. Are there large easily readable dials present on the stove or other appliances, with the "on" and "off" positions clearly marked?
21. Are refrigerators in good working order? Are refrigerators placed on 18-inch platforms to avoid bending over?
22. Are spaces for food storage adequate? Are shelves at eye level and easily reachable?
23. Is a sturdy stepladder present for reaching?
24. Are electrical circuits overloaded with too many appliances?
25. Are electrical appliances disconnected when not in use?
26. Are sharp objects (such as carving knives) kept in special holders?
27. Are cleaning fluids, polishes, bleaches, detergents, and all poisons stored separately and clearly marked?
28. Are kitchen chairs sturdy, with arm rests with high backs?
29. Is stove free from flammable objects?
30. Are pot holders available for removing pots and pans from the stove?
31. Is baking soda available in case of fire?

BATHROOM

32. Are there grab bars in the bath, in the shower, and around the toilet?
33. Are toilet seats high enough to get on and off of without difficulty?
34. Can the bathroom door be easily closed to ensure privacy? (Avoid locks.)
35. Are bathroom doorways wide enough for easy wheelchair and walker access?
36. Are there nonskid rubber mats in the bath, in the shower, and on the floor?
37. Is there good lighting in the area of the medicine cabinet?
38. Are internal and external medications stored separately? And safely (especially important with young grandchildren present in the house)?
39. Do medication containers have childproof tops? Are they labeled in large print? Is a magnifying glass present for reading medication instructions?
40. Have all outdated medications been discarded?
41. Do you notice any medications (both prescription and over-the-counter) that could cause adverse side effects or drug-drug interactions that the patient is unaware of?
42. Can the water temperature be easily regulated?
43. Are electrical cords, outlets, and appliances a safe distance from the tub?
44. Are razor blades kept in a safe place?
45. Is a first aid kit available?

BEDROOM

46. Is there adequate lighting from the bedside to the bathroom?
47. Are lights easily accessible? (If not, suggest keeping a flashlight by the bedside or using a flashlight for entry into dark rooms if light switch is not within easy reach.)
48. Are beds in good repair?
49. Are beds at the proper height to allow for easy transfer on and off without difficulty?
50. Do bedroom rugs have nonskid rubber backings?

Appendix

F

Assessment and Interventions for Patients at Risk to Falls

Goal/outcome: the patient will remain free of injury during hospital stay.
Nursing diagnosis: potential for injury (trauma)

Risk factors	Nursing interventions
1) History of Previous Falls	1) Assess previous pattern of falling and establish safety guidelines with patient and family.
	2) Orient to environment
	—Free environment from obstacles
	—Nurse call system demonstrated
	—Use of bathroom explained
2) Mental Status	1) Mental status assessment
Disoriented	2) Repeatedly reinforce activity limits and safety needs to patient/family
Confused	
Unable to make purposeful decisions	3) Involve family as much as possible
	4) Move patient closer to nurses' station
	5) Recommend safety belt if needed
	6) Assess need for sitter supervision
	7) Instruct sitter in individualized patient needs
3) Mobility Deficits	1) Assess patient's ambulatory status (have patient walk for you)
General debility	2) Provide for safe environment
Hemiparesis	—Bed in low position, brakes locked
Paraparesis	—No unnecessary furniture
Hemiplegic	—Side rails up if applicable
Paraplegic	—Nightlights—at bedside and in bathroom
Ataxia	—Nonskid footwear
Use of cane	—Call light (communication system) within easy reach and working
Use of crutches	—Assistive device in reach
Amputee	

From Spellbring A et al: Improving safety for hospitalized elderly, *Journal of Gerontological Nursing*, vol 14, no 2.
* This tool incorporates the nursing diagnosis: Potential for Injury. Risk factors to falls are the defining characteristics for the nursing diagnosis. The interventions are directed toward decreasing each risk factor. The outcome is to keep the patient free of injury during his length of stay. This tool can become a nursing standard to establish a protocol for a fall prevention policy.

The Fall Precaution Checklist incorporates the possible high risk areas for falls as well as safety interventions that can be implemented and documented. This flow sheet can be kept at the patient's bedside for use by all staff members. Due to the legal implications of this form if it is implemented, it needs to be piloted and approved for use in each institution.

Risk factors	Nursing interventions
4) Communication Deficits Dysarthric Aphasic No verbal response Foreign language	1) Assess patient's communication pattern 2) Establish effective communication system with patient. Use of visual aids, bells, etc. 3) Make frequent patient rounds 4) Provide interpreter for foreign language patient
5) Sensory Deficits Blind OS Blind OD Blind OU Use of glasses, contacts Blurred vision Postoperative eye	1) Assess vision in non-affected eye 2) Check effectiveness of eyeglasses 3) Poster in room indicating sensory deficit
6) Medications Diuretics Laxatives Barbiturates Tranquilizers Pain Meds Hypnotics Antihypertensives Eye gtts Sleeping Meds Anesthetics	1) Evaluate patient's medications—appropriate dosages 2) Assess risk of side effects particularly drug-associated hypotensive episodes—alert patients to side effects 3) Check for use of laxatives and diuretics 4) Be particularly aware of drug side effects in elderly or postop patients 5) Observe mobility patterns post-anesthesia
7) Urinary Alterations Urgency Frequency Use of BR at night	1) Assess usual pattern of urination 2) Plan individualized toileting schedule 3) Assess need for bedside commode, texas catheter, bed pan
8) Auditory Deficits Use of Hearing Aid Deaf (R) Ear Dear (L) Ear	1) Assess patient's ability to hear 2) Check effectiveness of hearing aid-batteries available 3) Speak as loudly as needed to communicate 4) Poster in room indicating sensory deficit
9) Improper Fitting Footwear	1) Check slippers for fit, safety, non-skid
10) Emotional Upset Loss of significant object	1) Mental status assessment 2) Evaluate patient's ability to interpret information given him/her
11) Presence of Orthostasis Hypotension	1) Determine history of problem 2) Teach patient to ambulate in stages 3) Elastic stockings 4) Teach patient to make position changes slowly

Appendix

G

Tinetti Gait and Balance Scale

Balance

Instructions: subject is seated in hard armless chair; the following maneuvers are tested.

1. Sitting balance

Leans or slides in chair = 0
Steady, safe = 1

2. Arise

Unable without help = 0
Able but uses arm to help = 1
Able without use of arms = 2

3. Attempts to arise

Unable without help = 0
Able, but requires more than one attempt = 1
Able to arise with one attempt = 2

4. Immediate standing balance (first 5 seconds)

Unsteady, staggers, moves feet & marked trunk sways = 0
Steady but uses walker, cane, or grabs for support = 1
Steady without support = 2

5. Standing balance

Unsteady = 0
Steady but wide stance (medial heel >4 inches apart)
or uses cane, walker, or other support = 1
Narrow stance without support = 2

6. Nudge (subject at maximum position with feet as
close together as possible; examiner pushes lightly on
subject's sternum with palm of hand three times)

Begins to fall = 0
Staggers, grabs but catches self = 1
Steady = 2

7. Eyes closed (at maximum position in #6)

Unsteady = 0
Steady = 1

8. Turn 360°

Discontinuous steps = 0
Continuous = 1
Unsteady (grabs, staggers) = 0
Steady = 1

From Tinetti M, Speechley M, and Ginter S: Risk factors for falls among elderly persons living in the community, New England Journal of Medicine, December 29, 1988.

9. Sit down

Unsafe (misjudges distance, falls into chair)	= 0
Uses arms or not a smooth motion	= 1
Safe, smooth motion	= 2

BALANCE SCORE: /16

Gait

Instructions: subject stands with examiner; walks down hallway at his/her "usual pace," then back at "rapid but safe" pace (using usual walking aid)

10. Initiation of gait (immediately after told to "GO")

Any hesitancy or multiple attempts to start = 0
No hesitancy = 1

11. Step length and height
    a. Right swing foot

Does not pass left stance foot with step = 0
Passes left stance foot = 1
Right foot does not clear floor completely with step = 0
Right foot completely clears floor = 1

    b. Left swing foot

Does not pass right stance foot with step = 0
Passses right stance foot = 1
Left foot does not clear floor completely with step = 0
Left foot completely clears floor = 1

12. Step symmetry

Right and left step length not equal (estimate) = 0
Right and left step appear equal = 1

13. Step continuity

Stopping or discontinuity between steps = 0
Steps appear continuous = 1

14. Path (estimate in relation to floor tiles; observe the excursion of one foot about 10 feet of course)

Marked deviation = 0
Mild/moderate deviation or uses walking aid = 1
Straight without walking aid = 2

15. Trunk

Marked sway or uses walking aid = 0
No sway but flexion of knees or back or spread arms = 1
No sway, flexion, use of arms or walking aid = 2

16. Walk stance

Heels apart = 0
Heels almost touching while walking = 1

GAIT SCORE: /12
TOTAL SCORE: /28

NAME: _____ CHART #: _____ DATE: _____

Appendix

H

Functional Assessment Stages (FAST) in Normal Aging and Alzheimer's Disease

Global deterioration scale	Clinical phase	FAST characteristics
1, No cognitive decline	Normal	No functional decrement—either subjectively or objectively—manifest.
2, Very mild cognitive decline	Forgetfulness	Complains of forgetting location of objects; subjective work difficulties.
3, Mild cognitive decline	Early confusional	Decreased functioning in demanding employment settings evident to co-workers; difficulty in traveling to new locations.
4, Moderate cognitive decline	Late confusional	Decreased ability to perform complex tasks such as planning dinner for guests, handling finances, and marketing.
5, Moderately severe cognitive decline	Early dementia	Requires assistance in choosing proper clothing; may require coaxing to bathe properly.
6, Severe cognitive decline	Middle dementia	(a) Difficulty putting on clothing properly (b) Requires assistance bathing; may develop fear of bathing (c) Inability to handle mechanics of toileting (d) Urinary incontinence (e) Fecal incontinence
7, Very severe cognitive decline	Late dementia	(a) Ability to speak limited to one to five words (b) All intelligible vocabulary lost (c) All motoric abilities lost (d) Stupor (e) Comatose

From Reisberg B, Ferris S, Anand R, et al: Clinical assessments of cognition in the aged. In Schamoian C, editor: Biology and treatment of dementia in the elderly, Washington, DC, 1984, American Psychiatric Press, Inc, pp 15-37.

Appendix

I

Global Deterioration Scale (GDS) for Age-Associated Cognitive Decline and Alzheimer's Disease

GDS stage	Clinical phase	Clinical characteristics
1 No cognitive decline	Normal	No subjective complaints of memory deficit. No memory deficit evident on clinical interview.
2 Very mild cognitive decline	Forgetfulness	Subjective complaints of memory deficit, most frequently in following areas: (a) forgetting where one has placed familiar objects; (b) forgetting names one formerly knew well. No objective evidence of memory deficit on clinical interview. No objective deficits in employment or social situations. Appropriate concern with respect to symptomatology.
3 Mild cognitive decline	Early confusional	Earliest clear-cut deficits. Manifestations in more than one of the following areas: (a) patient may have gotten lost when traveling to an unfamiliar location; (b) co-workers become aware of patient's relatively poor performance; (c) word and name finding deficits become evident to intimates; (d) patient may read a passage of a book and retain relatively little material; (e) patient may demonstrate decreased facility in remembering names upon introduction to new people; (f) patient may have lost or misplaced an object of value; (g) concentration deficit may be evident on clinical testing. Objective evidence of memory deficit obtained only with an intensive interview conducted by a trained geriatric psychiatrist. Decreased performance in demanding employment and social settings. Denial begins to become manifest in patient. Mild to moderate anxiety accompanies symptoms.

From Reisberg B, Ferris S, Anand R, et al: Clinical assessments of cognition in the aged. In Shamoian C, editor: Biology and treatment of dementia in the elderly, Washington, DC, 1984, American Psychiatric Press, Inc, pp 15-37.

GDS stage	Clinical phase	Clinical characteristics
4 Moderate cognitive de-cline	Late confusional	Clear-cut deficit on careful clinical interview. Deficit manifest in following areas: (a) decreased knowledge of current and recent events; (b) may exhibit some deficit in memory of one's personal history; (c) concentration deficit elicited on serial subtractions; (d) decreased ability to travel, handle finances, etc. Frequently no deficit in following areas: (a) orientation to time and person; (b) recognition of familiar persons and faces; (c) ability to travel to familiar locations. Inability to perform complex tasks. Denial is dominant defense mechanism. Flattening of affect and withdrawal from challenging situations occur.
5 Moderately severe decline	Early dementia	Patient can no longer survive without some assistance. Patient is unable during interview to recall a major relevant aspect of their current lives: e.g., their address or telephone number of many years, the names of close members of their family (such as grandchildren), the name of the high school or college from which they graduated. Frequently some disorientation to time (date, day of week, season, etc.) or to place. An educated person may have difficulty counting back from 40 by 4s or from 20 by 2s. Persons at this stage retain knowledge of many major facts regarding themselves and others. They invariably know their own names and generally know their spouses and children's names. They require no assistance with toileting or eating, but may have some difficulty choosing the proper clothing to wear.
6 Severe cognitive decline	Middle dementia	May occasionally forget the name of the spouse upon whom they are entirely dependent for survival. Will be largely unaware of all recent events and experiences in their lives. Retain some knowledge of their past lives but this is very sketchy. Generally unaware of their surroundings, the year, the season, etc. May have difficulty counting from 10, both backward and sometimes forward. Will require some assistance with activities of daily living, e.g., may become incontinent, will require travel assistance but occasionally will display ability to travel to familiar locations. Diurnal rhythm frequently disturbed. Almost always recall their own name. Frequently continue to be able to distinguish familiar from unfamiliar persons in their environment. Personality and emotional changes occur. These are quite variable and include: (a) delusional behavior, e.g., patients may accuse their spouse of being an impostor; may talk to imaginary figures in the environment, or to their own reflection in the mirror; (b) obsessive symptoms, e.g., person may continually repeat simple cleaning activities; (c) anxiety symptoms, agitation, and even previously nonexistent violent behavior may occur; (d) cognitive abulia, i.e., loss of willpower because an individual cannot carry a thought long enough to determine a purposeful course of action.
7 Very severe cognitive de-cline	Late dementia	All verbal abilities are lost. Frequently there is no speech at all—only grunting. Incontinent of urine; requires assistance toileting and feeding. Lose basic psychomotor skills, e.g., ability to walk. The brain appears to no longer be able to tell the body what to do. Generalized and cortical neurologic signs and symptoms.

Appendix

J

*Physical Self-Maintenance Scale (ADL)**

A. Toilet
   1. Cares for self at toilet completely; no incontinence.
   2. Needs to be reminded, or needs help in cleaning self, or has rare (weekly at most) accidents.
   3. Soiling or wetting while asleep, more than once a week.
   4. No control of bowels or bladder.
B. Feeding
   1. Eats without assistance.
   2. Eats with minor assistance at meal times, with help in preparing food or with help in cleaning up after meals.
   3. Feeds self with moderate assistance and is untidy.
   4. Requires extensive assistance for all meals.
   5. Does not feed self at all and resists efforts of others to feed him.
C. Dressing
   1. Dresses, undresses and selects clothes from own wardrobe.
   2. Dresses and undresses self, with minor assistance.
   3. Needs moderate assistance in dressing or selection of clothes.
   4. Needs major assistance in dressing but cooperates with efforts of others to help.
   5. Completely unable to dress self and resists effort of others to help.
D. Grooming (neatness, hair, nails, hands, face, clothing)
   1. Always neatly dressed and well-groomed, without assistance.
   2. Grooms self adequately, with occasional minor assistance (e.g., in shaving).
   3. Needs moderate and regular assistance or supervision in grooming.
   4. Needs total grooming care, but can remain well-groomed after help from others.
   5. Actively negates all efforts of others to maintain grooming.
E. Physical ambulation
   1. Goes about grounds or city.
   2. Ambulates within residence or about one block distance.
   3. Ambulates with assistance of (check one):
     (a) wheelchair (1. gets in and out without help; 2. needs help in getting in and out); (b) railing; (c) cane; or (d) walker.
   4. Sits unsupported in chair or wheelchair, but cannot propel self without help.
   5. Bedridden more than half the time.
F. Bathing
   1. Bathes self (tub, shower, sponge bath) without help.
   2. Bathes self, with help in getting in and out of tub.
   3. Washes face and hands only, but cannot bathe rest of body.
   4. Does not wash self but is cooperative with those who bathe him.
   5. Does not try to wash self and resists efforts to keep him clean.

* From Lawton MP: The functional assessment of elderly people, Journal of the American Geriatrics Society 19(6):465, 1971. Reprinted with permission from the American Geriatrics Society. Start by asking the patient to describe her/his ability to perform a given activity, e.g. feeding. Then ask specific questions as needed.

Appendix

K

Scale for Instrumental Activities of Daily Living (IADL)*

A. Ability to use telephone
  1. Operates telephone on own initiative: looks up and dials numbers, etc.
  2. Dials a few well-known numbers.
  3. Answers telephone but does not dial.
  4. Does not use telephone at all.
B. Shopping
  1. Takes care of all shopping needs independently.
  2. Shops independently for small purchases.
  3. Needs to be accompanied on any shopping trip.
  4. Completely unable to shop.
C. Food preparation
  1. Plans, prepares and serves adequate meals independently.
  2. Prepares adequate meals if supplied with ingredients.
  3. Heats and serves prepared meals, or prepares meals but does not maintain adequate diet.
  4. Needs to have meals prepared and served.
D. Housekeeping
  1. Maintains house alone or with occasional assistance (e.g., domestic help for heavy work).
  2. Performs light daily tasks such as dishwashing and bedmaking.
  3. Performs light daily tasks but cannot maintain acceptable level of cleanliness.
  4. Needs help with all home maintenance tasks.
  5. Does not participate in any housekeeping tasks.
E. Laundry
  1. Does personal laundry completely.
  2. Launders small items; rinses socks, stockings, etc.
  3. All laundry must be done by others.
F. Mode of transportation
  1. Travels independently on public transportation or drives own car.
  2. Arranges own travel via taxi but does not otherwise use public transportation.
  3. Travels on public transportation when assisted or accompanied by another.
  4. Travel limited to taxi or automobile, with assistance of another.
  5. Does not travel at all.
G. Responsibility for own medication
  1. Is responsible for taking medication in correct dosages at correct time.
  2. Takes responsibility if medication is prepared in advance in separate dosages.
  3. Is not capable of dispensing own medication.
H. Ability to handle finances
  1. Manages financial matters independently (budgets, writes checks, pays rent and bills, goes to bank); collects and keeps track of income.
  2. Manages day-to-day purchases but needs help with banking, major purchases, etc.
  3. Incapable of handling money.

*From Lawton MP: The functional assessment of elderly people, Journal of the American Geriatrics Society 19(6):465, 1971. Reprinted with permission from the American Geriatrics Society. Start by asking the patient to describe his/her functioning in each category, then complement with specific questions as needed.

Appendix

L

*Social Competence Activities**

ACTIVITIES IN THE HOME

Can you describe what your primary responsibilities have been in your home? Has this changed in recent weeks? If yes, in what ways?

e.g.: Who prepares the meals?
— If the patient does, ask if his health has affected this activity.
Who does the shopping?
— If the patient does, ask if his health has affected this activity.
Who does the laundry?
— If the patient does, ask if his health has affected this activity.
Who cleans the house?
— If the patient does, ask if his health has affected this activity.
Who does repairs around the house?
— If the patient does, ask if his health has affected this activity.
Who does the yard work?
— If the patient does, ask if his health has affected this activity.
Who runs errands?
— If the patient does, ask if his health has affected this activity.

WORK QUESTIONS

A. Do you work? That is, do you receive pay for the work you do? If yes:
(1) What kind of work are you presently doing?
(2) Are there some things at work you used to do that you aren't doing now?
B. If you don't work, did you stop working for pay because of illness? If yes:
(1) What kind of things do you do now that you think of as work (that is, things you are responsible for such as chores around the house, volunteer club duties)?
(2) Are there some things you used to do that you aren't doing now?
C. If you have never worked for pay or have not worked for pay for a considerable period of time unrelated to current illness:
(1) What kind of things have you done that you consider work (that is, things you are responsible for such as chores—yard work, repairs, cooking, cleaning, shopping—or volunteer work)?
(2) Are there some things you used to do that you aren't doing now?

RECREATIONAL AND SOCIAL ACTIVITIES

A. What kind of things do you do for recreation or just for fun? What about TV?
B. Has this changed in any way since your illness?
C. How much contact do you have with people not a part of your family, and where does this occur?
D. Do you keep in touch with your friends like you used to?
E. Are there things you'd like to do in the way of recreation or entertainment that you aren't doing right now?
F. What did you do (do you plan to do) on the most recent (upcoming) major holiday?

* Adapted from Benoliel JQ, McCorkle R, and Young K: Development of a social dependency scale, Research in Nursing and Health 3:3, 1980.

Appendix

M

Interdisciplinary Assessment Tool

Name _____ Age _____ Date of birth _____ Sex _____
Race _____ Religion _____ Marital status _____
Name of spouse/significant other _____ Phone # _____
Vital signs: Temp _____ Pulse _____ Resp _____ B/P _____ Ht _____
         Current wt _____ Usual wt _____ Ideal wt _____
Allergies: _____ Type of reaction _____
Food intolerances: _____
Smoker _____ Nonsmoker _____ Intolerance of smoke _____

Valuables:	Deposition:	Admitted:	Prosthesis:
_____ Money Amt _____	_____ Relatives	_____ Ambulatory	_____ Upper/lower dentures
_____ Rings	_____ Safe	_____ Wheelchair	_____ Contact lenses
_____ Watch	_____ Retained	_____ Stretcher	_____ Eyeglasses
_____ Other			_____ Hearing aid
			_____ Other: _____

Health status
Current complaints: _____
_____
Recent diagnostic testing: _____
Past medical and surgical conditions: _____
_____
_____
Family history of disease: _____
_____
_____

What the patient thinks will be accomplished by this hospitalization:
_____
_____

Current medications	Dose	Time of day
1.		
2.		
3.		
4.		
5.		

Adapted from the tool developed by the Missouri and Kansas Grantee Hospitals' Swing Bed Coordinators.

Review of systems

Date			Yes	No	and/or comments
	Glasgow Coma Scale:				
	Eyes: Open spontaneously	4			
	Open to verbal command	3			
	Open to pain	2			
	No response	1			
	Best motor response				
	Obeys verbal command	5			
	Localizes pain	4			
	Flexion—withdrawal	3			
	Flexion—abnormal (decorticate rigidity)	2			
	No response	1			
	Best verbal response				
	Oriented and converses	5			
	Disoriented & converses	4			
	Inappropriate words	3			
	Incomprehensible sounds	2			
	No response	1			
	TOTAL				
	Loss of taste				
	Loss of smell				
	Speech alterations				
	Sensation/touch/temperature				
	Tremors				
	Convulsions				
	Memory (long-term & short-term):				
	Strength				
	NR—no response	Rt arm			
	W—weak	Lt arm			
	S—strong	Rt leg			
		Lt leg			
	Headaches				
	Dizziness				

(Left margin vertical labels: Neurological, Head)

Continued.

Date		Yes	No	and/or comments
	Fainting			
	Head injuries			
	History of falls			
Neck	Pain			
	ROM			
	Lymphadenopathy			
Eyes	Blurred vision			
	Double vision			
	Peripheral vision loss			
	Tearing/exudate			
	Pain			
	Wears glasses/contact lens			
	Glaucoma			
	Cataracts			
	Ability to read			
Ears	Hearing deficit			
	Tinnitus			
	Earaches			
	Exudate			
	Cerumen			
Mouth/nose/throat	Nose bleeds			
	Sinusitis			
	Drainage			
	Deviated septum			
	Hoarseness			
	Dysphagia			
	Inflammation of throat/edema			
	Integrity of teeth			
	gums			
	buccal mucosa			
	Wears dentures			
Endocrine	Temperature sensitivity			
	Excessive hunger or thirst			
	Excessive dryness of skin			

Date		Yes	No	and/or comments
	Unusual hair growth			
	Thyroid enlargement			
Breast	Pain			
	Lumps			
	Discharge			
	Tenderness			
	Biopsies/surgery			
	Breast self exam			
Respiratory	Rate/regularity			
	Breath sounds			
	Rales			
	Wheezes			
	Rhonchi			
	Cough			
	Sputum: color, consistency			
	Pain			
	Dyspnea			
	Exertional dyspnea			
	Nasal flaring			
	Stridor			
	Retractions			
	Splinting			
	Tracheostomy			
	Activity intolerance			
Cardiovascular	Pacemaker			
	Pain/angina			
	Murmur			
	Palpitations			
	Rhythm			
	Color/cyanosis			
	Capillary refill			
	Edema			
	Pulse: peripherial/apical			

Continued.

Date			Yes	No	and/or comments
Skin	Hair				
	Nails				
	Skin color				
	Excoriation	1			
	Skin tear	2			
	Inflammation	3			
	Bruise	4			
	Suture lines	5			
	Growths	6			
	Rash	7			
	Pressure ulcer	8			
	Location				
	Size				
	Appearance				
	Color				
	Granulation tissue				
	Slough				
	Eschar				
	Clean				
	Dry/moist				
	Drainage				
	Odor				
Genitourinary	Urine: color/odor				
	Dysuria				
	Hesitancy				
	Frequency				
	Polyuria				
	Oliguria/anuria				
	Hematuria				
	Incontinence				
	Catheter				
	Stoma/ileal conduit				
	Venereal disease				
	Discharge: vagina/penis				
	Testicular mass				

Date		Yes	No	and/or comments
Reproductive	Circumcision			
	Last Pap smear			
	Menses onset			
	intervals			
	duration			
	LMP			
	cessation			
	Menopausal symptoms			
	Bleeding or pain with intercourse			
	Takes contraceptives			
Musculoskeletal	Muscle pain/cramps			
	ROM limitations			
	Contractures			
	Swollen or painful joints			
	Numbness/paralysis			
	Weakness			
	Back pain			
	Amputation			
	Previous trauma/fractures			
	Ambulates independently			
	Normal gait			
	Posture/balance			
	Walker/crutches/brace/cane			
	General strength			
	Fine motor function			
	Self transfer			
	Ability to climb stairs			
ADLs	Bathes self			
	Toilets self			
	Dresses self			
	Feeds self			
	Can prepare own meals			
	Can obtain own food			
	Can take own medication			

Continued.

Date			Yes	No	and/or comments
Emotional		Anxious			
		Fearful			
		Depressed			
		Uninterested			
		Suspicious			
		Dependent			
		Combative			
		Low self-esteem			
		Disrupted sleep			
		Usual sleeping patterns			
Patient teaching		Learning potential			
		Motivation			
		Learning needs			
Social/discharge planning		Transportation available			
		Family/significant other present			
		Financial resources			
		Lives alone			
		Physical/emotional handicaps			
		Conflicts with others			
		Significant losses			
		Regular social contacts			
		Noncompliance with recommended treatment			
		Family will be involved in care after discharge			
		Can call for help when needed			
		Observes safety practices			
		Suspected victims of abuse			
		Drug or alcohol problem			
		Anticipated setting for post-hospital care			
Activities		What do you do for fun?			
		Do you have a special interest or hobby?			
		Limitation in activities			
		Individual activity			
		Group activity			
		Friends/family visitors			
		Goals for activities			

Adapted from the tool developed by the Missouri and Kansas Grantee Hospitals' Swing Bed Coordinators.

Index

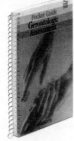
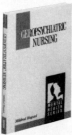
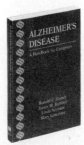
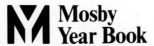